Complementary Therapies and the Management of Diabetes and Vascular Disease

Diabetes

dp

in Practice

Complementary Therapies and the Management of Diabetes and Vascular Disease

A Matter of Balance

Editor

Professor Trish Dunning

St. Vincent's Hospital, Melbourne, Australia

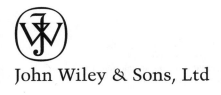

John Wiley & Sons, Ltd

Other Wiley Editorial Offices

John Wiley & Sons, Inc., 605 Third Avenue, New York, NY 10158-0012, USA

WILEY-VCH Verlag GmbH, Pappeallee3, D-69469, Weinheim, Germany

Jacaranda Wiley Ltd, 33 Park Road, Milton, Queensland 4064, Australia

John Wiley & Sons (Asia) Pte Ltd, 2 Clementi Loop #02-01, Jin Xing Distripark, Singapore 129809

John Wiley & Sons (Canada) Ltd, 6045 Freemont Blvd, Mississauga, Ontario L5R 4J3, Canada

Wiley also publishes its books in a variety of electronic formats. Some content that appears in print may
not be available in electronic books.

Library of Congress Cataloging-in-Publication data:

Complementary therapies and the management of diabetes and vascular disease / edited by
    Trish Dunning.
        p.   ;   cm.
Includes bibliographical references and index.
ISBN-13: 978-0-470-01458-5
ISBN-10: 0-470-01458-X
    1. Diabetes—Alternative treatment.   I. Dunning, Trish. [DNLM: 1. Diabetes Mellitus—therapy.
    2. Complementary Therapies—methods.   3. Vascular Diseases—therapy.   WK 815 C7367 2006]
RC661.A47C66 2006
616.4′62—dc22

                                                                                    2006016573

British Library Cataloguing in Publication Data

A catalogue record for this book is available from the British Library

ISBN-13 978-0-470-01458-5
ISBN-10 0-470-01458-X

Typeset in 10.5/13pt Times by Integra Software Services Pvt. Ltd, Pondicherry, India
Printed and bound in Great Britain by Antony Rowe Ltd, Chippenham, Wiltshire
This book is printed on acid-free paper responsibly manufactured from sustainable forestry
in which at least two trees are planted for each one used for paper production.

Contents

6 Essential Oils (Aromatherapy)   **125**
Trish Dunning

7 Counselling and Relaxation Therapies   **158**
Sue Cradock and Chas Skinner

8 Energy Therapies   **179**
Geraldine Milton

Preface

Medicine, perfume and herbalism co-existed synergistically until the late 1800s. The rise of modern chemistry processes, laboratory techniques, and scientific principles enabled modern medicines to be developed and led to the separation of these modalities. 'Scientific medicine' emerged as the dominant system. Health systems usually evolve in societies to meet prevailing health needs, which is reflected in the current move to reconcile complementary and conventional approaches to more effectively meet the current needs of the public. The World Health Organization's (WHO) *Traditional Medicine Strategy 2002–2005* is a working document reflecting some of these issues, which is being implemented in a number of countries. The WHO Strategy is sensitive to the differences between countries and regions.

Complementary therapies have a strong consumer-driven following. Research indicates that more than 17 per cent of people with diabetes attending ambulatory services in the UK and at least 25 per cent in Canada and Australia use complementary therapies. In the USA, people with diabetes are 1.6 times more likely to use complementary therapies than non-diabetics. People with diabetes commonly use nutritional therapies and supplements, aromatherapy, massage, herbs, meditation, and spiritual counselling to complement conventional diabetes management regimens, to control unpleasant symptoms and to manage diabetes complications and other concomitant diseases such as arthritis, and intercurrent illnesses such as 'the common cold'. Interestingly, the International Diabetes Federation adopted the Yin Yang as the symbol of World Diabetes Day in 2003.

People often use complementary therapies because they are dissatisfied with the way conventional medicine manages chronic diseases (not holistic) and because they feel disempowered in consultations with conventional practitioners. Complementary therapy use is associated with higher education, poor health and philosophical congruence with complementary therapy philosophy.

Complementary therapies elicit a range of reactions, from uncritical acceptance to extreme scepticism, yet their popularity continues to grow globally. Given the high rate of complementary therapy use, conventional practitioners can no longer afford to ignore or adopt judgemental attitudes towards complementary therapies. Many conventional practitioners now incorporate complementary therapies into their practice and refer to or collaborate with complementary practitioners. New terms such as 'integrative medicine', 'integrated medicine' and 'complementary and alternative medicine' have emerged to reflect the move towards reintegration. However, understanding and working with complementary therapies and their potential to improve health care is a slow process that depends on quality research, policy-makers, individual practitioners and consumers as well as health systems.

'Complementary therapies' is a general term that covers a broad range of therapies and is preferable to 'alternative', 'natural' and 'non-scientific' because these terms could also be applied to a great many conventional medicines and because it suggests complementary therapies can enhance and be used with other therapies, including conventional medicines. However, one must respect the terms used in specific countries, for example, Africa, South East Asia and the Western Pacific use 'traditional medicine'. Several definitions of complementary therapies exist. Most indicate a focus on prevention, well-being, and supporting the body's intrinsic capacity for self-healing mentally, physically and spiritually. Some definitions also indicate the boundaries between complementary and conventional practices are not fixed, to reflect the changing nature of health-care delivery.

The speed of change is compelling. Complementary therapists from different backgrounds meet in joint forums and also meet frequently with conventional practitioners. Articles about complementary therapies often appear in reputable peer-reviewed journals, although the focus is often still on adverse events such as drug/herb interactions leading to hypo/hyperglycaemia, trauma and burns to neuropathic feet rather than positive benefits such as symptom management, stress management and improved quality of life, which indirectly affect metabolic parameters. Complementary therapy units are included in conventional health professional education programmes and research centres have been established in major universities and teaching hospitals throughout the world.

Prince Charles (2000) noted in a guest editorial in the *British Medical Journal* that he was encouraged by the British Medical Association's more tolerant attitude towards complementary therapies. Prince Charles has long been a proponent of complementary therapies. In February 2004, *The Sunday Times* announced that the Queen had appointed a doctor who used alternative therapies, as the new royal physician.

Many conventional practitioners do not have a good understanding of complementary therapies, their potential benefits for people with diabetes or the safety issues involved. Likewise, many complementary therapists have limited understanding about diabetes and the issues that need to be considered when recommending complementary therapies to people with diabetes. The aim of the editor and contributors is to produce an informative evidence-based book that will help health professionals understand the complementary therapies people with diabetes commonly use, their potential benefits, possible adverse events, how they can be safely integrated, and to suggest clinical practice guidelines for the safe combination of complementary and conventional therapies in diabetes management.

The traditional healing practices of many cultures are reflected in the book. Some, such as Chinese medicine, are well known, others such as Australian Aboriginal healing practices are less well known. Migration means cultural diversity is a global phenomenon and one can expect to encounter a diverse range of health-care approaches in almost all countries.

It is hoped that this book will be of interest and practical help to both conventional practitioners and people with diabetes.

TRISH DUNNING
Melbourne, June 2006

Foreword

Diabetes and vascular diseases such as coronary heart disease are both common and serious; about half of us will die because of them. Effective prevention and treatment are, therefore, very important and in the past few decades, we have made considerable progress towards these aims. At the same time, complementary therapies have experienced a surprising comeback. I say comeback because virtually all of them have a long tradition of use, much longer than most conventional approaches. Some enthusiasts believe that this fact alone proves their effectiveness and safety – I am not one of them. History of usage, while interesting and perhaps useful for formulating hypotheses, is a far cry from scientific proof.

The tension between experience and evidence dominates much of complementary medicine today. It is also well reflected in this book. Its authors are keenly aware of the need for evidence but sometimes seem to struggle when trying to summarise it. The problems they encounter are obvious: there are mountains of anecdotes but data from clinical trials are usually scarce and often flawed. Critical assessment, an approach that is standard in mainstream medicine, remains unusual in complementary medicine. All too often, criticism is seen as destructive rather than a constructive precondition of progress.

This book represents an important step in the right direction. Not only is it timely, it also advances complementary medicine in more than one way: it summarises the existing evidence succinctly, and it clearly points out the many areas where the evidence is weak or even non-existent. We should use this knowledge wisely; as patients or clinicians, we ought to exercise caution, as researchers, we must fill the often huge gaps in our current understanding, and, as decision-makers, we should consider investing in the further study of this fascinating area. In all, two things seem painfully obvious: progress can only come from thoughtful but rigorous research, and double standards are a disservice to everyone.

PROFESSOR EDZARD ERNST
Exeter, UK

List of Contributors

Russell Banks Royal Melbourne Institute of Technology, Melbourne, Australia

Lesley Braun Melbourne, Australia

Leon Chaitow London, UK

Sue Cradock Queen Alexandra Hospital, Portsmouth, UK

Gary Deed Carina, Victoria, Australia

Rocco Di Vincenzo Melbourne, Australia

Trish Dunning St. Vincent's Hospital and University of Melbourne, Melbourne, Australia

Devaka Fernando Sherwood Forest Hospitals NHS Trust and University of Sheffield, UK

Heather McDonald Australian Institute of Aboriginal and Torres Strait Islander Studies, Sydney, Australia

Geraldine Milton Seaford, Victoria, Australia

Paula Mullins St Thomas' Hospital, London, UK

Liza Oates Monash University, Australia

Kylie A. O'Brien Department of Medicine, Monash University, Victoria, Australia

Mohan Pawa Fieldway Medical Centre, Surrey, UK

Chas Skinner University of Southampton, Southampton, UK

Charlie Changli Xue Royal Melbourne Institute of Technology, Melbourne, Australia

Acknowledgements

I am grateful to the management of John Wiley & Sons for commissioning this book and entrusting its growth and development to my care. Special thanks are due to Joan Marsh, Executive Commissioning Editor of Wiley & Sons and the Project Editor, Fiona Woods, for their support and advice.

I am grateful to Australian Scholarly Publishing for permission to reproduce Tables 6.1, 6.2 and 6.3 in Chapter 6; Elsevier for permission to use the material in Table 3.2 in Chapter 3; Dr A.W. Fuhr and Activator Methods International Ltd for permission to reproduce the photograph of the Activator in Chapter 16; Colette Heimowitz, M.Sc. VP, Education, Research Atkins Health and Medical Information Services for permission to reproduce the Atkins pyramid and Mohan Pawa and Heather McDonald for allowing us to use the photographs appearing in Figures 2.1 and 12.1, respectively.

The significant contribution of all the people who wrote chapters for the book must be acknowledged and I thank them most sincerely for sharing their knowledge and coping with my 'nagging'. I sincerely thank Dr E. Ernst for agreeing to write the Foreword.

This book is dedicated to people with diabetes who choose to incorporate complementary therapies into their health management plans and to the health professionals who care for them.

Most important of all, my thanks go to my family, including all the four-legged ones, but, especially, my husband John, the wind beneath my wings.

1 Introduction to Diabetes

Gary Deed and *Trish Dunning*

1.1 Incidence and Prevalence of Diabetes

The dramatic increase in the incidence and prevalence of type 2 diabetes and obesity is an alarming health concern. Despite increased awareness of the value of eating a healthy diet and undertaking regular physical activity, the incidence of type 2 diabetes has not been reduced. In fact, diabetes is a serious and growing global health problem. The Centre for Disease Control and Prevention (2006) described diabetes as an 'epidemic of our time that threatens to spiral out of control unless early, focused preventative actions are taken'. The challenge for health professionals and governments encompasses economic, social, and health planning in developed nations as well as in newly developed or developing countries, irrespective of culture or location.

Worldwide, the number of people with diabetes has tripled since 1985 (*Medical and Health Annual Encyclopaedia Britannica*, 1999), which supports earlier predictions of the global epidemic nature of diabetes in the first quarter of the twenty-first century. Type 2 diabetes is among the top ten leading causes of death in Westernised societies (Moutet *et al.* 1990). The number of people with type 2 diabetes throughout the world is expected to double by 2030 according to a recent study carried out by the WHO in collaboration with universities in Scotland, Denmark and Australia (Wild *et al.* 2004). Type 2 diabetes represents a huge challenge because of the total number of diagnosed cases as well as those at potential risk. It is expected to exceed 220 million people worldwide by 2010, thus doubling in 10 years.

Currently, at least 15.7 million adults in the United States, >8 per cent of the adult population, have diabetes and the incidence is outpacing population growth (ADA Position Statement 2006). In addition, American children as young as 7 and 8 show many of the signs of insulin resistance syndrome (IRS) related to early onset obesity (Freedman and Dietz 1999). Type 2 diabetes and its complications now claim 300,000 lives in the United States each year, incurring expenses of over $130 billion to the health-care system. Wild *et al.* (2004) projected the number of Americans diagnosed with diabetes would reach 29 million by 2050.

Complementary Therapies and the Management of Diabetes and Vascular Disease Editor Trish Dunning
© 2006 John Wiley & Sons, Ltd.

Besides the mortality associated with diabetes, there are high health costs and disease burden to individuals resulting from the long-term complications and the unremitting nature of diabetes self-care. Complications can negatively impact on the individual's quality of life and mental health, see Chapter 7.

The International Diabetes Institute (IDI) predicted diabetes would affect 1.5 million Australians by the year 2010 primarily due to the increasingly overweight and physically inactive population and the cultural mix that includes several cultural groups known to be at high risk of developing type 2 diabetes. Estimates from a national survey, the Australian Diabetes and Obesity and Lifestyle Study (AusDiab) undertaken in 1999–2000, show Australia is quickly approaching one million people with diagnosed type 2 diabetes, approximately 7.5 per cent of the Australian population (Dunstan *et al.* 2002). AusDiab shows the following:

- An estimated 7.5 per cent of the population (938,700 Australians) aged > 25 have type 2 diabetes.
- Type 2 diabetes affects 8.0 per cent of Australian males, 7.0 per cent of Australian females and approximately 50 per cent of these are not aware they have diabetes. The increase in prevalence is occurring faster and earlier among males than females.
- The prevalence increases with increasing age, from 0.3 per cent among people aged between 25–34 to 23.7 per cent among those over 75.
- In eight years from 1990–1998, type 2 diabetes increased by 70 per cent in the 30–39 year age group, which demonstrated an increased incidence in younger people.
- 16.1 per cent of the population has either impaired glucose tolerance or impaired fasting glucose, known risk factors for diabetes.

1.2 Overview of Diabetes

Diabetes mellitus is a serious, chronic, currently incurable disease that manifests in several forms, the most common of which are type 1 and type 2 diabetes and gestational diabetes. It is primarily a disorder of carbohydrate, protein and fat metabolism arising from a lack of or resistance to insulin. The common metabolic consequence of untreated diabetes, regardless of type, is persistent hyperglycaemia and frequently hyperlipidaemia, which reflect cellular inability to ultilise glucose efficiently as an energy source. Various metabolic derangements occur as a consequence of the inability to utilise glucose and result in the classic symptoms of diabetes and the acute metabolic consequences such as ketonaemia and metabolic acidosis and hyperosmolar states. In the longer term, metabolic changes and accompanying inflammation lead to complications such as coronary heart disease, stroke, kidney disease and neuropathy.

People with diabetes frequently consult complementary practitioners or self-initiate complementary therapies to manage diabetes and its physical and mental complications as well as other comorbidities and intercurrent illnesses. In addition, they often use them in preventative health plans, see Chapter 2. Therefore, it is important to determine whether people with diabetes use complementary therapies and why they use them, rather than assuming it is only to control blood glucose.

Signs and symptoms of diabetes

Hyperglycaemia occurs as a result of the underlying metabolic abnormalities of glucose homeostasis and is responsible for the symptoms. The symptoms are usually pronounced in type 1 diabetes but may be absent in type 2:

- frequent urination – polyuria and/or nocturia and usually glycosuria;
- excessive often unquenchable thirst – polydipsia;
- lethargy;
- weight loss;
- frequent, and poorly resolving infections;
- visual changes.

Classification of diabetes

The classification of diabetes and diagnostic criteria were revised in 1997 in a partnership between the American Diabetes Association (ADA) and the World Health Organization (WHO). The terms type 1 and type 2 diabetes replaced insulin-dependent and non-insulin dependent diabetes respectively. Most countries subsequently adopted the revised classification by the Expert Committee on the Diagnosis and Classification of Diabetes Mellitus in 1997. The main types of diabetes are:

- type 1, which is further divided into two forms:
  - immune-mediated diabetes that occurs as a consequence of autoimmune destruction of the insulin-producing beta cells of the pancreas;
  - idiopathic diabetes, which has no known aetiology.
- type 2, which is associated with relative insulin deficiency and insulin resistance;
- gestational diabetes, which occurs during pregnancy.

Impaired glucose homeostasis is a stage between normal glucose homeostasis and diabetes, and is a significant risk factor for cardiovascular disease. Two forms exist: impaired fasting glucose and impaired glucose tolerance. In these states the plasma glucose is higher than normal but lower than commonly accepted diagnostic criteria.

Other types listed in the 1977 classification include diabetes associated with other disease processes such as endocrine disorders (Cushing's disease, acromegaly), and pancreatic diseases (cancer, pancreatitis), and drug- or chemical-induced diabetes, for example, steroid-induced diabetes. Genetic defects of beta cell function such as maturity Onset Diabetes of the Young (MODY) and of insulin action also occur. MODY should not be confused with type 2 diabetes occurring in young people as a consequence of the lack of adequate physical activity and obesity.

Diagnosis

Normal blood glucose ranges between ~3–6 mmol/L. Diabetes is diagnosed on the basis of presenting symptoms and/or elevated blood glucose levels. Where symptoms are not present, abnormal fasting blood glucose (>7 mmol/L) needs to be demonstrated on at least two occasions. When symptoms are present, an elevated blood glucose level is usually diagnostic. Elevated urine glucose is no longer an accepted diagnostic criteria for diagnosing diabetes.

In some cases, an oral glucose tolerance (OGTT) test may be necessary, for example, equivocal random blood glucose levels and a strong family history of diabetes especially during pregnancy. OGTT must be performed under test conditions and not undertaken when the individual is acutely ill, uraemic, in the postoperative period, or when the individual has been immobile for more than 48 hours. Usually a 75 g glucose load is used and the diagnosis is determined on the 2-hour glucose level. The diagnostic criteria are shown in Table 1.1.

Type 1 diabetes

Type 1 diabetes culminates in metabolic derangements and the classic symptoms, which occur as a result of progressive insulin deficiency, which usually develops over a long prodromal stage during which the beta cells of the pancreas are gradually destroyed. Type 1 accounts for between 7–10 per cent of diagnosed cases of diabetes. The most common cause is autoimmune pancreatic islet cell destruction. The basis of the destruction has been the subject of a great deal of research (the search for a cure).

The aetiology appears to be multifactorial. Associations between viral illnesses and nutritional intake of foods such as milk and potatoes have been noted and investigated as causes. However, the association between these potential causal factors is relatively weak, difficult to reproduce, and complicated by many

Table 1.1 Criteria for diagnosing diabetes based on World Health Organization guidelines. Fasting plasma glucose is preferred but all three tests are used. The levels shown are venous plasma glucose levels. Capillary blood glucose is ~10–15 per cent higher than venous blood. Diagnosis of diabetes is not usually made on the basis of capillary blood or urine glucose tests.

Diabetes stage	Fasting plasma glucose in mmol/L	Random plasma glucose in mmol/L	Oral glucose tolerance test in mmol/L at 2-hours
Normal	<6.1		<7.8
Impaired glucose tolerance	Impaired fasting glucose >6.1 and <7.		>7.8 and <11.1
Diabetes	>7	>11.1 and symptoms	>11.1

confounders (Gale 2005). Recent epidemiological research suggests the rate of progression of the beta cell destruction may be a significant factor in the age at onset of type 1 diabetes ('accelerator hypothesis'). Higher body mass index (BMI) was associated with younger age of onset of type 1 diabetes in a large cohort (n = 9248) of German and Austrian children (Knerr et al. 2005). Thus, weight gain may be a risk factor for early onset of both type 1 and type 2 diabetes.

The onset of type 1 diabetes commonly occurs in childhood and adolescence but can occur in adults. Type 1 can also present for the first time in older people, however, the onset may be slower and the symptoms less pronounced, which delays diagnosis and treatment. Type 1 also occurs in a small number of people after pancreatic trauma or pancreatitis. Insulin is required from diagnosis to replace the lack of insulin.

Type 2 diabetes

The majority of people with diabetes have type 2, which is due to the inability of insulin to maintain glucose homeostasis (insulin resistance) even in the presence of high levels of insulin (hyperinsulinaemia), which is often a feature in the early stages. Insulin secretion occurs in two phases: an initial spike when glucose enters the blood stream and stimulates insulin release, the first phase, then a second less pronounced spike, the second phase. Loss of the first phase often occurs in type 2 diabetes but the beta cells respond to insulin secretagogues such as sulphonylureas (Dornhorst 2001).

Type 2 diabetes is associated with elevated fasting blood glucose, and reduced glucose utilisation post prandially. Type 2 diabetes develops as a result of a genetic predisposition and environmental factors (Turner and Clapham 1998). Significantly, type 2 diabetes is often 'silent' and is diagnosed when the individual presents with a diabetes-related complication such as heart disease. The causes of type 2 diabetes are related to changes in cellular responses to what would otherwise be adequate levels of insulin (insulin resistance). The areas of current research include changes in metabolic hormones associated with or which occur as a consequence of obesity (Vettor et al. 2001).

Type 2 diabetes is insidious and associated with progressive beta cell failure, which means a majority of people with type 2 may eventually require insulin. The majority of people with type 2 diabetes are over the age of 55 years, have central (truncal/abdominal) obesity, and a sedentary lifestyle. People over 45 years with a genetic history of diabetes in a close family member, or current hypertension or heart disease are most at risk of type 2 diabetes. Table 1.2 shows a simple self-administered risk factor check used by Diabetes Australia in diabetes awareness campaigns. However, in many countries, type 2 diabetes is starting to occur at an earlier age and appears to be associated with the rise of obesity in children and young adults.

Table 1.2 Type 2 Diabetes Tick Test (Reproduced with kind permission from Diabetes Australia www.diabetesaustralia.com.au). This is a self-administered health prevention initiative of Diabetes Australia. If people tick more than one positive response they are advised to discuss their health with their doctor to determine whether they have type 2 diabetes.

- I am over 45 and have high blood pressure
- I am over 45 and am overweight
- I am over 45 and one or more members of my family has diabetes
- I am over 55
- I have heart disease or have had a heart attack
- I had high blood sugar levels while I was pregnant (gestational diabetes)
- I have had a borderline high blood sugar test
- I have polycystic ovary syndrome and am overweight
- I am over 35 and am a Pacific Islander or from an Asian cultural background or from the Indian sub-continent

Insulin resistance

Insulin resistance is a pre-diabetic stage known variously as the metabolic syndrome, syndrome X, syndrome X and the insulin resistance syndrome (IRS). Insulin resistance and hyperinsulinaemia improve with increased activity and weight loss. The classic features of IRS are:

- central obesity: increased body mass index and waist hip ratio;
- hyperinsulinaemia;
- impaired utilisation of glucose;
- reduced glucose storage as glycogen;
- elevated fasting and post-prandial blood glucose;
- hyperlipidaemia, which inhibits insulin signalling and reduces intracellular glucose transport;
- reduced fibrinolysis;
- hypertension;
- endothelial dysfunction;
- inflammatory changes that affect the insulin receptor activity;
- systematic low grade chronic infection;
- athersclerosis.

Central obesity is a significant risk factor for cardiovascular disease, and weight gain after young adulthood represents an additional risk independent of initial weight (Hubert *et al.* 1983). Low oestrogen levels after menopause in women with diabetes may compound weight gain, make it more difficult to exercise and increase the cardiovascular risk (Poehlman and Tchernof 1998). A recent study indicates coffee consumption improves glucose-tolerance and reduces the risk of type 2 diabetes but the specific components of coffee exerting the glucose-lowering effect are unknown but are independent of the coffee preparation method but the clinical implications are unclear (*Diabetes Care* 2006, 29: 398–403).

Gestational diabetes

Gestational diabetes refers to IGT occurring during pregnancy, affecting approximately 3 per cent of pregnancies. The exact cause remains unknown but insulin resistance due to placental hormones has been suggested. Current recommendations are that all pregnant women should be screened between 24 and 28 weeks gestation followed by an OGTT if the screening test is abnormal. Opinions vary about whether a 50 g or 75 g glucose load should be used. If the blood glucose cannot be controlled by diet and activity, insulin will be needed.

The aim is to maintain the glucose in the normal range to reduce the risks of hyperglycaemia to the mother and baby. These include macrosomia (large infant body weight) complicating labour and necessitating caesarian section, respiratory distress in the newborn and neonatal hypoglycaemia. The blood glucose usually returns to normal after the baby is born but ~40 per cent of women develop type 2 diabetes in later life. Thus a follow-up OGGT is recommended 6–8 weeks after delivery and regular screening thereafter to enable early detection and treatment of diabetes.

1.3 Management Strategies

The basis of managing type 2 diabetes is by improving metabolic control through physical activity and dietary changes. However, glucose-lowering medicines, and, if necessary, insulin, are prescribed as the disease advances. Commonly used glucose-lowering medicines include:

- sulphonylureas that enhance insulin secretion from beta cells;
- meglitinides that augment insulin secretion;
- biguanides that inhibit hepatic glucose production and increase glucose uptake in muscles and reduce triglycerides and LDL cholesterol levels;
- thiazolidinediones (TZD) that improve insulin sensitivity in muscle and to some extent in the liver and reduce triglyceride levels;
- alpha-glucosidase inhibitors that inhibit the action of glucose oxidase in the gut, thereby delaying glucose absorption into the blood stream;
- insulin, which comes in several forms: rapid acting, short acting, intermediate acting, and long acting. The rapid or short-acting insulins are often combined with longer-acting insulins to achieve 24-hour glycaemic control. Insulin is administered by subcutaneous injection using a range of devices. Insulin pumps, which can be programmed to continuously deliver a small amount of insulin into the subcutaneous tissue (basal) and bolus doses with meals, are becoming more widely used but they are expensive. Inhaled insulin is emerging as an alternative to short acting insulin for some people. During surgery and acute illness, for example, ketoacidosis (DKA), clear short-acting insulin is often administered intravenously.

Sometimes combinations of glucose-lowering medicines are required. In addition, a range of other medicines are needed to manage diabetes complications, for example, antihypertensive and lipid-lowering agents, and comorbidities such as arthritis, and intercurrent illnesses. Thus, the medicine regimen can be complicated and should be reviewed on a regular basis.

In some cases insulin and glucose-lowering medicines are used together in type 2 diabetes. Insulin is also required when women with type 2 diabetes become pregnant and often when type 2 diabetes develops following gestational diabetes later in life. Insulin is sometimes used on a temporary basis in type 2 diabetes, for example, during intercurrent illness or surgery and managing hyperosmolar states.

Glucose-lowering medicines can have significant side effects, for example:

- Hypoglycaemia (sulphonylureas and TZDs). Hypoglycaemia increases the risk of trauma, falls and affects mental health and quality of life.
- Weight gain (sulphonylureas and TZDs).
- Gastrointestinal symptoms such as bloating and nausea (biguanides and Alpha-glucosidase inhibitors).
- Lactic acidosis (Metformin) is more likely in patients with severe renal impairment (GFR < 40 ml/minute), myocardial infarction, and intercurrent illnesses that cause hypoxia. Metformin should not be used when these conditions are present (Holstein and Stumvoll 2005). Metformin is also associated with vitamin B_1 malabsorption (Bauman *et al.* 2000).
- Liver toxicity: the early forms of TZDs were associated with liver failure but it rarely occurs with newer agents. The liver function is usually monitored initially when TZDs are commenced.

1.4 Management Targets and Regimens

The generally accepted metabolic management targets are shown in Table 1.3. The frequency of testing depends on the specific parameter. For example HbA_{1c} is usually monitored at three monthly intervals but blood pressure should be checked at each consultation. Fasting lipids, microalbuminuria, foot assessment to detect peripheral neuropathy and vasculopathy, and eye examinations should be undertaken at least yearly but may be undertaken less or more frequently depending on the age of the individual, their risk factors for inadequate metabolic control, and the results of previous examinations and investigations.

In addition to these complication monitoring processes, people with diabetes undertake regular blood glucose self-monitoring, test for ketones during illness and are generally responsible for their care, as already indicated. Self-care is hard work and initial and ongoing diabetes education and support are essential, see Chapter 7. Although assessing mental health and quality of life, and undertaking structured medication reviews that include complementary medicines are not usually included in management regimens, they are important and affect metabolic outcomes. Therefore, these issues should be included in diabetes annual reviews. Recently, mental health screening questions were included in the Australian National Diabetes Information Audit and Benchmarking tool, (ANDIAB).

Table 1.3 Current metabolic targets that need to be monitored on a regular basis. (National Health and Medical Research Council 2004). These targets may vary around the world and need to be adjusted to individual needs and especially for children and older people.

Management parameter	Target
Blood glucose	Fasting 4–6 mmol/L
HbA$_{1c}$	≤7 per cent
Lipids	
• Cholesterol	• <4 mmol/L
• LDL	• <2.5 mmol/L
• HDL	• >1.0 mmol/L
• Triglycerides	• <2.0 mmol/L
Blood pressure	<130/80 mm Hg
Weight BMI	≤25 kg/m^2 where practical
Urinary albumin excretion	<20 μg/min in a timed overnight collection or <20 mg/L in a spot collection. Albumin/creatinine ratio: women <3.5 mg/mmol and men 2.5 mg/mmol
Physical activity	At least 30 minutes walking or similar activity at least 5 days/week

The general management aims are to do the following:

- Achieve metabolic targets within the capacity of the individual without producing unnecessary hypoglycaemia or other adverse events. Hypoglycaemia causes a considerable amount of distress to people with diabetes and their families and can put the individual and other people at significant risk. It is not unusual for people to run their blood glucose high to avoid hypoglycaemia. Health professionals often do not appreciate or under-rate the physical and psychological effects of hypoglycaemia or the level of fear it engenders.
- Control hyperglycaemic symptoms and symptoms associated with complications such as pain.
- Follow a regular healthy diet and exercise plan.
- Stop smoking, which contributes to vascular risk factors as well as many cancers.
- Support the individual to set achievable management goals to maintain quality of life.
- Undertake regular complication risk assessment and treatment when indicated.

1.5 Short-term Complications

The short-term complications of diabetes include:

- ketoacidosis (DKA) due to insufficient insulin, which primarily occurs in type 1 diabetes due to intercurrent illnesses but can occur in type 2 during serious illnesses such as septicaemia or myocardial infarction. It may be the presenting feature at the initial diagnosis of type 1 diabetes.

- hyperglycaemic hyperosmolar non-ketotic states (HONK), which often occur in older people during illness. HONK also occurs in diagnosed type 2 diabetes.
- intercurrent illnesses such as colds and flu, which predispose individuals to DKA and HONK;
- hypoglycaemia in insulin-treated individuals and those taking oral glucose-lowering agents.

1.6 Long-term Complications

Two landmark studies, the Diabetes Control and Complications Trial (DCCT) in type I (1993) and the United Kingdom Prospective Diabetes Study (UKPDS) (1998) in type 2, demonstrated the importance of controlling blood glucose and blood pressure respectively, to reduce the complications of diabetes. The complications of all forms of diabetes include small blood vessel damage (microangiography), which particularly affects the eyes, kidneys and neural tissue. Common manifestations include retinopathy and nephropathy. Large blood vessel damage (macroangiography) and dyslipidaemia are significantly associated with increased mortality from coronary diseases, peripheral vascular disease, and stroke.

Table 1.4 Common long-term complications of diabetes.

Condition	Complication
Nephropathy	Diabetic nephropathy Chronic renal failure End stage renal disease requiring dialysis Affects medicine excretion
Retinopathy	Diabetic retinopathy Glaucoma Cataract
Neuropathy (peripheral and autonomic)	Peripheral: Neuropathic pain, which affects quality of life Foot pathology such as changed gait that predisposes the individual to trauma, ulcers, amputation and fall Autonomic: Gastroparesis Atonic bladder Silent myocardial infarction Postural hypotension, which increases falls risk Erectile dysfunction
Cardiovascular disease	Coronary artery disease Cerebrovascular disease Peripheral vascular disease
Pregnancy-related complications	Birth defects Macrosomia Neonatal hypoglycaemia Interventions such as forceps and caesarian deliveries.

Myocardial infarction is often 'silent' (asymptomatic) in type 2 diabetes, which delays treatment and increases the associated morbidity and mortality. All people with diabetes should be treated as if they have known cardiovascular disease (Tabibiazar and Edelman 2003). The American Diabetes Association (ADA) recommends including cardiac stress tests when the individual has two or more cardiovascular risk factors as well as for people with microalbuminuria, and sedentary people about to commence an exercise programme (ADA 2006). Table 1.4 shows the common the long-term complications associated with diabetes.

The long-term complications are associated with prolonged hyperglycaemia measured by HbA_{1c} (glycosylated haemoglobin) and hypertension and the associated abnormalities (Diabetes Control and Complications Trial 1993; United Kingdom Prospective Study 1998). The current HbA_{1c} target is <7.0 per cent. The causes of long-standing hyperglycaemia are multifactorial and include genetic predisposition, free radical oxidative damage, protein glycosylation, and endothelial changes. In addition, lower socio-economic status, psychological issues that lead to lack of motivation, emotional distress, poor eating habits and depression, inadequate knowledge on the part of the person with diabetes and the health professionals caring for them, have been implicated (DeVries *et al*. 2004).

1.7 Psychological Aspects

The diagnosis of diabetes affects people in many different ways depending on their age, knowledge and beliefs about diabetes, locus of control, available support, culture and the knowledge, beliefs and attitudes of the health professionals who care for them, see Chapter 7. Many people go through an initial grieving stage as they come to terms with the diagnosis and may re-grieve when they develop a complication.

Self-care is necessary and expected with the availability of modern technological devices to test blood glucose and blood ketones. The individual is also expected to problem-solve and adjust their treatment to accommodate fluctuations in these parameters. Inadequate self-care is associated with poorer health outcomes, more frequent admissions to emergency departments or hospital, low self-esteem, and increases the risk of short- and long-term complications (Cieckanowski *et al*. 2000).

Depression is common and is associated with the burden of diabetes, which puts a strain on relationships, and can create shock and guilt. The stigma of having diabetes is still an issue in many social circumstances, as are uncertainty about the future, loss of control, and past negative experiences with health professionals (Caven *et al*. 2001). Signs and symptoms of depression in the person with diabetes include disinterest, reduced confidence, lack of energy, changes in sleep and eating patterns, and self-neglect, including diabetes self-care. These negative psychosocial factors and symptoms can result in hyperglycaemia, which further lowers mood.

1.8   Diabetes Management Requires Integrated Approaches

The sobering incidence and prevalence data previously discussed emphasise the fact that a best practice approach to managing diabetes involves addressing the needs of people with diabetes and those of health professionals in an integrated manner. In addition, diabetes management is regarded as requiring a team approach that includes relevant health professionals and places the person with diabetes in a central role. In other words, provide holistic care. In this context, 'holism' refers to providing care in the context of the whole person and respecting the fact that each person is a unique individual (Vickers 1996).

A philosophical basis of many complementary approaches is the belief that 'the body has the capacity to heal itself' and the role of health professionals is to support the healing process. Such a philosophy is very close to the emerging modern diabetes person-centred management philosophy.

1.9   People with Diabetes' Needs, Capacities and Resources

At the centre of integrated management is the person with diabetes making choices about their health and informed decisions about the interventions they choose to use. Research shows that people with chronic illnesses often choose to use both conventional and complementary medicine (Astin 1998; Bausell *et al.* 2001; Pettigrew *et al.* 2004). The reasons for using complementary therapies and the frequency of use are discussed in Chapter 2.

The research emphasises the fact that people with chronic illnesses, including diabetes, do not share the intellectual dichotomy that often exists in conventional health professional training. They appreciate the ability to make choices and adapt both systems to their lives. The choice of using complementary medicine is often based on the belief that it is 'more congruent with their own values, beliefs, and philosophical orientations toward health and life' (Afridi and Khan 2003).

The general public, including people with diabetes, is increasingly knowledgeable about health issues and available health-care choices and has high expectations of health professionals and services. However, they may be overly optimistic about the safety of many therapies, under-estimate or not be informed about the risks, or not attribute unwanted effects to treatments (Ernst 1996).

1.10   Health Professionals' Needs

There is a need to establish professional education programmes that encompass all aspects of diabetes and its manifest complications using sound evidence-based principles. Integrating these twin aspects in a therapeutic process has shown that people who are assisted to develop networks of trust, gain access to preventive education, and then use appropriate interventions based on this knowledge, have better disease-related outcomes such as improved HBA_{1c} and significantly lower complication rates (Afridi and Khan 2003). The challenge for health professionals is to facilitate the process of developing team care and 'networks of trust'. Until recently, most people took the advice of non-professional sources such as friends, and Internet sites and the media; fewer than 50 per cent seek advice from a health professional (Giveon *et al.* 2003; Lanski *et al.* 2003).

Some of the challenges for health professionals that have emerged in the literature include: Patients not asking about complementary therapy use; patients receiving or perceiving negative responses from conventional practitioners when they disclose their complementary therapy use; and lack of knowledge about complementary therapies (conventional practitioners) and about conventional care (complementary practitioners) (Giveon *et al.* 2003), see Chapter 2.

Significantly, lack of communication between practitioners from the two approaches can lead to confusion and increases the risk of adverse outcomes. However, these factors are changing, especially in primary care settings where practitioners are often exposed to questions related to complementary therapies and their usefulness, and where there is an increasing number of referrals to complementary practitioners and vice versa (Crock *et al.* 1999; Hall and Giles-Conti 2000; Van Haselen *et al.* 2004). Likewise, there is an increasing amount of credible research and literature that can help health professionals negotiate the complex and diverse field of 'complementary therapies' and identify their role and scope in diabetes care, see Chapter 4. It is no longer appropriate to consider conventional and complementary care as two separate paradigms (Ernst 1996).

1.11 Integration – Is It Possible?

Chapter 4 discusses issues surrounding integrating the two approaches and suggests some strategies for combining conventional and complementary approaches. Thus, in summary, there is evidence that people with diabetes achieve better outcomes if they are well educated about their diabetes, its management, complications, and monitoring, including and encompassing complementary therapies. A significant improvement in health professional education is required, and could include non-judgemental history taking related to complementary therapies, education about common complementary modalities, and how to access relevant information. Conversely, complementary practitioners require similar education about conventional management approaches. Practice guidelines have also been suggested as a way to assist safe integration (Yeh *et al.* 2002; Mehrotra *et al.* 2004; Giveon *et al.* 2004).

This book is one attempt to address some of the educational needs of health professionals caring for people with diabetes in the twenty-first century who are working within a changing society where people with diabetes no longer want to be defined by disease-focused reductionistic terms such as 'diabetics', or descriptions such as the 'diabetic foot'. These practitioners *will* be sharing patients with complementary practitioners, which leads to questions about the 'sanctity, integrity and power of the therapeutic relationship' such that 'the medical profession can no longer just be the possessor of knowledge.' In fact, this book is a move towards the pluralism, harmonisation, and integration desired by Lewith and Bensoussan in the *Medical Journal of Australia* (Bensonssan *et al.* 2004).

Professor Cohen in the same journal outlined the practical nature of the process of integration. He suggested most general practitioners have patients with chronic illness who could benefit from the services of complementary practitioners and virtually all complementary practitioners have patients who require access to mainstream diagnosis and therapy. Collaboration requires shared respect, trust, and education. Importantly, the dangers of not integrating care include delaying or depriving people of safe and effective management and increase the potential for harmful interactions (Cohen 2004).

1.12 Complementary Therapies

Not all Complementary and alternative medicine (CAM) practitioners agree on the principles of diseases but most encompass three ideals: (1) treatment should be as natural as possible; (2) it should be holistic; and (3) it should promote general well-being. Most ascribe to vitalism in some way, for example, terms such as vital force, life energy, and the body's ability to heal itself. Some complementary therapies are more effective and safer than others.

Until recently there has been limited quality research into complementary therapies, because, as in other areas, funding is difficult to access, research expertise and research mentors are lacking, and there is limited infrastructure to support research. A great deal of the available research is difficult to interpret due to methodological flaws, poor reporting, and a great deal is not conducted in the manner the particular therapy is practised (Vickers 1996). However, many complementary therapies have a long history of safe traditional use that provides a firm foundation for future research. There is no doubt there are complementary practitioners with idealistic, extremist views, just as there are conventional practitioners who are sceptical about complementary therapies (Bratman 1997).

1.13 Summary

The book encompasses the principle that people with diabetes are essential members of the health care team who require support to achieve better health outcomes for an increasingly prevalent global epidemic. The book provides readers with a definition of complementary and alternative medicine and discusses some of the evidence to support the integration of some complementary therapies into modern diabetes management. The book provides an in-depth insight into commonly used complementary therapies and their application in the management of people with diabetes. By exploring and understanding such accumulated knowledge, health professionals may be able to provide relevant information to help people make informed choices that match their life expectations, not just our more disease-focused management regimens.

References

Afridi MA, Khan MN. Role of health education in the management of diabetes mellitus. *J Coll Physicians Surg Pak.* 2003; **13**(10): 558–561.

American Diabetes Association. Standards of medical care in Diabetes–2006. *Diabetes Care* 2006; **29**: S4–42.

Astin A. Why patients use alternative medicine: results of a national study. *Journal American Medical Association* 1998; **279**(19): 1548–1553.

Bauman W, Shaw S, Jayatilleke J, Spungen A, Herbert V. Increased intake of calcium reverses vitamin B_{12} malabsorption induced by Metformin. *Diabetes Care* 2000; **223**(9): 1227–1231.

Bausell R, Lee W, Berman B. Demographic and health-related correlates to visits to complementary and alternative medical providers. *Medical Care* 2001; **39**(2): 190–196.

Bensoussan A, Lewith G. Complementary medicine research in Australia. *Complementary and Alternative Medicine* 2004; **181**(6): 331–333.

Bratman S. *The Alternative Medicine Sourcebook*. Lincolnwood: Lowell House, 1997.

Caven D, Fosbury J, Tigwell P. Psychology in diabetes – why bother? *Practical Diabetes International* 2001; **18**(7): 228–229.

The Centre for Disease Control and Prevention. 2006; www.cdc.gov/nccdphp/dnpa/ press/archive/twinepid.htm (accessed February 2006).

Cieckanowski P, Caton W, Russo W. Impact of depressive symptoms on adherence, function and costs. *Archives of Internal Medicine* 2000; **160**: 3278–3285.

Cohen M. CAM practitioners and "regular" doctors: is integration possible? *Medical Journal of Australia* 2004; **180**(12): 645–646.

Crock R, Jarjoura D, Polen A, Rutecki G. Confronting the communication gap between conventional and alternative medicine: a survey of physicians' attitudes. *Alternative Therapies Health Medicine* 1999; **5**(2): 61–66.

DeVries J, Snoek F, Heine R. Persistent poor glycaemic control in adult type 1 diabetes: a closer look at the problem. *Diabetic Medicine* 2004; **21**: 1263–1268.

Diabetes Care. Coffee reduces the risk of developing type 2 diabetes. *Diabetes Care* 2006; **29**: 398–403.

Diabetes Control and Complications Trial Research Group. The effect of intensive insulin treatment of diabetes on the development and progression of long term complications in insulin dependent diabetes mellitus. *New England Journal of Medicine* 1993; **329**: 977–986.

Dornhorst A. Insulinotrophic meglitinide analogues. *Lancet* 2001; **358**(9294): 1709–1716.

Dunstan D, Zimmet PZ, Welborn TA, De Courten MP, Cameron AJ, Sicree RA, Dwyer T, Colagiuri S, Jolley D, Knuiman M, Atkins R, Shaw JE. The rising prevalence of diabetes and impaired glucose tolerance: the Australian Diabetes, Obesity and Lifestyle Study. *Diabetes Care* 2002; **25**(5): 829–834.

Ernst E. *Complementary Medicine: An Objective Appraisal*. Oxford: Butterworth Heinemann, 1996.

Freedman D, Dietz W. The relation of overweight to cardiovascular risk factors among children and adolescents: the Bogalusa Heart Study. *Paediatrics* 1999; **103**(6): 1175–1182.

Gale E. Spring harvest? Reflections on the rise of type 1 diabetes. *Diabetologia* 2005; **48**: 2445–2450.

Giveon S, Liberman N, Klang S, Kahan E. A survey of primary care physicians' perceptions of their patients' use of complementary medicine. *Complementary Therapies in Medicine* 2003; **11**(4): 254–260.

Giveon SM, Liberman N, Klang S, Kahan E. Are people who use "natural drugs" aware of their potentially harmful side effects and reporting to family physician? *Patient Education and Counselling* 2004; **53**(1): 5–11.

Hall K, Giles-Corti B. Complementary therapies and the general practitioner: a survey of Perth GPs. *Australian Family Physician* 2000; **29**(6): 602–606.

Holstein A, Stumvoll M. Contraindications can damage your health – is metfomin a case in point? *Diabetologia* 2005; **48**: 2454–2459.

Hubert HB, Feinleib M, McNamarn PM, Castelli WP. Obesity as an independent risk factor for cardiovascular disease: a 26-year follow-up of participants in the Framingham Heart Study. *Circulation* 1983; **67**(5): 967–968.

Knerr I, Wolf J, Reinehr T, Stachow R, Grabert M, Scober E, Rascher W, Holl R. The "accelerator hypothesis": relationship between weight, height, body mass index and age at diagnosis in a large cohort of 9248 German and Austrian children with type 1 diabetes. *Diabetologia* 2005; **48**: 2501–2504.

Lanski S, Greenwald M, Perkins A, Simon H. Herbal therapy use in a pediatric emergency department population: expect the unexpected. *Pediatrics* 2003; **111**(5 Pt 1): 981–985.

Lewith G, Bensoussan A. Complementary and alternative medicine – with a difference. *Medical Journal of Australia* 2004; **180**(11): 585–586.

Medical and Health Annual Encyclopaedia Britannica. Chicago: Encyclopaedia Britannica Inc. 1999.

Mehrotra R, Bajaj S, Kumar D. Use of complementary and alternative medicine by patients with diabetes mellitus. *National Medical Journal of India* 2004; **17**(5): 243–245.

Moutet J, Kangambega-Nouvier P, Donnet J, Pileire B, Eschvege E, Patterson A. Diabetes mellitus and public health in Guadeloupe. *West Indian Medical Journal* 1990; **39**(3):139–143.

National Evidence-Based Guidelines for the Management of Type 2 Diabetes Mellitus prepared by the Australian Centre for Diabetes Strategies, Prince of Wales Hospital, Sydney, for the Diabetes Australia Guideline Development Consortium.

Pettigrew A, King M, McGee K, Rudolph C. Complementary therapy use by women's health clinic clients. *Alternative Therapies Health Medicine* 2004; **10**(6): 50–55.

Poehlman E, Tchernof A. Traversing the menopause: changes in energy expenditure and body composition. *Coronary Artery Diseases* 1998; **9**: 799–803.

Tabibiazar R, Edelman S. Silent ischemia in people with diabetes: a condition that must be heard. *Clinical Diabetes* 2003; **21**: 5–9.

Turner N, Clapham C. Insulin resistance, impaired glucose tolerance and non-insulin dependent diabetes pathologic mechanisms and treatment: current status and therapeutic possibilities. *Progress in Drug Research* 1998; **51**: 33–94.

United Kingdom Prospective Study (UKPDS 33, 34). Intensive blood glucose control. *Lancet* 1998; **352**: 837–853, 854–865.

Van Haselen R, Reiber U, Nickel I, Jakob A, Fisher P. Providing complementary and alternative medicine in primary care: the primary care workers' perspective. *Complementary Therapies in Medicine* 2004; **12**(1): 6–16.

Vettor R, Milan G, Rossato M, Federspil G. Review article: adipocytokines and insulin resistance. *Pharmacological Therapies* 2005; **22**(Suppl 2): 3–10.

Vickers A. *Massage and Aromatherapy: A Guide for Health Professionals.* Chapman and Hall, London, 1996.

Wild S, Roglic G, Green A, Sicree R, King H. Global prevalence of diabetes: estimates for the year 2000 and projections for 2030. *Diabetes Care* 2004; **27**: 1047–1053.

Yeh G, Eisenberg D, Davis R, Phillips R. Use of complementary and alternative medicine among persons with diabetes mellitus: results of a national survey. *American Journal of Public Health* 2002; **92**(10): 1648–1652.

2 Complementary Therapy Use

Mohan Pawa

2.1 Introduction

The general public is increasingly demanding and using complementary therapies. Consequently a wide range of health-care options are available in most countries. Likewise, the complexity of the types of therapies available and therefore the use are increasing, partly due to international travel and migration and international communication systems such as the Internet. The terminology surrounding complementary therapies is confusing and changing. From the 1970s until the 1990s they were known as 'traditional', 'alternative', 'natural', 'fringe medicine', 'unorthodox', 'unscientific', and 'unconventional'. Current terminology reflects the changes that have occurred in the past ten years and the increasing tolerance if not acceptance with which they are regarded, for example, 'complementary medicine', 'complementary therapies', and 'complementary and alternative medicine' (CAM). However, some countries such as Africa and the Western Pacific and South East Asia regions still use the term 'traditional' (World Health Organization (WHO) 2002).

2.2 Defining Complementary Therapies

The term 'complementary therapies' is actually an umbrella term that encompasses more then 300 different modalities. CAM is defined in various ways:

> Group of diverse, medical and health care systems, practices and products that are not presently considered to be part of conventional medicine.
>
> (National Center for Complementary and Alternative Medicine USA)

Complementary Therapies and the Management of Diabetes and Vascular Disease   Editor Trish Dunning
© 2006 John Wiley & Sons, Ltd.

A broad domain of healing resources and their accompanying theories and beliefs, other than those intrinsic to the politically dominant health system of a particular society or culture in a given period. They include all practices, ideas self-defined by their users as preventing or treating illness or promoting health and well being. The boundaries within and between complementary and the dominant systems are rarely sharp or fixed.

(Cochrane Collaboration and US National Institute of Health)

Diverse health practices, approaches, knowledge and beliefs incorporating plant, animal, and/or mineral-based medicines, spiritual therapies, manual techniques and exercise applied singularly or in combination to maintain well-being, as well as to treat, diagnose or prevent illness.

(WHO 2002)

Therapies which can work alongside and in conjunction with orthodox medical treatment

(British Medical Association)

All the above definitions share the common theme that CAM is diverse and encompasses various health practices or approaches, which are self-defined by the users and applied on their own or in combination with conventional medicines. The two systems can be separate with one system dominant but also they can complement each other.

Table 2.1 Commonly used complementary therapies. The list is derived from the literature and the personal experience of the authors. Therapies * indicate herbs and/or supplements may be used.

---

*Acupuncture
*Aromatherapy
*Ayurveda
Chiropractic
*Herbal medicines and supplements
*Homeopathy
Humour
Kinesiology
Manipulative therapies
*Massage
Meditation
Music
*Naturopathy
*Nutritional therapies (nutraceuticals)
Reflexology
Reiki
Therapeutic touch and holistic touch
Pet therapy

As well as a range of definitions of CAM, there is a range of ways they are categorised or grouped. For example, the US NIH divided CAM into five main categories:

1. Alternative medical systems such as Chinese medicine and Ayurveda. Chinese medicine was known as 'traditional Chinese medicine' until recently.
2. Mind–body therapies.
3. Biological-based systems such as herbal medicine, which is sometimes known as phytomedicine. Herbal medicine encompasses the major herbal traditions: Chinese, Kampo (Japanese), Ayurveda (India), North American Indian, and European.
4. Manipulative and body therapies such as massage and chiropractic.
5. Energy therapies.

These are general categories. Some CAM fit into more than one category, for example, aromatherapy: the essential oils are part of phytotherapy but the application method may be massage, which falls within the manipulative therapy category. Commonly used CAM are shown in Table 2.1. Some CAM, such as Chinese medicine and Ayurveda, have a long history of traditional use; others such as Bowen therapies are more recent. Most do not have the same scientific basis as conventional medicine.

2.3 What Is Traditional Use?

'Traditional use' encompasses evidence found in herbal monographs, and historical sources often accumulated over centuries, which represents a synthesis of the accumulated wisdom of experts, which is the lowest form of evidence in conventional health care. The type of traditional evidence is an important consideration. In a hierarchy of traditional evidence, monographs could be considered to be better evidence than consensus recommendations, case history reports, textbooks and CAM conference reports (Kraft 2005).

Other methods of determining the value of traditional use evidence include:

- geographical distribution of use. The wider the global use, the higher the 'evidence';
- consistency of documented use from an historical context;
- terminology such as accurate classification of plants by using botanical names;
- type of documentation and its relevance to particular societies. Some cultures have written documents, others are based on oral traditions. Both are open to inaccurate translation and interpretation.
- use according to the traditional methods, precautions, doses and dose intervals. Modern extraction and preparation methods may change some of the traditional aspects of some CAM, for example, the composition of herbal medicines and essential oils.
- traditional indications for use and any modifications as a result of modern information and research (Kraft 2005).

These issues need to be considered when evaluating the safety and efficacy of CAM and its application for specific individuals.

2.4 Philosophical Basis of CAM

Each CAM has its own philosophical basis but there are some common core elements:

- Self-care and prevention are important components of health.
- The body has the capacity to heal itself. In this context, healing does not refer to curing but to a process combining physical, mental, emotional, and spiritual aspects to achieve a balance respecting the values of each component.
- The patient plays a central role in their care.
- The practitioner assists the healing process by selecting and administering appropriate treatments in consultation with the patient.
- Balance and harmony are essential to health.
- The presenting symptoms are a guide to the location of the imbalance and may suggest management strategies, for example, see Chinese medicine discussed in Chapter 11.
- The aim of management strategies is to restore balance.
- Physical, psychological and spiritual factors are intricately linked and imbalance in one of these aspects creates imbalance in another.
- Ill health is an opportunity for positive change.

Many of these issues apply to conventional care and are appropriate to diabetes management, although the terminology used in the conventional health-care system is different. For example, current diabetes care emphasises patient-centred care and empowerment as being integral to achieving optimal outcomes.

2.5 Frequency of CAM Use

General

The decision to use CAM is complex and depends on a number of issues such as health beliefs and the experience and the advice of significant others (Braun *et al.* 2005). People often use more than one CAM and frequently combine CAM and conventional therapies. The WHO provides some general global CAM usage statistics, which are shown in Table 2.2 but does not provide any diabetes-specific data. The information that is available suggests CAM use is multifactorial and that people rarely abandon conventional care. Instead they consider their health-care options and mix and match to achieve their health goals (Thomas *et al.* 1991; Eisenberg *et al.* 1998). They also choose CAM that are congruent with their personal values and beliefs, which are multifactorial and can result from past experiences including those with conventional care and CAM (Astin 1998).

Over 50 per cent of the Australian population uses some form of CAM (MacLennan *et al.* 1996) and public spending on CAM far exceeds that spent on conventional pharmaceutical medicines. Usage is similar in the USA where

Table 2.2 Frequency of use of complementary and alternative therapies derived from the World Health Organization Traditional Medicine Strategy 2002. These figures probably underestimated the true frequency of use at the time they were collected and may not accurately reflect current use.

Country	Frequency of use (%)
Africa	~80
Australia	*52
Belgium	31
China	40
France	49
Japan	~60
Switzerland	46
United Kingdom	#24
United States	> 42

Source: * Derived from Complementary Therapies in the Australian Health Care System (2003). # Derived from a BBC Survey.

CAM expenditure increased to 45.2 per cent, between 1990 and 1997, exceeding out-of-pocket expenditure for all US hospitals, which represents a total of over US $21 billion. Furthermore, visits to CAM practitioners exceed total visits to all US primary care sources (Eisenberg *et al*. 1998). A recent UK survey of CAM use showed that 48 per cent of the population had tried CAM and over 10 per cent had consulted a CAM practitioner in the last year (Thomas *et al*. 2001).

The European Research Initiative on Complementary and Alternative Medicine (EURICAM) indicated that patients increasingly consult CAM practitioners and use CAM therapies either in conjunction with conventional medicines or as an alternative, often because of the side effects associated with conventional medicines, which they find difficult to live with. Some patients find conventional treatments are not effective. Patients in many European countries seek a more ecological and holistic view of health.

The shift in demand has engendered a great deal of debate and frequently adverse and judgemental comments by conventional practitioners who often have little knowledge of CAM. Some legitimate concerns arise from the limited evidence base for many CAM therapies. In order to resolve some of the debate, EURICAM advised the European Union (EU) to provide research funding to evaluate the role of CAM in the EU.

In the UK, researchers from the Royal London Homoeopathic Hospital examined patients' reasons for using CAM in the National Health Service in UK, including the nature and duration of their main health problem. Sharples *et al*. (2003) distributed questionnaires to examine the impact of CAM on people's main health problem, satisfaction with clinical care, and compliance with conventional medicines (n = 499). Some 63 per cent of respondents had lived with their main problem for more than five years: most had musculoskeletal problems (32 per cent); 90 per cent were satisfied with their conventional care, and 81 per cent indicated their main problem had improved on using CAM. Significantly, 29 per cent of the

262 taking conventional medicines stopped taking them after starting CAM and 32 per cent reduced their conventional medicine doses. The researchers concluded that conventional medicine does not meet the needs of some patients and that CAM could wholly or partly replace conventional medicines in some cases.

Rolniack *et al.* (2004) found 47 per cent of a convenience sample of 174 patients attending an emergency department in an urban Catholic hospital in the USA used CAM, especially prayer, music therapy and meditation and one-third did not disclose their CAM use. Rolniack *et al.* did not find any sociodemograpic predictors of CAM use, but users were more likely to have a chronic condition. It is not clear whether diabetes was among the chronic conditions in this study but the association between chronic disease and CAM use is consistent with other research. Interestingly, Honda and Jacobson (2004) found an association between specific personality domains, coping strategies and social support and CAM use among adults, which might predict CAM use.

Older people often use chiropractic, herbal medicines, relaxation, vitamin supplements and religious and spiritual healing (Foster *et al.* 2000). People in Foster *et al.*'s study who regularly consulted their primary conventional practitioners were more likely to consult a CAM practitioner but the majority did not disclose their CAM use. Adolescents are also likely to use CAM.

Braun *et al.* (2005) surveyed adolescents between 12 and 18 years attending an urban clinic (n = 401) and found two-thirds used CAM and most were females. Half indicated they made their own health decisions but parents made health decisions for 27 per cent, but CAM users were likely to have been influenced by family members or friends. Some 25 per cent were taking at least one conventional medicine. Common therapies used were herbal medicines, dietary supplements, massage, chiropractic, spiritual therapy, aromatherapy, yoga and tai chi mainly to control pain, reduce stress and boost their immune system or generally improve their health. Similar to the older CAM users in Foster *et al.*'s (2000) study, Braun *et al.*'s respondents did not disclose their CAM use. Interestingly, 71 per cent reported never being asked about CAM, which is worrying considering the frequent reminders to conventional practitioners in a range of publications about the need to ask about CAM use. It is not clear whether people with diabetes were included in either of these studies.

People often seek CAM for specific health concerns such as pain. Haetzman *et al.* (2003) identified high use of CAM therapies among people with chronic pain in a survey of 840 individuals in the UK, and the percentage of people consulting CAM and conventional practitioners increased with increasing pain severity. The prevalence of CAM use in Haetzman *et al.*'s study is higher than previously reported for chronic pain management (Andersson *et al.* 1999). Most used CAM in conjunction with conventional pain management strategies. It is unclear whether people with diabetes were included in either of these studies but diabetic complications such as peripheral neuropathy are associated with significant levels of pain, see Chapter 15.

People also use CAM for serious conditions. For example, 45 per cent of 308 people with cardiac disease attending ambulatory care centres used CAM

(Abramson 2005) and were more likely to inform their general practitioner than their cardiologist about their CAM use. Like Braun *et al.*'s cohort, Abramson's subjects indicated their doctors did not ask about CAM use. The majority had received CAM information from the lay press and friends, although 21 per cent had received information from their doctors. CAM use was associated with increasing age, high income, and high levels of education. Abramson's study raises concern about the potential interactions between herbal and conventional medicines in a group of patients likely to be taking multiple medicines and which is likely to include people with diabetes, because cardiovascular disease is the leading diabetes-related complication and cause of death, see Chapter 1.

Gozum and Unsal (2004) found a high use of herbal medicines in a random sample of 385 older community-dwelling women in Turkey. Herbal medicine users were not significantly different from non-users, but those women who had difficulty performing activities of daily living, poor self-reported health, chronic conditions including diabetes, and made frequent visits to physicians used herbal medicines more frequently. Herbal medicines in Turkey are usually prescribed by traditional healers, many of whom are older women, which may have influenced the women in Gozum and Unsal's study.

Despite continued widespread CAM use, there is some limited evidence that 'herbal supplement' use could be levelling out in the USA. In a survey of 8500 adults, Kaufman (2005) found more people were taking herbs and supplements in 2002 than in a previous survey three years earlier but attributed the increase to a high usage of the antioxidant lutein. When lutein use was excluded, supplement use was similar with approximately 14 per cent of mostly older people taking supplements. Older people may be particularly at risk of adverse events since the incidence of diabetes and its complications, and comorbidities, and the need for conventional medicines, are likely to be higher. Interestingly, many older people consider supplements to be natural and harmless and do not view them as medicines (Stupay and Siversten 2000).

Health professional S'1 CAM use

The general public and people with diabetes are not the only people who use CAM. Health professionals also use CAM personally and consult CAM practitioners, incorporate CAM into their practice, recommend CAM to patients, or refer patients to CAM practitioners. Ernst *et al.* (1994) indicated 95 per cent of German physicians, 54 per cent of 89 Israeli physicians, and 73 per cent of 200 Canadian physicians use CAM personally, especially younger physicians, and consider it moderately effective. Likewise, Berman (1998) found the longer physicians had been in practice, the less favourable their views of CAM were. Practitioners in Berman's study considered biofeedback, counselling and diet and exercise to be more 'legitimate' than other therapies.

Conventional practitioners using CAM come from all practice areas but general practitioners (GP) and nurses are the most frequent users. Visser and Peters (1990) indicated that GPs were more pragmatic about CAM use than hospital doctors and that conventional practitioners view therapies such as manipulation, counselling and massage as conventional therapies, which makes it difficult to classify CAM. Some conventional practitioners come from cultures where CAM therapies predominate and thus have traditional experience of CAM and accept the efficacy and benefit of some CAM; others see CAM as an income stream (Sharma 1992) because health insurers reimburse some CAM-related costs in many countries. Likewise, CAM training is offered as a component of many conventional education programmes and CAM-related publications appear in an increasing number of conventional journals (Ernst 1996 p ix).

Researchers from the Royal London Homoeopathic Hospital conducted a survey to assess primary care workers' perception of the need to integrate CAM and suggestions about how it could be integrated into primary care, via a postal survey of 149 general practitioners (GP), 24 nurses and 32 other primary care team members (n = 205) (Haselen *et al.* 2004). Of these, 171 respondents stated that 68 per cent of referrals to CAM practitioners were initiated on the request of the patient: 58 per cent because they felt conventional therapies were ineffective; 32 per cent had more than one reason. Haselen *et al.* concluded that there is considerable interest in CAM among primary care professionals and many are already referring patients to or recommending referrals to CAM practitioners, mostly in response to patient demand. Most respondents favoured integrating at least some CAM therapies into conventional primary care. The findings also suggest there is an urgent need to educate/inform primary care health professionals about CAM.

Helmrich *et al.* (2001) used focus groups to investigate the beliefs and attitudes of nurses to non-pharmacological pain management (n = 37) from medical, surgical, palliative, and critical care areas in two Australian hospitals. Participants indicated non-pharmacological pain management offers some advantages to general well-being and could alleviate pain until conventional medicines took effect. The nurses indicated a lack of organisational support hindered their use. They used a range of CAM therapies including massage, relaxation, distraction, heat, aromatherapy, acupuncture and imagery. CAM pain management strategies are discussed in Chapter 15. Likewise, Tracey *et al.* (2005) found the majority of a random sample of 726 critical care nurses in the USA felt CAM was a beneficial legitimate form of care and wanted more information about CAM.

Diabetes health professionals use or recommend CAM to people with diabetes. For example, Sabo *et al.* (1999) surveyed 2,850 American diabetes educators about their CAM use and achieved a response rate of 829. A range of therapies such as physical activity, diet, laughter and humour, relaxation therapy, prayer, meditation and massage were used or recommended regularly. There were gender differences between the sexes with respect to the type of therapies used. Females were more like to use/recommend relaxation, music therapy and humour while males were more likely to use/recommend homeopathy and megavitamins, however, there were only a few males in the study. Older respondents with years of diabetes education experience were more likely to use/recommend CAM. It is not clear whether the educators using CAM had relevant qualifications.

In a smaller survey of 38 Australian diabetes educators, Dunning (2003) found 16 reported using CAM in patient care to manage stress, relieve pain and improve well-being and 27 used CAM for personal health care. Five reported 'improved' HbA_{1c} levels and reduced doses of glucose-lowering medicines as a result of CAM. Only one respondent had a CAM qualification, which raises concern about their CAM knowledge and competence. This is a small study and needs to be interpreted with caution. The studies by Sabo *et al.* and Dunning suggest diabetes educators may be using/recommending CAM to their patients in some way.

People with diabetes and CAM use

Some people with diabetes use CAM to improve glycaemic control but they also use it for a range of other reasons, such as prevention, to manage distressing symptoms such as pain associated with complications, and to improve their quality of life. Some of the therapies they use are effective and beneficial, others are ineffective and may be harmful. Therefore, it is important that people who use CAM should inform their conventional practitioners about their CAM use. However, conventional practitioners have a responsibility to enquire about CAM use from their patients, see Chapter 4. Bhardwaj (1975) studied attitude towards different systems of medicine among physicians and head of the households in four villages in the Indian Punjab and reported that traditional remedies had a modest but not insignificant role within the context of total health care and chronic disease without any serious health threats.

Leese *et al.* (1997) found 17 per cent of people with diabetes attending an outpatient clinic in the UK used CAM. In Canada Ryan *et al.* (1999) found 25 per cent and in Australia Dunning found that between 17–25 per cent of people with diabetes in outpatient settings used a range of CAM therapies, usually in combination with conventional therapies, thought they were beneficial. Usage was similar among people with type 1 and type 2 diabetes. Egede *et al.* (2002) extracted data from a US medical expenditure survey and estimated that people with diabetes are 1.6 times more likely to use CAM than non-diabetics and suggested diabetes is an independent predictor of CAM use in people over 65 years.

Yeh *et al.* (2003) undertook a systemic literature review of herbs and dietary supplements to assess the efficacy and safety and effects on glycaemic control among patients with diabetes. They observed that many chemicals used in modern conventional medicines have plant origins, for example, Metformin was derived from the flowering plant *Galega officinalis* (goat's rue or French lilac). Vitamin and mineral supplements are commonly used for primary or secondary disease prevention, but information about the efficacy and safety of herbs, vitamins or other dietary supplements for diabetes management is conflicting. Quality randomised control trial (RCT) with Jadad scores of three or more are available for *Cocinia sativam*, Ginseng species, *Bauhinia forficate* and *Myrcia unifora*. Less rigorous RCT evidence exists for *Allium cepa, Ocimum sanctum, Ficus carica, Silibum marianum, Opunita streptacanta. Gymnema sylvestre* and *Momordica charantia*, see Chapter 9.

Pawa (1991) conducted a study of CAM use among Indo-Asians people with type 2 diabetes living in the UK for his MSc thesis to determine the relationship among beliefs, knowledge and glycaemic control. He interviewed 30 Asians with type 2 diabetes from the Indian subcontinent visiting Ealing General Hospital outpatient clinic about their diabetes-related knowledge, beliefs, and behaviour with a view to understanding variations in blood glucose control. Some 57 per cent of respondents used herbal medicines and other traditional therapies, some in conjunction with prescribed glucose-lowering conventional medicines. Only 16 per cent of respondents informed their doctor or other health professionals about their CAM use. This finding is consistent with other studies reported in the literature. A common reason for not informing doctors about CAM use was a concern that conventional health professionals might not be familiar with CAM herbal medicines or may advise the patient to stop taking them.

Commonly used herbal medicines were Kerela in the form of a vegetable or juice, Jamun juice or Methi seeds. Many people with type 2 diabetes bring the traditional remedies, including herbal medicines, from their countries of origin when they go on holidays overseas or import them when they migrate, often on the suggestion of a family member. The influence of family members on CAM use in Pawa's study is consistent with the literature.

People also used a variety of fixed combinations, which had four to five common ingredients, some with glucose-lowering effects. The Central Council for Research in Ayurveda and Sidha (Ministry of Health and Family Welfare) helped Pawa locate relevant publications from their libraries and other educational research centres. Many of the articles identified the glucose-lowering effects of combined preparations but very few observed such effects in single herbs. A number of plants and their extracts have been tested in diabetic animal models (rat, rabbit, guinea pig and rhesus monkey) in South-East Asia. Over 150 herbs and their isolates were tested but only a limited number had glucose-lowering properties. Figure 2.1 depicts a selection of fixed combination and other traditional glucose-lowering remedies identified in Pawa's study.

In Figure 2.1, Madhu dosantak, the wooden tumbler, is made from the wood of *Pterocarpus marsupium* from the family Papillonaeceae. In rural areas of the Chhatisgarh region of Madhya Pradesh many people with diabetes fill the tumbler with water, leave it overnight and drink the water the next morning. Saifi *et al.* (1971) obtained authenticated samples of the wood and finely powdered them to produce an alkaloidal fraction. The alcohol extract was administered into the peritoneal cavity of adult albino rabbits and the blood glucose was measured every hour for three hours. A significant drop in blood glucose occurred, 23.3 per cent in one hour, 29.9 per cent in two hours, and 33.3 per cent in three hours. In contrast, blood glucose increased in the control group: 23.3 mg, 29.9 mg, 33.3 mg at one, two and three hours, respectively. Harnath *et al.* (1958), Joglekar *et al.* (1959) and Gupta (1963) recorded mild to moderate hypoglycaemic effects in animals using similar extracts in earlier studies.

Salacia macrosperma (Saptarangi) is commonly used plant. Arora *et al.* (1973) boiled pulverised leaves and roots in 16 times their volume of water to obtain

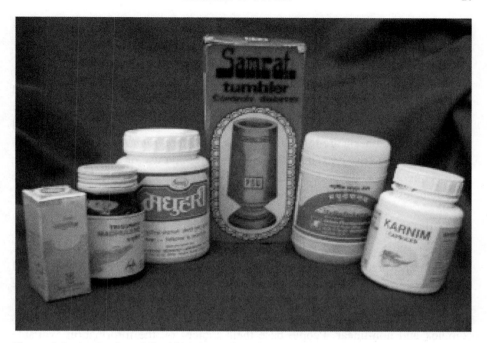

Figure 2.1 A selection of fixed blend propriety glucose lowering formulations used in the UK (Pawa 1999). The main ingredients in each formulation are shown. Madhu Dosantak: Wooden cup Madhu Hari: Gudmar, Karela Beej, Jamun, Guthi, Neem Patra, Shilajeeta, Amba Haldi. Madhulene: Gudmar, Jamun Guthi, Neem Patra, Shilajeet. Karnim: Karela, Neem Patra, Tulsi Kutu. Jambrulin: Jamungiri, Biu Patra, Gudmar, Neem Patra, Shilajeet. Madhu Mehari: Tribang Bhasam, Gudmar, Camun Giri, Karela, Shilajeet. Ayshu–82: Gudmar, Karela, Jamun, Mango Giri, Shilajeet.

a decoction containing 1 gm of the crude herb. The decoction was administered orally at a dose of 1gm/kg body weight to rabbits weighing between 1.25 and 1.75 kg. Blood glucose was measured at baseline after an 18-hour fast and four hours after the decoction was administered. Four different samples from different experiments were used to compare the glucose-lowering effects with Tolbutamide. A significant drop in blood glucose occurred four hours after administering the decoction in all samples. The greatest fall was in the Tolbutamide group.

Sivprakasam *et al.* (1982) studied the hypoglycaemic effect of commonly used herbal preparations as a Sidha remedy. Chooranam or Kadal azhinjii contains Chinnensis Syn Saptrangi and Triphia tablets, which contain *Terminlia chebula, Termanalia bellerica* and *Phyllanthus embelica*. Five hundred mgs of Kadal azhinjil Chooranam taken twice per day and Triphla tablets 25 mg three times per day were administered in water to 25 patients with diabetes whose blood glucose fell by 40–50 per cent after 120 minutes (Sivpraksam *et al.* 1982). The researchers suggested that the combination increased the renal threshold for glycosuria, which disappeared sooner than the fall in blood glucose. These are old, mostly animal studies and may not be transferable to humans. Likewise, some of the glucose-lowering conventional medicines employed as comparators are no longer used in some countries because more effective agents are available.

Herbal medicines commonly used to manage blood glucose in the Philippines include: Ampalaya leaves, Apdo ng tilapia, Balat ng Kamachilli, Caimito fruis, Cogon leaves, Eucalyptus leaves, Neem leaves and Ugat ng makahiya, as well as herbs such as banana and *Allium sativum* to control hypertension. A list of traditional Indonesian plant remedies is available in Tagalog and English. Herbal medicines in Indonesia are regulated by *The Traditional and Alternative Medicine Act* 1997. Despite these examples of health profession use of and belief in CAM, there is ongoing debate about its use, safety and benefits generally, and for people with diabetes.

2.6   Profile of Likely CAM Users

Although the preceding literature provides important information about CAM users, there is no definite prototype or predictor of CAM use and there may be differences between people using different types of CAM. As can be seen above, the decision to use CAM or conventional medicine or a combination of both is complex and non-linear. People base their choices on the information available to them at the time, which is likely to be derived from a number of sources as well as the advice of significant others such as family and health professionals. In general, CAM users appear to do the following:

- consider their health-care options and mix and match to suit their needs. One concern with this approach is that they also often self-diagnose, which may delay effective appropriate treatment and lead to suboptimal health outcomes.
- have a cultural preference for CAM;
- hold philosophies similar to those of CAM but their philosophies are not dissimilar to conventional therapy users;
- be in poor health and often have chronic diseases such as diabetes or limitations to usual activities of daily living, which affects their quality of life and mental well being;
- use CAM for specific problems such as managing symptoms rather than for general problems or curing diseases, for example, as adjuncts to conventional therapies for chronic diseases but they are more likely to consult conventional practitioners for acute life-threatening illnesses (Thomas *et al.* 2001; Lewith and Chan 2002).
- be committed to the environment;
- be well educated and financially secure;
- most likely be female and older;
- often have suffered a traumatic life event, for some people, the diagnosis of diabetes is a traumatic event;
- have limited access to conventional medicines.

Importantly, CAM users are not fearful of or dissociated from conventional medicine and do not usually 'shop around' for health-care options. However, they do have different constructs of CAM and conventional therapies.

People selecting homeopathic remedies are concerned about the invasive techniques, 'toxic medicines', and lack of a spiritual perspective of conventional medicine compared with those only consulting GPs (Furnham and Bhagrath 1992). Furnham and Foley (1994) also compared homeopathy users with a cohort of people consulting GPs and found homeopathy users were more critical about the efficacy of conventional medicine, believed their health would improve with homeopathic remedies, were more self-aware and tried harder to maintain their health and believed in self-empowerment (Lewith and Chan 2002).

Lewith and Chan found CAM users (n = 10) used 21 constructs to describe CAM compared with 38 used by non-CAM users (n = 10). CAM users but not non-CAM users used the constructs: adverse reactions, holism, intervention, effectiveness, individuality and the body boundary, whereas only two CAM constructs were mentioned by non-CAM users: 'not done in hospital' and 'medication versus procedure'. However, both groups suggested similar issues were important when considering conventional therapies: cure was the most important dimension, then invasiveness, and third, chemically based. Interestingly, effectiveness, cost, individuality, and interventions were considered to be less important by both CAM and non-CAM users and the lack of quality evidence was considered to be more relevant to CAM than conventional therapies.

Sometimes people with diabetes use CAM intermittently to improve their blood glucose profile before their routine visits to conventional practitioners (Day 2005). These studies highlight the importance of determining why people use CAM therapies rather than assuming they are only used to control blood glucose levels. Likewise, the way people measure 'effectiveness' needs to be determined. They are likely to consider how the results are likely to affect them personally, rather than generalisable evidence.

2.7 Culture, Health Beliefs and CAM

The *Social Sciences Encyclopedia* (1990) defines culture as the way people live their lives. Culture consists of conventional patterns of thoughts and behaviours as well as values, beliefs and rules of conduct, which are passed from one generation to the next generation through learning rather than biological inheritance. Four basic characteristics have been applied to culture:

1. It is learned, not biologically inherited.
2. It is shared by all the members of the same cultural group.
3. It develops and adapts according to the environment.
4. It is dynamic and constantly evolving.

Helman (2001) described culture as:

A set of guidelines that is inherited by an individual as a member of a particular society and that tells them how to view the world, how to experience it emotionally and how to respond in it, its relation to other people, to supernatural forces or gods and to natural environment.

Culture also provides a pathway through which guidelines are transmitted to the next generation using symbols, language, art and rituals. Hence culture has an important influence on many different aspects of people's lives including their beliefs, behaviours, perceptions, emotions, rituals, diet, dress, body image, and particularly attitudes towards issues such as health, illness and pain. Therefore, it is hard to predict how people will react to illness, death, and misfortune without understanding the culture they grew up in or acquired and through which they perceive and interpret their world.

Culture also offers an explanatory model of the factors that influence people's perception about CAM use. Culture and health beliefs are an enormous subject and beyond the scope of this chapter but a brief overview of the way culture and health beliefs influence people's CAM use is relevant. The human body is more than just a physical organism fluctuating between health and illness. People also have a social as well as a physical reality, a focus and a set of beliefs about their social and psychological significance, and the structure and functions of their bodies. The shape and size of the adornments they wear are the ways of communicating and informing individuals about their position in the society.

Many sociologists have used the term 'body image' to describe the ways individuals conceptualise and experience their bodies, consciously and unconsciously. Fisher (1968) suggested body image includes: 'his [a person's] collective attitudes, feelings and fantasies about his body' as well as 'the manner in which a person has learnt to organise and integrate his body's experiences'. Thus, the culture people grow up in teaches them how to perceive and interpret the changes that occur in their bodies and their health behaviours, for example, it may help explain why people use CAM on the recommendations of family and friends in the studies cited earlier.

Body image is acquired as a part of growing up in a particular family, culture and society but there are individual variations. It also includes beliefs about the optimal body shape and size, clothing, body decorations, beliefs about boundaries, inner structure and functioning. These are important considerations with respect to weight control and diabetes, especially type 2. However, culture changes occur, commonly because of factors such as globalisation and the influence of the media and the Internet. Therefore, one should be pragmatic about CAM use in body alterations especially in people with diabetes or family history of type 2 diabetes.

Various theories have been developed to explain the structure, clinical importance and functioning of the body. A common element in many theories is the need for harmonious balance among the elements or forces within the body, for example, the humoral theory, which originated in ancient China and India, Humoral theory was described by Hippocrates in 460 BC and refers to four liquids or humours; blood, phlegm, yellow bile, and black bile. When these four humours are balanced, the body is healthy; imbalance of any one of the four results in ill health. Diet, the environment and the season of the year can affect the balance. Managing imbalance or disease relies on restoring the optimal balance among the humours, which might require interventions such as diet or medicines. Thus, humoral medicine remains the basis of lay beliefs about the health and illness in much of Latin America, the Islamic cultures and is a component of Ayurvedic and Chinese medical systems, see Chapters 10 and 11.

Food is more than just a source of nutrition, it plays major part in individuals' life and is deeply embedded in the social, religious and economic aspect of most countries. Various cultural classifications and theories about food exist in the literature, including sacred and profane foods as part of many religious traditions. Profane foods are considered dangerous to health. In addition, parallel food classifications exist, for example, Harwood (1971) observed an example of parallel foods among the Puerto Ricans in New York City where diseases, foods and medicines were grouped into cold and hot categories: hot (*caliente*) and cold (*frio*). These categories do not mean the temperature of the food is cold or hot but refers to the effect it has in or on the body.

Arthritis, colds, menstrual periods, and joint pains are cold diseases, while constipation, diarrhoea rashes, tenesmus and ulcers are hot diseases. Hot medicines are aspirin, castor oil, penicillin, cod liver oil, iron and vitamins; cold medicines are bicarbonate soda, mannitol, nightshades and milk of magnesia. Hunt (1976) described the hot–cold classification system among some Asian immigrants living in Britain including Hindus and Muslims. Ilnesses were treated by restoring the balance of hot and cold forces within the body, for example, a febrile illness was treated with cold foods such as rice, green gram and buttermilk.

Aslam *et al.* (1976) found traditional beliefs about health were prevalent among Asians living in Britain and one-fifth consulted traditional healers in Britain. Likewise, Bhopal (1986) conducted a community-based interview with Asians living in Glasgow and found knowledge of herbal remedies, the healer and cultural concepts such as the hot–cold theory was prevalent. Illness was attributed to hot and cold imbalances. When Asian peoples returned to their countries of origin, they frequently consulted an Asian healer. Asian healers were not consulted as frequently in Glasgow because there were fewer healers in practice at the time of the study.

Various foods have been used as medicines to treat illness and restore the balance of the internal forces of the body. The effect of medicines on human physiology and emotional status depends not only on the established pharmacological properties; other factors such as personality and social or culture background can either enhance or reduce the effects and are probably responsible for the various responses that occur, including the placebo effect.

Similarly, economic and market forces concerned with producing, advertising and selling medicines as well as the social climate also play a major part in people's decision to use health care and specific therapies. Most of the Indian population still lives in rural areas and rely heavily on CAM to manage chronic diseases due to their inability to access adequate health-care services, the cost involved, and health beliefs where chronic diseases are still perceived to be the consequence of a curse or evil forces. Conventional therapies are often inaccessible or viewed as unsatisfactory, therefore, CAM remains popular.

Other models include the Health Belief Model, which has been widely studied in a range of conditions including diabetes in the past two decades. Bhardwaj (1975) studied attitudes towards different medicine systems in four Punjabi villages in India and found that generally there was an increasing preference for modern medicine to achieve quick cures in the acute stages of illness but traditional medicines were still popular to manage chronic diseases because they were presumed to be more effective and safe. They also interviewed physicians and the heads of households and their views supported the reports of the villagers regarding the comparative curative aspects of the indigenous modern medicines.

Dissatisfaction with conventional medicines can also influence people's choice of health care. Little is known about how CAM should be integrated into conventional, but the issues need to be explored in light of the increasing use of CAM especially in primary care, see Chapter 4.

2.8 Reported Adverse Events Associated with CAM

The general risks and safety issues surrounding CAM medicines are discussed in Chapter 3 and other specific risks and benefits are discussed in the relevant chapters. A number of adverse events associated with CAM use and diabetes are described in the literature. These include:

- Stopping insulin by four people with type 1 diabetes, three of whom developed ketoacidosis and one life-threatening weight loss and hyperglycaemia (Gill *et al.* 1994).
- Infection and burns to neuropathic legs caused by moxibustion and cupping, therapies used in Chinese medicine (Ewins *et al.* 1993).
- Severe bruising following an aromatherapy massage given by the wife of a man with diabetes on anticoagulant therapy. It is difficult to determine whether the bruising was caused by the essential oils or the pressure of the massage itself, see Chapter 6.
- Hypoglycaemia with CAM glucose-lowering medicines especially when they are combined with conventional glucose-lowering medicines but also when they are used by non-diabetics (Dunning *et al.* 2001).
- Toxicity including kidney damage from contaminated and incorrectly labelled CAM products.
- Electrolyte disturbances such as hypokalaemia from using potassium supplements concomitantly with ACE inhibitors.
- Hypotension.
- Hypertension.
- Allergies.

2.9 Summary

CAM use is a complex issue. Conventional practitioners need to consider CAM use in all people with diabetes and recognise they may not be using CAM solely to manage blood glucose levels. Importantly, many conventional practitioners also use CAM for personal reasons, and in the care of patients or refer them to CAM practitioners.

References

Abramson. Frequency of CAM use among cardiac patients. *American Heart Association Scientific Session* 2005; Abstract 2520.

Amos A, McCarthy D, Zimmet P. The rising global burden of diabetes and its complications: estimate and projections to the year 2010. *Diabetic Medicine* 1997; **14** (Suppl 5): S1–S85.

Andersson H, Ejlertsson G, Leden I, Schertsen B. Impact of chronic pain on health care seeking, self-care and medication. *Journal of Epidemiology and Community Health* 1999; **53**: 503–509.

Arora RB, Mishra KS, Seth SDS. A study on hypoglycaemic effect of Septarangi. *Journal of Research of Indian Medicine* 1973; **8**(4): 17–20.

Aslam M, Davies S, Fletcher R. Compliance in medicine by immigrants. *Nursing Times* 1976; **75**(22): 931–932.

Astin J. Why patients use alternative medicine: results of a national survey. *Journal of the American Medical Association*. 1998; 279.

Berman B, Singh B, Hartnoll S, Reilly D. Primary care physicians and complementary-alternative medicine: tracing, attitudes and practice patterns. *Journal of American Board of Family Practice* 1998; **11**: 272–281.

Bhardwaj S. Attitudes towards different systems of medicines: a survey of four villages in Punjab India. *Social Science and Medicine* 1975; **9**: 603–612.

Bhopal R. Bhye Bhaddi™: a food and health concept of Punjabi Asians. *Social Sciences and Medicine* 1986; **23**(7): 687–688.

Braun C, Bearinger L, Halcon L, Pettingell S.: Adolescents use alternative therapies for pain relief. *Journal of Adolescent Health* 2005; **37**: 76–81.

Day C. Are herbal remedies of use in diabetes? *Diabetic Medicine* 2005; **22**: 1–21.

Dunning, T. Complementary therapies and diabetes. *Complementary Therapies in Nursing and Midwifery* 2003; **2**: 74–80.

Dunning T, Chan S, Pendek R. A cautionary tale of the use of complementary therapies. *Diabetes in Primary Care* 2001; **3**(2): 39–43.

Egede L, Ye X, Zheng D, Silverstein M. The prevalence and pattern of complementary and alternative medicine use in individuals with diabetes. *Diabetes Care* 2002; **25**: 324–329.

Eisenberg D, Davis RB, Ethener SL, Scott A, Wilkey S, Van Rompey M, Kissler RC. Trends in alternative medicine use in the United States 1990–1997. *Journal of the American Medical Association* 1998; **280**(18): 1569–1575.

Eisenberg O, Kessler R, Foster C. Unconventional medicine in the United Kingdom: patients, practitioners and consultants. *Lancet* 1993; **346**: 542–545.

Ewins D, Bakker K, Youn M, Boulton A. Alternative medicine: potential dangers for the diabetic foot. *Diabetic Medicine* 1993; **10**: 988–992.

Fisher S. Body image. In: Sills D (ed.) *International Encyclopedia of the Social Sciences*, pp. 113–116. London: Free Press/Macmillan, 1968.

Foster D, Russell P, Hamel M, Eisenberg, D. Alternative medicine use in older Americans. *Journal of the American Geriatrics Society* 2000; **48**: 156–165.

Furnham A, Bhagrath R. A comparison of health beliefs and behaviours of clients of orthodox and complementary medicine. *British Journal of Clinical Psychology* 1992; **32**: 237–246.

Furnham A, Foley J. The attitudes and behaviours of patients of conventional vs complementary (alternative) medicine. *Journal of Clinical Psychology* 1994; **50**: 458–469.

Gill G, Redmond S, Garratt F, Paisley R. Diabetes and alternative medicine: cause for concern. *Diabetic Medicine* 1994; **11**: 210–213.

Gozum S, Unsal A. Use of herbal therapies by older, community-dwelling women. *Journal of Advanced Nursing* 2004; **46**(2): 171–178.

Gupta S. Effect of *Gymnema sylvestre* and *Pterocarpus marsupima* on glucose tolerance in albino rats. *Indian Journal of Medical Science* 1963; **17**: 501.

Haetzman M, Elliott A, Smith B, Hannaford P, Chambers W. Chronic pain and the use of conventional and alternative therapy. *Family Practice* 2003; **20**(2): 147–154.

Harnath P, Rao R, Anjaneyalu R, Ramauattan J. Studies on hypoglycaemic and pharmacological properties of some stibleane. *Indian Journal of Medical Science* 1958; **12**: 85.

Harwood A. The hot–cold theory of disease: implications for treatment of Puerto Rican patients. *Journal of the American Medical Association* 1971; **216**: 1153–1158.

Helman C. *Culture Health and Illness*, 4th edn. Oxford: Butterworth Heinemann, 2001.

Helmrich S, Yates P, Nash R, Hobman SA, Poulton V, Berggren L. Factors influencing nurses' decisions to use non-pharmacological therapies to manage patient's pain. *Journal of Advanced Nursing* 2001; **19**(1): 27–35.

Honda K, Jacobson J. Use of complementary and alternative medicine among United States adults: influences of personality, coping strategies, and social support. *Preventative Medicine* 2004; **40**: 46–53.

Hunt S. The food habits of Asian immigrants. In: *Getting the Most out of Food*. Van den Berghs & Jurgens, 1976, pp. 15–51

Joglekar G, Choudhury N, Aiman R. Effect of plant extract on glucose absorption in mice. *Indian Journal Physiology and Pharmacology* 1959; **3**: 76.

Kaufman Herbal supplement use levelling off in the US. *Archives of Internal Medicine* 2005; **165**: 261–286.

Leese G, Gill G, Horton G. Prevalence of complementary medicine use within a diabetic clinic. *Practical Diabetes International* 1997; **14**(7): 207–208.

Lewith G, Chan J. An exploratory qualitative study to investigate how patients evaluate complementary and conventional medicine. *Complementary Therapies in Medicine* 2002; **10**: 69–77.

MacLennan A, Wilson D, Taylor A. Prevalence and cost of alternative medicine in Australia. *Lancet* 1996; **347**: 569–573.

Pawa M. A study of the relationship between beliefs, knowledge and glycaemic control in Asians with type II diabetes mellitus. Unpublished Master of Science thesis, 1991.

Rolniak S, Browning L, MacLeod B, Cockley P. Complementary and alternative medicine use among urban ED patients: prevalence and patterns. *Journal of Emergency Nursing* 2004; **30**(4): 388–394.

Ryan E, Pick M, Marceau C. Use of alternative therapies in diabetes mellitus. Proceedings of the American Diabetes Association meeting, San Diego, USA, 1999.

Sabo C, Michael S, Temple L. The use of alternative therapies by diabetes educators. *The Diabetes Educator* 1999; **25**(6): 945–954.

Sadikot SM, Nigam A, Das S, Bajaj S, Zargar AH, Prasannakumar KM, Sosale A, Munichoodappa C, Seshiah V, Singh SK, Jamal A, Sai K, Sadasivrao Y, Murthy SS, Hazara DK, Jain S, Mukherjee S, Bandyopadhay S, Sinha NK, Mishra R, Dora M, Jena B, Patra P. The burden of diabetes and impaired glucose tolerance in India using the WHO 1999 criteria: prevalence of diabetes in India study (PODIS). *Diabetes Research and Clinical Practice* 2004; **66**: 301–307.

Saifi AQ, Shindhe S, Kavishwar WK, Gupta SR Study in hypoglycaemic effect of septarangi. *Journal In Res. In Indian Medicine* 1971; **6**(2): 156–165.

Sharma U. *Complementary Medicine Today; Practitioners and Patients.* London: Routledge, 1992.

Sharples F, van Haselen R, Fisher P. NHS patients' perspective on complementary medicine: a survey. *Complementary Therapies in Medicine* 2003; **11**(4): 243–248.

Sivprakasam K, Kalavathy K, Yasodha R, Veluchamy G. Hypoglycaemic effect of commonly used herbs for Sidha. *Journal Res. Ay. Sid.* 1982; **5**(1–4): 25–32.

Thomas KJ, Nicholl JP, Coleman P. Use and expenditure on complementary medicine in England: a population-based survey. *Complementary Therapies in Medicine* 2001; **9**: 2–11.

Tracey M, Lingquist R, Savik K, Letanuki S, Srdelbach S, Kreitzer M, Berman B. Use of complementary and alternative therapies: a national survey of critical care nurses. *American Journal of Critical Care* 2005; **14**: 404–445.

Van Haselen RA, Reiber U, Nickel I, *et al. Complementary Therapies in Medicine* 2004; **12**(1): 6–16.

World Health Organization (WHO). *Traditional Medicine Strategy 2002–2005.* Geneva: WHO, 2002.

Yeh GY, Eisenbergh, DM, Kaptchuk TJ, Phillips RS. Systemic review of herbs and dietary supplements for glycaemic control in diabetes. *Diabetic Care* 2003; **26**: 1277–1294.

3 Complementary Medicine and Safety

Lesley Braun

3.1 Introduction

The aim of this chapter is to provide an overview of the safety issues associated with complementary therapies; issues and adverse events relating to specific therapies are discussed in the relevant chapters. A chief concern of the public when they consider the various therapies or medicines available is whether they will provide potential benefits; safety is often assumed. One Australian study found that 90 per cent of complementary medicine (CM) users assumed CM products were safe compared to 65 per cent of non-users. In the same study, respondents felt CM was or should be subject to the same standards as prescribed medicines (MacLennan *et al.* 2002). Similar perceptions about CM product safety is held in the UK (Sharples *et al.* 2003).

The perception that all complementary medicines are safe at all times is often based on the assumption that they are 'natural' and natural products are inherently safe. The argument that CM is natural is simplistic and not well thought out, because nature provides us with many examples of unsafe substances such as the naturally occurring poisons hemlock, jimsonweed and oleander. The public also assumes that possible adverse effects and toxicities will be listed on product labels. If no adverse effects or toxicity is listed on a label, people assume the product is safe. In Australia, some warnings are required on labels, however, complementary medicines are not accompanied by comprehensive consumer medicine information (CMI) in the same way as many conventional medicines.

Importantly, CM users tend to have poorer health than the general community and do not use CM because they are dissatisfied with conventional health care (Austin 2001), see Chapter 2. People use CM because it is congruent with their own values, beliefs and philosophical orientations towards health and life, which raises the possibility of people receiving care from both complementary and conventional practitioners. Dual care is not necessarily dangerous and can produce significant benefits when it is well coordinated. However, if the health-care practitioners

Complementary Therapies and the Management of Diabetes and Vascular Disease   Editor Trish Dunning
© 2006 John Wiley & Sons, Ltd.

involved recommend various medicines and treatments and remain unaware of what the other practitioners recommend, a potentially unsafe situation can arise. The prospect of interactions, adverse reactions leading to misdiagnosis, induction of withdrawal effects, and misleading pathology investigation results are examples of unwanted outcomes that can arise when combined care is not coordinated.

Some conventional practitioners are aware that adverse reactions and interactions are possible with CM; however, it is uncertain whether they have the confidence, knowledge and access to relevant resources to be able to appropriately advise patients. One study that investigated whether physicians were aware of the side effects, medicine interactions and contraindications of ten commonly used herbs, found physician knowledge was poor and likely to put patients and themselves at risk. One question asked the physicians to match ten herbs to their relevant side effects. The average number of correct responses was 1.32 with a standard deviation of 1.39 (Silversten and Spiegel 2001).

It is essential for both clinicians and patients to recognise that every medicine or therapy has the potential to cause harm. The ideal in clinical practice is to combine

Table 3.1 Potential harms associated with the using complementary medicines.

Potential harm	Definition
Delay in diagnosis	If a patient has avoided or delayed seeking medical advice because they are self-treating with a complementary medicine or their complementary medicine practitioner has not referred them to a medical practitioner for early/correct diagnosis
Adverse effects	Increased risk of adverse reactions with inappropriate use of complementary medicine products or patient's self-selecting complementary products without professional advice. Increased risk if products used are not manufactured to pharmaceutical grade quality.
Medicine interactions	Increased risk of medicine interactions when patients self-select complementary products without professional advice; do not disclose their use of complementary products to their pharmacist or their health care professionals do not disclose use of pharmaceutical medicines to their complementary practitioner
Financial cost	If an expensive medicine or therapy is not providing benefits and a patient continues to use it, the continued use places an unnecessary financial burden on the patient
Lost opportunity to treat	Failure to undertake a treatment with proven benefits, when the current treatment being used is ineffective
False hope of a cure	When cure is unlikely, the use of any medicine or therapy, which is associated with false hope may delay important considerations such as attending to 'unfinished business'

knowledge of the medicine, knowledge of the disease, experience of both, and knowledge of the patient and their individual circumstances when recommending medicines and other care. In the case of CM, gaining a working knowledge of the most popular medicines and therapies is essential to avoid unsafe recommendations and promote beneficial ones, see Chapter 4. Table 3.1 lists some of the potential harms associated with using CM. It should be noted that most of these concerns also apply to conventional medicine.

Safety is a complex issue. Many of the safety issues surrounding CM also apply to conventional medicine and fall into several inter-related categories:

- patient
- practitioner
- product
- the environment in which care is delivered including the health system.

3.2 Practices

It is important to distinguish between the practice of CM and the complementary medicines, products and procedures CM practitioners use. In addition, CM practice includes the discipline-specific skills that CM practitioners are trained to use, thus education also plays a role. CM education often encompasses a philosophy and rationale for the diagnosis and utilisation of specific therapeutic techniques such as massage, chiropractic, osteopathy and acupuncture. It may also involve prescribing and dispensing medicinal substances such as vitamins, minerals or food supplements, pre-manufactured herbal or homeopathic medicines or prescribing, and in some cases compounding herbal preparations specifically for individuals.

Although the prescription of herbal and homeopathic products clearly falls under the aegis of CM, vitamin and mineral supplements are widely employed by conventional practitioners who often prescribe nutritional supplements to address deficiency states. CM practitioners also recommend nutritional supplements for deficiency states but they also take into account subclinical deficiencies and use nutritional supplements as preventative agents, see Chapter 5.

3.3 Risks and safety

CM practice is associated with similar risks to those in conventional practice. These risks include:

- incorrect prescribing, for example, poor treatment choice, inappropriate doses or dose intervals, and inappropriate duration of treatment;
- negligent practice such as using non-sterile acupuncture needles or ceasing appropriate medical therapy;
- misdiagnosis, for example, failing to detect an abnormality, which causes progression of the underlying disease;

- failing to refer, which can occur if the practitioner is not aware of the limits of their knowledge and competence;
- failing to explain the relative risks as well as the benefits to patients (Myers and Cheras 2004).

Appropriate training, education, access to accurate and timely information and experience can improve safety. A large amount of credible information is available through professional organisations, journals, seminars, and conferences, as well as online to both complementary and conventional practitioners. In addition, collaboration between practitioners based on shared respect and trust provides another important avenue to improve the safety of patients. In particular, collaboration can minimise the risk of delaying or depriving patients of safe and effective treatment, both conventional and complementary, and reduce the risk of adverse events.

In Australia, integration is currently being supported by government initiatives such as the new Medicare Plus package, as well as initiatives from organisations such as the Australian Medical Association (AMA), the Royal Australian College of General Practitioners (RACGP) and the Australasian Integrative Medicine Association (AIMA) see Chapter 4. Similar initiatives are occurring in other countries.

3.4 Adverse Events

Products

Adverse reactions to any dietary, environmental or medicinal substance, even placebo, are possible. Product-related adverse events might occur due to a number of factors such as poor manufacturing practices, adulteration including with conventional medicines, inaccurately identified raw materials, and non-sterile techniques. Product manufacture is regulated in some countries but people still use products that do not comply with the regulations, for example, when they purchase them from other countries.

Definitions of adverse events

Safety information about potential adverse events is derived from a variety of sources such as post-marketing surveillance, spontaneous reporting schemes, laboratory and animal studies, anecdotal reports, theoretical reasoning, and increasingly, research studies. Adverse medicine-related events (ADR) occur due to intrinsic or extrinsic factors, which are discussed later in the chapter. In addition, medicine-related toxicity may be:

- an acute allergy, which occurs very soon after the medicine is applied or administered;
- short term, which takes between three and 12 months to manifest;
- long term, which occurs over years and which represents a cumulative effect.

A number of definitions of 'adverse event' can be found in the literature. For example, Pierlaissi (2003) defined adverse events as unintentional, identifiable injuries that occur as a result of medicine mismanagement rather than the disease process. Medicine errors are likely to occur when a planned action is not completed as intended, the incorrect medicine is used, or the management plan is not appropriate to achieve the management aim. The term 'adverse event' is often used to refer to preventable, systemic problems rather than health professional or patient performance; however, a serious adverse event could directly result from these causes or they can contribute to the ADR depending on the event. Alternatively, adverse events are defined as all noxious and unintended responses to a dose of a medicinal product. A serious adverse event is life-threatening, which means the patient could die and hospitalisation is required, or length of time spent in hospital is prolonged because of the event. Some serious ADRs cause significant disability, congenital abnormalities, birth defects, or death.

The World Health Organization (WHO) defined an adverse drug reaction (ADR) as a 'response to a medicine which is noxious and unintended that occurs at doses normally used in humans'. Alarmingly, the rate of ADR-related hospital admissions is increasing and accounts for considerable morbidity, mortality, and extra costs.

Some factors that can lead to ADRs are inappropriate medicine doses or dose intervals, inappropriate medicine combinations, and using medicines when they are contraindicated. In addition, some patient factors such as frailty, younger and older age, and kidney or liver disease increase the risk of ADRs. People taking multiple medicines, typically older people and oncology patients, are at increased the risk. Unfortunately, most ADRs occur in people who are prescribed treatment according to relevant guidelines and accepted practice (Burgess et al. 2002).

The amount of published literature on conventional medicine-related ADRs is overwhelming and consists of anecdotal reports (30 per cent) as well as formal studies and randomised controlled trials (35 per cent) (Aronson et al. 2002). However, very few formal CM ADR studies are available and relatively little has been published in the peer-reviewed literature. Therefore, there is often insufficient information to help practitioners make a rational decision about the relative risks, thereby presenting one of the great difficulties of clinical practice.

In Australia, anticoagulant, anti-inflammatory, and cardiovascular medicines feature prominently in preventable, high impact ADRs, which collectively make up over one-half of all ADRs reported (Runciman et al. 2003). One review of 14 Australian studies showed that ADRs occurred in 2.4–3.6 per cent of hospital admissions, which translates to at least 80,000 medication-related hospital admissions each year (Roughead 1999).

Pirmohamed et al. (2004) conducted a prospective observational study at two large general hospitals in Merseyside, England, which identified that 6.5 per cent of hospital admissions were related to an ADR where the ADR directly led to the admission in 80 per cent of cases. The median bed stay was eight days, accounting for 4 per cent of the hospital bed capacity, which equates to a projected annual cost of such admissions at £466 million (US $800 million or Aus$1093 million).

Once again, the medicines most commonly implicated in these ADRs were anti-coagulants, non-steroidal anti-inflammatory medicines and diuretics. The most common ADR was gastrointestinal bleeding.

Although ADRs associated with CM products are possible, relatively few reports have been collected through spontaneous post-marketing surveillance systems. The Uppsala Monitoring Centre (UMC) is the coordinating centre for the WHO International Drug Monitoring Programme. It holds the most extensive database of adverse reactions to herbal medicines in the world and collects data from national centres in 72 countries. Over the past 20 years, 11,716 suspected herbal case reports have been collected compared to over three million individual case safety reports on pharmaceutical medicines (www.who-umc.org).

The most commonly reported non-critical ADRs from the highest to the lowest incidence were: pruritis, urticaria, rash, erythematous rash, nausea, vomiting, diarrhoea, fever, abdominal pain and dyspnoea. The most common critical ADRs in order of frequency were: face oedema, hepatitis, angiodema, thrombocytopenia, hypertension, chest pain, convulsions, purpura, dermatitis and death.

The Adverse Drug Reactions Advisory Committee (ADRAC) database in Australia consists of suspected adverse reactions to medicines reported since the 1st November 1972. Only 1112 reports related solely to CM products until 19th April 2005. This is reassuring when one considers that in 2000, MacLennan *et al.* identified approximately 52 per cent of the population used at least one non-medically prescribed complementary medicine excluding calcium, iron, and prescribed vitamins, which amounts to approximately 10 million CM users. Several explanations could account for the relatively few complementary medicine ADR reports. One explanation is that non-prescription medicines (over the counter medicines or OTC) including CM products are inherently safe because of pre-market safety checks and the intrinsic safety of the ingredients deemed suitable to be included in OTC medicines. Another factor is under-reporting, which is a major problem for both CM and conventional ADR reporting. In the specific case of CM, CM practitioners, as well as the staff of CM medicine retail outlets such as health food store and pharmacies may not always have direct or easy access to ADR reporting schemes. Likewise, they may not be:

- aware of ADR reporting schemes or processes;
- qualified to consider the possibility of ADRs;
- motivated to report any adverse events that come to their notice.

In addition, herbal medicine consumers may not be motivated to report ADRs to their physician, as one English study suggests (Barnes *et al.* 2004). Alternatively, they may not consider the possibility that the symptoms they experience could be related to their medicines.

Unfortunately, reports of adverse effects of herbal medicines often cause controversy and a great deal of media hype and are usually single case reports with incomplete data. For example, one systematic review, which assessed information from four electronic databases, located 108 cases of suspected medicine–herb interactions. However, 68.5 per cent were classified as 'unable to be evaluated' because of inadequate documentation. Only 13 per cent were described as 'well-documented' and the authors of the review considered 18.5 per cent were 'possible' interactions (Fugh-Berman and Ernst 2001).

Overall, adverse reaction reports should be viewed as a starting point. They indicate that a safety issue may have arisen but until causality can be established, it is difficult to know whether the ADR can realistically be attributed to a medicine or whether other factors are also implicated. In the case of herbal medicines, the product in question should be analysed and authenticated to ensure that they are not contaminated or adulterated and to correctly identify the botanical source of the product. This is particularly important when the product suspected of causing the ADR has not been manufactured under a strict code of Good Manufacturing Practice (GMP), which might arise when products are purchased on the Internet or imported from countries that do not have a GMP or other relevant regulations in place.

One limitation of the pre-existing spontaneous post-marketing surveillance systems is that they do not provide an estimate of the prevalence of ADRs associated with specific complementary medicines, which makes it difficult for clinicians to determine whether the incident they encounter is rare, idiosyncratic or common or even whether it is likely to be associated with the product. The difficulty occurs because CM products are not listed on the National Health Scheme and people outside the CM industry often do not know specific usage figures. Knowing how many doses of the specific product are sold in a defined period and the number of ADRs reported over the same period could provide a general guide to the incidence, help practitioners put case reports into context, and assess the relevance of the ADR to their individual patient.

3.5 Intrinsic and Extrinsic Factors

Adverse events can be intrinsic or extrinsic. Intrinsic factors relate to the active ingredients within a product. In the case of an herbal product, the herb itself is considered intrinsic, whereas extrinsic factors relate to product characteristics resulting from poor manufacturing process and quality control such as contamination and adulteration. Adverse reactions can arise from variability in naturally occurring active/toxic constituents due to:

- growing conditions;
- using inherently toxic herbs that cause toxicity;
- overdose of herbs;
- medicine–herb interactions especially with medicines with a narrow therapeutic index.

Alternately, extrinsic factors rather than the active ingredient in the medicine can cause adverse reactions. Adverse reactions are differentiated into two main classes: type A and type B reactions.

Type A reactions

More than 80 per cent of ADRs causing admission or occurring in hospital are type A reactions. These are dose-related, predictable from the known pharmacology of the medicine and therefore potentially avoidable (Routledge *et al.* 2004). Frail, older patients who are also likely to be receiving a combination of medicines, and those with altered hepatic or renal function are most at risk of type A reactions. Both of these factors apply to many people with diabetes. In addition, even younger people with diabetes are likely to be taking several medicines, which increases their risk of both type A and type B reactions.

An example of a type A adverse reaction to an herbal medicine is elevated blood pressure and fluid retention associated with the continuous use of high dose herbal liquorice containing glycyrrhizin. Glycyrrhetinic acid, a compound found in the herb liquorice, inhibits 11beta-hydroxysteroid dehydrogenase, thereby reducing catabolism of corticosteroids (Heilmann *et al.* 1999). As a result, corticosteroid elimination is reduced and activity prolonged. If continued for sufficient time, a state of pseudohyperaldosteronism can develop. Pseudohyperaldosteronism has been observed clinically and can be avoided by recommending patients do not use high dose liquorice herbal products for longer than two weeks. Many people with diabetes require at least one and often more antihypertensive agents, which increases the risk.

Type B reactions

Type B reactions are idiosyncratic, difficult to predict and not dose-related. Often they are immunologically mediated and comprise 6–10 per cent of ADRs to pharmaceutical medicines (Myers and Cheras 2004). Factors that increase the risk of type B reactions are polypharmacy, altered renal or hepatic function, chronic alcohol intake and malnutrition. Females are also at slightly higher risk than males.

An example of a type B adverse reaction is *Compositae* dermatitis, which is an allergic contact dermatitis caused by exposure to allergens from the *Compositae* or daisy group of plants and plant extracts. Some examples of common plants that belong to the compositae family are: arnica (*Arnica montana*), chamomile (*Chamomilla recutita*), marigold (*Calendula officinalis*), echinacea (*Echinacea spp.*), tansy (*Tanacetum vulgare*), feverfew (*Tanacetum parthenium*), and yarrow (*Achillea millefolium*). The most important allergens in the *Compositae* family are sesquiterpene lactones (SL), which are present in the oleoresin fraction of leaf, stem, flower and possibly pollen (Gordon 1999). The condition is most frequently seen in middle-aged and older people and typically starts in summer and disappears in the autumn or winter. The dermatitis manifests as eczema and can develop by exposure to airborne particles, direct topical application such as cosmetics, perfumes, essential oils, or oral ingestion of allergenic components.

Immunologically-mediated reactions to medicines

These reactions do the following:

1. Require a period of sensitisation. Thus, some time may elapse before the connection between the medicine and the reaction is recognised.
2. Occur in a small proportion of the population.
3. Occur with medicine doses far below the therapeutic range.
4. Subside after the medicine is discontinued in most instances (Gruchalla 2000).

Idiosyncratic reactions are rare, however, they can occur in response to any substance, including CM supplements.

3.6 Pre-market Safety Mechanisms

The regulation of complementary medicines varies greatly between countries and is influenced by ethnological, medical, and historical factors. In Australia, a number of important safety measures occur before complementary medicines can be sold and these are designed to reduce the risk of adverse effects. Australia has an international best-practice, risk-based regulatory system that encompasses both complementary and pharmaceutical medicines (Braun and Cohen 2005). The Therapeutic Goods Administration (TGA) regulates the system, which aims to ensure the safety and quality of products and truthful labelling of therapeutic goods. The TGA acts to ensure that all CM products are produced according to the code of GMP and licences, and audits manufacturers. Penalties are in place for manufacturers found to be in breach of the regulations.

All products are entered onto the Australian Register of Therapeutic Goods (ARTG) and allocated an Aust L number if considered low risk (most CM products) or Aust R number if considered high risk (prescription drugs) or low risk with a high-level claim. Products with either an Aust L or Aust R number have been evaluated for safety and quality whereas those with an AUST R number have also been evaluated for efficacy. In the case of CM products, the TGA recognises evidence from traditional sources and accepts that if a substance has been used with good effect and apparent safety for generations, it may be considered safer than a newly created substance that has never existed in nature. The scheduling system is another indicator of the potential of a substance to cause harm or be open to abuse. Most complementary medicine products are unscheduled and available over the counter. Table 3.2 lists the rational use of CM products.

In the United States, the Food and Drug Administration (FDA) treats dietary supplements as foods and enacted the Dietary Supplement Health Education Act (DSHEA) in 1994 in order to formalise a number of regulatory statutes designed to ensure continued public access to these products. Under this system, nutraceutical manufacturers are responsible for ensuring product safety and that any therapeutic claims for a product are substantiated by adequate evidence and that product label information is 'truthful and not misleading'. The DSHEA distinguishes foods from dietary supplements by requiring every supplement to be clearly labelled

Table 3.2 The rational use of complementary medicine products: factors to consider

Factors to consider	Rationale
Products without an AUST L or AUST R number *should not be used*	The quality of the product cannot be guaranteed as it is not known whether it was made under Australian GMP standards
Be informed and seek unbiased information	Marketing/sales and company information is not sufficient
Do not rely on label claims alone	Although Australian manufacturers must hold the evidence to support the claims made on a product label, often the label claims do not provide enough information to make an informed judgment
Do not rely on the doses recommended on the label	Australian manufacturers tend to state the lowest effective dose on the label to ensure that a patient's general requirements will be met; however, in practice, practitioners will prescribe a dose to meet the individual's needs – this may be higher than label doses yet still be within safe limits
Take care when high risk medicines are involved	Such as those with a narrow therapeutic index and many anticancer drugs – screen for interactions. In the case of herbal medicines, any product containing St John's wort (*Hypericum perforatum*) should be considered higher risk – screen for interactions.
Take care with people considered to be at higher risk of adverse reactions	The elderly, children, people with altered renal or liver function, when multiple drugs are being taken, people with depression, atophy or malnutrition
Ensure that all health professionals involved in a patient's care are aware of CM use	Effective communication will foster appropriate and safe use
Do not assume all health care professionals have the knowledge to monitor safe CM use	Few have had formal training to be aware of the safety issues involved or have access to evidence-based safety data
Know the manufacturer and supplier details	If in doubt about a product, call the manufacturer or supplier for more information
Know the prescriber's details (if relevant)	The original prescriber may have valuable information about the patient and the medicine – this may help you come to an informed opinion
Medicines should be stored appropriately	Appropriate storage will depend on the patient's circumstance (e.g. at home, hospital or in a hospice), level of vigilance and the type of medicine used

Source: Adapted with permission, from Braun, L., Cohen, M. 2005, *Herbs and Natural Supplements: An Evidence Based Guide*. Sydney: Elsevier, Table 11, p. 44.

and include a Supplement Facts Panel listing all the ingredients (Brownie 2005). Although the FDA has no regulatory control over what dietary products are brought onto the market, it can remove a product after it reaches the market if it can prove that it has violated the regulations governing product safety, information, labelling, or claims. To withdraw a product, the FDA must also prove that the product places the consumer at 'significant or unreasonable risk'.

The European Union process for licensing products is determined for each product and is based on evidence of quality, safety and efficacy. Much of the traditional and, where it exists, research evidence, is documented in monographs such as the German E Commission monographs and the European Scientific Cooperative on Phytotherapy (ESCOP) monographs. These are examples only and health professionals are advised to be familiar with the systems in place in their own countries, see Chapter 4.

3.7 Preventing Adverse Medicine Reactions

In order to promote patient safety and prevent ADRs, open communication based on trust and mutual respect is crucial between patient and physician and among all other health care professionals involved in the patient's care. One way of achieving this is for CM practitioners to label all dispensed herbal medicines with the botanical names of the herbs included in the product, together with suggested doses and dose intervals, the date of manufacture, and practitioner contact details. A regular medicines review by both conventional and complementary practitioners will provide further opportunities to identify potential ADRs, encourage patients to inform their conventional practitioners about their CM use, promote patient compliance, and ensure that the appropriate medicines are being taken safely.

In all fields of clinical practice, continuing education for practitioners is essential to ensure they are up-to-date with the latest research findings about the efficacy and safety of all the management strategies they use. An important adjunct to education is access to accurate and timely medical and complementary medicine resources and having a network of experts or informed colleagues for consultation and reference.

Patients also play an important role in promoting a beneficial and harm-free outcome and should ensure that they understand the benefits and potential risks associated with their management and be confident that they know how to take/use products appropriately. Printed patient information is another valuable communication tool that can promote patient safety. It should provide patients with a clear explanation about the medicine being recommended and encourage them to report a suspected adverse event to their practitioners. When problems do arise, practitioners need to be aware of their professional responsibility to report suspected adverse medicine reactions. The important aspects of an adverse medicine event report are listed in Table 3.3.

Ultimately, safety is a complex issue that involves both 'likelihood' and 'consequence'. Good clinical practice requires careful consideration of the

Table 3.3 Important components of an adverse reaction case report.

Patient demographics – male/female, age, social history if relevant
Suspected product details – formula as stated on label including fillers and excipients, batch number, expiry date and Aust L or Aust R number.
Details of the person making the report.
Manufacturer details
Relevant medical history
Other medications and treatments (including herbal and natural medicines)
Dose used, duration of use and administration form
Date and time of onset
Adverse effects – description of signs and symptoms
Outcome of event
Information regarding rechallenge, if applicable
Presence of confounding variables, e.g. additives?

likelihood of an adverse event and the potential severity of the consequence and then making a decision as to whether a treatment should proceed.

3.8 Safety of CM and Diabetes Management

Most often, CM practices and medicines are used as adjuncts to conventional approaches in diabetes management. This can produce beneficial outcomes such as an improved sense of well-being, a reduction in symptoms and risk of future disease and may even lower doses of conventional medicines to be used in some instances. However, adverse reactions and unwanted interactions are possible, therefore, combined use should be monitored and guided by a health-care professional, see Chapter 9.

Complementary medicines commonly used to regulate blood glucose levels or prevent or treat diabetic complications are discussed in Chapters 9, 10, 11 and 12. Where they are known, the common uses and adverse reactions are also listed. Interactions are included in table 3.1 however; most are speculative and have not been confirmed in formal studies. They are listed to alert practitioners to the possibility that a safety issue might arise and should be interpreted accordingly. Additionally, the clinical significance of any known or suspected adverse effect or interaction often relates to the dosage used, chronicity of use and administration route and these issues need to be taken into account.

References

Aronson J, Derry S, Loke Y. Adverse drug reactions: keeping up to date. *Fundamental of Clinical Pharmacology* 2002; **16**: 49–56.
Astin J. Why patients use alternative medicine: results of a national study. *Journal of American Medical Association* 1998; **279**: 1548–1553.
Barnes J, Mills S, Abbot N, Willoughby M, Ernst E. Different standards for reporting ADRs to herbal remedies and conventional OTC medicines: face-to-face interviews with 515 users of herbal remedies. *British Journal of Clinical Pharmacology* 1998; **45**: 496–500.

Brownie S. The development of the US and Australian dietary supplement regulations: what are the implications for product quality? *Complementary Therapies in Medicine* 2005; **13**: 191–198.

Burgess C, Holman C, Satti A. Adverse drug reactions in older Australians, 1981–2002. *Medical Journal of Australia* 2005; **182**: 267–270.

Fugh-Berman A, Ernst, E. Herb–drug interactions: review and assessment of report reliability. *British Journal of Clinical Pharmacology* 2001; **52**: 587–595.

Gordon L. Compositae dermatitis. *Australasian Journal of Dermatology* 1999; **40**: 123–128.

Gruchalla R. Understanding drug allergies. *Journal of Allergy Clinical Immunology* 2000; **105**: S637–S644.

Heilmann P, Heide J, Hundertmark S, Schoneshofer M. Administration of glycyrrhetinic acid: significant correlation between serum levels and the cortisol/cortisone-ratio in serum and urine. *Experimental Clinical Endocrinology and Diabetes* 1999; **107**: 370–378.

MacLennan A, Wilson D, Taylor A. The escalating cost and prevalence of alternative medicine. *Preventative Medicine* 2002; **35**: 166–73.

Myers S, Cheras P. The other side of the coin: safety of complementary and alternative medicine. *Medical Journal of Australia* 2004; **181**: 222–225.

Pirmohamed M, James S, Meakin S, Green C, Scott A, Walley T, Farrar K, Park B, Breckenridge A. Adverse drug reactions as cause of admission to hospital: prospective analysis of 18 820 patients. *British Medical Journal* 2004; **329**: 15–19.

Roughead E. The nature and extent of drug-related hospitalisations in Australia. *Journal of Quality in Clinical Practice* 1999; **19**: 19–22.

Routledge P, O'Mahony M, Woodhouse K. Adverse drug reactions in elderly patients. *British Journal Clinical Pharmacology* 2004; **57**: 121–126.

Runciman W, Roughead E, Semple S, Adams R. Adverse drug events and medication errors in Australia. *International Journal of Quality in Health Care* 2003; **15** (Suppl 1): i49–i59.

Sharples F, van Haselen, R, Fisher P. NHS patients' perspective on complementary medicine: a survey. *Complementary Therapies in Medicine* 2003; **11**: 243–248.

Silverstein D, Spiege 1 A. Are physicians aware of the risks of alternative medicine? *Journal of Community Health* 2001; **26**: 159–174.

4 Integrating Complementary and Conventional Therapies

Trish Dunning

4.1 Introduction

Change is the hallmark of progress. Change is implied in the definitions of complementary therapies given in the Preface and Chapter 2, and certainly applies to most health systems where change is occurring rapidly. The history of health care suggests every great health tradition has evolved to resolve the health problems peculiar to the particular setting and time, that is, society and health care influence each other. The current global move to integrate complementary and conventional care is an attempt by the general public, particularly those with chronic conditions, health professionals and in some cases governments, to address modern health problems (World Health Organization (WHO) 2002; Cohen 2004). The current health period could be called the 'age of chronic diseases', since they predominate in many countries.

No single health professional group has a monopoly on health. Complementary and conventional practitioners have similar goals: to provide optimal health care. Integrating conventional and complementary therapies could provide more options to help people live with chronic diseases such as diabetes (Caspi *et al.* 1999) and create an optimal healing environment (Marshall *et al.* 2004). People with chronic pain, cardiovascular disease, mental health problems and gastrointestinal disturbances often seek integrated care. Many of these comorbidities are complications of diabetes. Cohen (2004) stated:

> There is an imperative for collaboration, as most GPs have chronically ill patients who could benefit from the services of CAM [complementary and alternative] practitioners, and virtually all CAM practitioners have patients who require access to mainstream diagnosis and therapy.

Common ground needs to be identified in order to achieve effective integration. Although the history and theory underpinning complementary and conventional

---

Complementary Therapies and the Management of Diabetes and Vascular Disease   Editor Trish Dunning
© 2006 John Wiley & Sons, Ltd.

therapies are different, there are commonalities. For example, they both focus on providing holistic care for individuals within their society, advocate prevention, and aim to treat the underlying causes of ill health. Therefore, conventional practitioners need to acknowledge that complementary therapies can make an important contribution to health care and complementary therapists need to acknowledge that conventional practitioners also provide holistic care. Both groups need to acknowledge the deficiencies of their particular approach and decide where the strengths of one can support the other to offer balanced care.

The pathway to complementary care is neither linear nor simple, see Chapter 2. We live in an 'information age' and people have access to a great deal of health-care information from many sources, both accurate and inaccurate. Likewise, a variety of health-care options are available in most countries, and health consumers are aware of their right to be involved in decisions about health care. In fact, people with diabetes are expected to be active participants in their care, and health professionals promote empowerment, patient-centred care, concordance, and the 'expert patient'. In such a climate people are more likely to seek alternatives. In addition, people are likely to use a range of therapies to create their own form of 'complementary care', although they rarely totally reject conventional medicine. However, complementary or traditional medicine may be more accessible and affordable in some countries (WHO 2002).

4.2   What is Integration?

Terms such as 'integrative', 'integrated medicine/care' and 'complementary and alternative therapies (CAM)' are beginning to be used more widely to describe the combination of complementary and conventional care as conventional practitioners and government agencies recognise and respond to consumer demands for complementary therapies. Indeed, it would be irresponsible 'not to be aware of and discuss proven alternatives [with patients]' (Phelps 2004). Shortall *et al.* (1996) defined clinical integration as: 'The extent to which patient services are co-ordinated across people, functions, activities and sites so as to maximise the value of services delivered to patients.' The definition is appropriate to integrating conventional and complementary therapies even though Shortall was not specifically referring to complementary therapies. The WHO (2002) defined three levels of integration to describe the degree to which complementary therapies are officially recognised in health systems:

1. *Integrative*, where it is officially recognised and incorporated into all areas of health care, such as national medicine policies, product regulatory processes, utilisation in hospitals and the community and reimbursed under insurance systems, for example, China.
2. *Inclusive*, where it is recognised but not fully integrated into health delivery systems.
3. *Tolerant* where the health system is entirely based on conventional health care.

Integration probably actually occurs on two levels: at an individual patient level, considering the person within their relevant society, and at a policy level (Whittenmore 2005). Marshall *et al.* (2004) discussed the notion of creating optimal healing environments, which are consistent with complementary definitions of healing as a dynamic process that includes transformation and involves the individual's entire system (Dossey 2003). It is also consistent with current conventional diabetes empowerment management strategies, as already indicated.

4.3 Concerns about Integration

Concerns are related to five main issues:

1. the safety of the consumer based on their history, the clinical assessment, and available treatment and considering their personal choice of therapies;
2. the knowledge and competence of health professionals delivering care, which includes conventional practitioners delivering complementary therapies;
3. the evidence for particular management strategies to help health professionals decide which therapies could be effective in particular situations;
4. the safety and quality of the products;
5. organisational issues such as policies, guidelines, and communication, collaboration and referral systems.

These concerns need to be considered by individual countries, service providers and patients in order to determine how future health-care systems will operate. Consideration also needs to be given to the fact that the general public has not abandoned conventional care, but it does have very high expectations of what it can deliver, including demands for 'cures'. People expect conventional doctors to prescribe medicines for almost every illness, regardless of whether other more suitable options are available.

Integration suggests the best complementary and conventional strategies are combined to achieve optimal care. The debate about whether complementary therapies are 'an unproven form of medicine', or a viable option/addition to conventional management has not been resolved. Tension between the two approaches increased with the emergence and gradual dominance of 'scientific care' (conventional care), which implied complementary approaches were 'unscientific'. Although conventional care is still dominant, many nurses, doctors and other health professionals include complementary therapies such as massage, hypnosis, biofeedback and aromatherapy in their practice, and integrated clinics have been established to meet community demand, especially in primary care (Cohen 2004).

Some conventional practitioners believe 'all complementary therapies have to offer is more tools beyond drugs and surgery' and 'conventional medicine is the proper and only way to provide high quality care' (Caspi *et al.* 1999). Some are concerned about the 'miracle cures' they believe complementary therapy practitioners offer (Elisha 2005). Such stereotyping is counter-productive and is unlikely to assist people with diabetes make appropriate choices.

Although Dr Michael Wooldridge and Dr Karen Phelps in Australia and Prince Charles in the UK helped place complementary therapies in the public forum by indicating that 'to ignore the role of complementary therapies in the face of increasing community use is arrogant', opposition to their use and scepticism about their benefit and safety continue. Cooperation among health professionals is important to the success of integrated care and to achieving optimal clinical outcomes. At present, complementary therapies are often 'tacked on' to conventional management without defining the expected clinical outcomes or monitoring the effects of the therapy or combination of therapies. Despite these concerns, hospitals are increasingly beginning to provide complementary options for patients or at least accepting the patient's choice to use them (Cohen and Ruggie 2003).

Complementary therapists are concerned about the potential loss of their holistic philosophical basis, and that a therapy might no longer be 'complementary' if it is integrated into conventional care. While these concerns may be well founded, continuing with the current system will continue to result in uncoordinated care, patients not informing conventional practitioners they use complementary therapies, and health professionals using complementary therapies in an ad hoc manner. As a consequence, the risk of adverse events could increase, costs to individual patients and health systems are likely to increase, and the difficulties appropriately attributing outcomes will continue.

Conventional practitioners are concerned about the legal, ethical and practical issues that could arise if complementary therapies are used alone or combined with conventional therapies. Their concerns include:

- deciding who is responsible for coordinating the care and taking overall responsibility for the patient's health care;
- the importance of informing the individual about the risks and benefits of each conventional and complementary therapy or combination of therapies;
- whether individuals are informed about conventional therapies when they only consult a complementary practitioner and vice versa;
- concerns that complementary practitioners only advise patients to consult a conventional practitioner when the complementary therapy does not produce the expected results or the condition deteriorates (Elisha 2005);
- whether the conventional doctor is responsible for providing 24-hour care when a person elects to use a complementary therapy;
- ensuring complementary therapists are competent, appropriately qualified and accountable for their practice;
- establishing and maintaining good communication and referral processes between all health care providers and the patient;
- the fact that many pharmacies, supermarkets and health food shops stock complementary products, which means people can self-diagnose, self-treat and purchase products without the benefit of appropriate advice. Many complementary therapists share this concern;

- complementary practitioners prescribing and selling products, which represents a conflict of interest and raises ethical issues.

These concerns arise from the following:

- the need to ensure processes are in place to protect the health and safety of the public and individuals;
- the right of people to make informed choices about their health and how it is managed;
- the need for the public and many health professionals to be aware of and use relevant appropriate complaints mechanisms and procedures;
- the ethical responsibilities of all health providers including practitioners, manufacturers and distributors/sponsors towards health care;
- having a consistent approach to health care to ensure standards of care are developed, met and maintained. These include standards for education, research, regulation and self-regulation (Complementary Therapies in the Australian Health System 2003).

Thus integration concerns issues that affect local, national and international, primary care and hospital services, complementary and conventional practitioners, regulators, manufacturers, distributors and advertisers. Currently evidence-based care based on systematic reviews of 'good' evidence, the need to ensure the increasing amount of new research is incorporated into care where relevant, and the need to contain costs, dominate health care.

4.4 Benefits of Integration

Integration could enhance health and healing and emphasise the importance of the patient–health professional relationship, prevention strategies and healthy lifestyle including diet, exercise and stress management, and psychological well-being (Snyderman and Weil 2002). These factors are central to achieving optimal diabetes and cardiovascular outcomes (Marshall *et al.* 2004).

Metabolic disturbance is a complex phenomenon consisting of physical and psychological parameters; therefore, the integrated approach has much to offer to help people with diabetes achieve the stringent metabolic targets required for optimal diabetes management, provided their needs and safety are not put at risk. *The UK Integrated Health Care Report* suggested management priorities for integrated services including stress-related disease, functional conditions, musculoskeletal disorders and chronic pain. A number of delivery mechanisms were suggested, and processes for determining the quality of integrated care based on structure, process and outcome standards, the appropriateness of care and accessibility, acceptability, equity, effectiveness and efficiency.

Despite these potential benefits, integration currently occurs largely on the basis of public demand and is often based on the traditional use of many therapies rather than on a strong research basis. Funding is a key issue for both conventional and complementary care as well as integrated care. Even where usefulness, safety and benefit are demonstrated, funding is often not available or is only provided in the short term.

The plea for integration and equitable access to complementary therapies is not limited to the public. Bensoussan and Lewith (2004) stated they believe the Australian government has 'a social and ethical obligation to respond appropriately to community needs' and pointed out complementary therapies have potential applications in preventative care and chronic disease management, both of which are applicable to diabetes and cardiovascular disease. In particular, complementary therapy users demonstrate a commitment to their own self-care, which is the key to effective diabetes management.

However, integration and collaboration require respect and trust on both sides (Cohen 2004). In Australia, funding systems, such as Medicare Plus, are ideally suited to integrated diabetes care since they were established to ensure comprehensive, collaborative care for people with complex needs, including those with diabetes. Some multidisciplinary clinics provide or refer patients to complementary practitioners. In countries such as China, integration of Western and Chinese medicine is well established. In addition, some private health insurance companies in some countries provide rebates for a range of complementary therapies, depending on the level of cover the individual holds.

Statements from professional organisations such as the Australian Medical Association (AMA) address the need to consider integrated complementary/conventional care because of the risks associated with continuing to provide separate health-care systems, for example, delay in appropriate care and accurate diagnosis when patients only consult complementary practitioners and adverse events such as interactions and trauma.

However, integration is not a simple process. Key issues include:

- defining what the public needs and expects of health care;
- objective assessment of the current system to determine why people seek complementary health care, recognising that patients do not necessarily have the same goals or measure outcomes the same way as health professionals;
- supporting research into complementary and integrated health care. As evidence of safety and benefit emerges, it becomes ethically difficult to ignore their place in health care (Australian Government 2004);
- including common core elements in the education curricula of all health professionals. However, where this does occur in nursing and medicine, students are often unable to use the therapies they learn because of 'the system' (Bettiens 1998);
- providing appropriate and accurate information about both approaches to patients and health professionals;
- supporting complementary therapy professional organisations to develop and maintain self-regulatory programmes that include curricula design and ongoing professional development and research;
- determining the most effective integrated models and their cost benefits, which requires resources to determine standards and general outcome measures;

- determining suitable outcome measures of integrated diabetes management. These should include emotional, spiritual and social outcomes and not only focus on achieving metabolic targets, which are already defined.
- effective adverse event monitoring.

4.5 Obstacles to Integration

Although there is growing evidence that integrating complementary and conventional medicine is desirable and is actually occurring, obstacles remain. These include educating and regulating complementary practitioners, differences in the terminology used in the two systems and globally, equity of access for patients, research and research funding and the requirements of evidence-based care, reimbursement and funding procedures for complementary therapies, and medico-legal issues.

Another challenge to integration is the perceived differences between the philosophies of the two systems, particularly the notion of healing (complementary) as distinct from curing (conventional). Healing is concerned with the wholeness of being while curing is concerned with the wholeness of body (Schuster 1997). While there is an increasing trend to consider psychological and quality of life issues in diabetes management strategies, the spiritual aspects are still largely ignored. However, it is incorrect to conclude that integration automatically leads to holistic care. Some complementary therapists, especially in the research and academic fields, emphasise symptom management rather than holism. In addition, when they consider 'diabetes management', the main focus is often on 'anti-diabetic' therapy rather than the whole range of issues that need to be managed. Others believe the need to treat 'the individual rather than the disease' makes it difficult to use established guidelines that focus on an 'average person'.

Complementary therapies are rarely documented in conventional patient health records. In fact, some aged care facilities have copious separate forms to document complementary therapies, which actually highlight their separateness.

4.6 How Can Integration Be Achieved?

There are many opinions about the best way to integrate the two approaches safely, including what constitutes an appropriate integrated framework that addresses stakeholders', concerns and an agreed definition of 'complementary therapies' (WHO 2002). Integration is an evolving process and is occurring differently in the world generally and in specific countries and areas of countries. The key elements of integration include:

- Reaching agreement about integration.
- Identifying existing:
  - health systems, policies and protocols;
  - information, communications and referral patterns;
  - registers and databases;

- prescribing patterns;
- processes for annual patient health reviews including medicines review.
- Developing a suitable infrastructure that:
  - is flexible;
  - has common protocols and care pathways underpinned by evidence that supports/facilitates clinical judgement rather than replaces it;
  - includes common assessment and evaluation procedures that address physical, psychological, spiritual, environmental, cultural and individual aspects of care (holism);
  - puts the person at the centre of care;
  - recognises existing co-ordinated and shared care models of care that could be adapted to include complementary therapies;
  - involves interdisciplinary care and intercollegiate meetings, education programmes, case discussions.
- Defining roles, responsibilities and scope of practice of practitioners.
- Identifying appropriate standards of integrated care.
- Identifying, undertaking and supporting complementary therapy and integrated therapy research, audit quality improvement and evaluation studies to determine aspects such as safety and efficacy, dose and dose intervals, cost benefit, and patient and practitioner satisfaction. Research could be a key aspect of education and professional development programmes, especially for complementary therapists (Jackson and de Jong 1999), which includes developing research priorities and could include whole systems such as Chinese medicine and Ayurveda (Meyers 2004).
- Deciding which general and disease-specific outcomes need to be monitored, including adverse events and the appropriate monitoring methods.
- Ensuring quality ingredients are used in complementary medicines and that they are appropriately labelled and marketed so that therapeutic claims can be evaluated. In some countries such as Australia, complementary medicines are regulated under the same system as conventional medicines. The Australian complementary health industry is likely to change as the recommendations made following the review of *Complementary Medicines in the Australian Health System* (2003) are implemented. Likewise, the Modernised Chinese Medicine International Association (MCMIA), established in 1998 by the Chinese government, has begun a programme to standardise herbal preparations to improve their quality and safety (Fox and Lau 2005).
- Using a Quality Use of Medicines framework that places the emphasis on prevention and using non-medicine options first (National Strategy for the Quality Use of Medicines 2002).
- Ensuring the patient is informed about and understands the benefits and risks involved. In some cases the potential effects on other people in the vicinity may need to be considered, for example, vapourising essential oils in an open area.

Complementary and conventional practitioners will need to establish professional partnerships and collaborative care and referral processes, which requires individual health professionals to develop a working knowledge about combined complementary and conventional care, the benefits and risks, being aware of the limitations of their own knowledge and competence, and developing non-judgemental attitudes. A key issue is having systematic methods of documenting and communicating care and evaluating outcomes, both positive and negative, and methods of interprofessional communication.

4.7 Current Integrative Models

Several integrative models currently exist including the Ornish model (Faas 2001) complementary therapy centres located within general hospitals staffed by complementary and conventional practitioners, and in primary care settings where GPs and complementary therapists provide a truly integrated model of care. Many conventional practitioners in these settings are qualified in therapies such as nutritional medicine, acupuncture, herbal medicine, homeopathy and Chinese medicine.

Bettiens (1998) described several models for delivering complementary care in the UK:

- general practice models where GPs or nurses use complementary therapies, independent complementary therapy practitioners on NHS-funded premises, or private referral to complementary therapy practitioners. These processes apply in fund-holding and non-fund holding practices.
- GPs provide complementary therapies after attending courses. These GPs establish a network of colleagues for referral purposes.
- complementary centres such as the London Homeopathic Hospital, which has defined standards for complementary therapies;
- complementary therapies delivered in specific trusts or centres such as outpatient settings, palliative care, ICU and cardiothoracic units;
- charitable projects;
- ad hoc or 'add on' especially in acute care.

Similar models occur in other countries such as integrated clinics in hospitals and primary care. In Australia, in 1997, 20 per cent of GPs actively practised at least one complementary therapy and almost 50 per cent were interested in complementary therapy training (Cohen 2004). These figures are likely to have increased since then. While it is difficult to estimate the proportion of people with diabetes accessing complementary therapies independently or from complementary health care programmes, it is likely to be significant given the frequency of use, see Chapter 2.

4.8 Regulatory Issues

The increasing use of complementary therapies raises concerns about litigation. These risks can be reduced if practitioners practise within the relevant legislation, follow processes for regulating practice and self-regulate their practice according to Codes of Professional Conduct and Ethics, appropriate standards, and relevant policies and guidelines. Most complementary therapies therapists are not regulated under the law. Many have stringent self-regulatory mechanisms in place that include the level of education required, requirements for continuous professional development, and in some cases evidence of recent first aid training, including cardiopulmonary resuscitation. Like mandatory regulation, voluntary regulation requires organisational expertise and appropriate funding.

One concern, however, is that not everyone describing him or herself as a 'complementary therapist' undergoes accredited training or joins a professional association, which in some cases could be because they do not meet the stringent professional requirements, especially educational requirements. Like conventional practitioners, complementary therapists are concerned when complementary therapy organisations set up self-credentialling process without some form of peer review. This concern was highlighted in a recent court case in Australia where a 37-year-old man died of kidney disease after a detoxification programme carried out under the care of a naturopath whose qualifications were obtained through a 'dubious operator' (Woods 2005). Such behaviour not only puts the public at risk but also brings those complementary therapists, who are appropriately qualified and practise responsibly, into disrepute.

The main aim of regulation is to manage risk. Debate about whether complementary therapies should be regulated has arisen because of the risks associated with specific therapies, the quality of products, and the standard of practitioner education (New South Wales Health 2002; Complementary Medicines in the Australian Health System 2003; Woods 2005). Some of these risks are generic such as the patient not accessing or stopping conventional treatment, others are specific such as herb–medicine interactions, serious allergy to an essential oil, and complementary practitioners not recognising serious health problems and not referring or referring the person too late for appropriate management. For example, a baby boy died receiving treatment from a homeopath who did not recognise the child had a congenital heart defect (MJA 2004). Complementary therapy safety issues are discussed in Chapter 3.

Conventional practitioners, products and services are regulated through a number of Acts and regulations. Medicines and other therapeutic goods are controlled in various ways depending on existing regulatory systems, see Chapter 3. At present, many governments do not have the constitutional powers to regulate complementary practitioners to the same extent as conventional practitioners. An exception in Australia is Chinese medicine practitioners in the state of Victoria who are regulated under the *Chinese Medicine Registration Act* 2000 (Vic). Professor Eden, Director of the Natural Therapies Unit at the Royal Women's Hospital, Sydney, suggested it might be possible to regulate complementary therapies by an independent organisation similar to the National Heart Foundation (Woods 2005) but the suggestion has not been widely discussed.

Office of Complementary Medicines in Australia

Legislation underpinning the regulation of complementary therapies and the formation of the Office of Complementary Medicine (OCM) was proclaimed in Australia in April 1999. The OCM focuses on regulating complementary therapies in a transparent manner and forming links with complementary practitioners, industry, academics and consumers. The responsibilities of the OCM include evaluating complementary medicines data in order to assess whether it is safe to register or list the complementary medicines and providing advice to the Minister for Health, the Therapeutic Goods Association (TGA) and the Complementary Medicines Evaluation Committee (CMEC) as part of the regulatory process. Some complementary therapies also need to comply with the Food Standards of Australia (FANZ). The TGA works closely with FANZ with respect to products at the food/medicine interface such as vitamins and supplements. In some cases Health Acts also apply to these products. More regular assessment of therapeutic claims for complementary medicines, and clarification of the place of complementary medicines in the National Medicines Policy and Quality Use of Medicines framework are likely to occur. Currently, harmonisation procedures concerning medicines are being developed and implemented between Australia and New Zealand.

United Kingdom and other countries

In the UK, herbs, homeopathic substances and essential oils are considered to be medical products if they are used for therapeutic purposes (Medicines Control Agency, Medicines Act 1968). Two sets of regulations apply, *Control of Substances Hazardous to Health* 1994 (COSHH) and *Chemical Hazards Information Packaging* 1996 (CHIPS) through the Medicines and Healthcare Products Regulatory Agency (MHRA). These regulations are currently under review. Under the COSH and CHIPS regulations, substances are classified into categories such as very toxic, toxic, harmful, irritant, corrosive, and flammable, according to their chemical safety. Some substances are more hazardous than others based on their LD_{50} rating (the point at which 50 per cent of test animals die). In this context, 'hazard' refers to the potential to cause harm, and 'risk' refers to the likelihood that harm will occur in the circumstances of the use. Consideration is given to how the substance is handled, duration of exposure, and individual susceptibility when determining the hazard rating. Hazard ratings and labels differ among countries and health professionals are advised to become familiar with the system in their own countries.

Other relevant regulatory bodies and relevant Acts in the UK include the Medicines Control Agency, the *Health and Safety at Work Act* 1974, Consumer Protection Acts, the Council of Complementary and Alternative Medicine (CCAM), and the British Complementary Medicine Association (BCMA), which represents 78 complementary therapy organisations, training schools and research foundations. The main aim of the BCMA is to safely integrate complementary therapies into the health system. In addition, specific complementary therapy organisations such as the International Federation of Aromatherapists and the Aromatherapy Organisations Council have developed professional documents such as standards of practice and codes of conduct.

The House of Lords Report (2000) recommended reforming regulatory processes of unlicensed herbal remedies in the UK. The MHRA subsequently proposed reforms in these areas. The consultation document is available on the MHRA website: www.mhra.gov.uk as Consultation Letter MLX 299 (accessed March 2005). Other bodies include the Office of Alternative Medicine in the USA. The USA has contributed a significant amount of funding to complementary therapies, but the same level of support is not available in other countries (Fluhrer 2002), and the National Centre for Complementary medicine in Europe.

On a local level, practitioners could maintain a portfolio of current, relevant information in areas where complementary therapies are used that does the following:

- Lists the herbal therapies, homeopathic substances and essential oils used in the care of people with diabetes and classifies them according to their potential to cause serious adverse events (hazard rating). This information can be obtained from reputable texts, journals, safety data sheets, product manufacturers, product suppliers and producers, and relevant regulatory organisations.
- Indicates the type of person most likely to be harmed by the product or particular administration methods and/or combination therapy, for example, burns to neuropathic legs from cupping. This might include related hazards such as fire hazard for some products such as essential oils.
- Indicates any particular assessment that needs to be undertaken before the therapies are used.
- Evaluates the potential level of risk associated with particular products and patients, considering existing guidelines and the actual risk, taking account of hazard and risk ratings and the findings of the individual patient assessment.
- Decides whether any particular risk reduction strategies are required, for example, not using some herbal medicines or essential oils concomitantly with anticoagulant medicines, adjusting complementary as well as conventional medicines for surgery, and protecting neuropathic feet.
- Establishes standardised processes and guidelines.
- Ensures knowledgeable and competent practitioners deliver the treatment within the limits of their knowledge and competence and scope of practice.
- Decides which outcomes need to be monitored and use appropriate outcome measures (Fowler and Wall 1998).

Self-regulation

While complementary therapies may not be statutorily regulated, most reputable complementary therapy associations encourage transparent, accountable self-regulation, particularly where medicines are part of the therapeutic options.

Self-regulation largely occurs through professional associations and encompasses accountability and responsibility and scope of practice. These are key aspects of the duty of care that applies to all health professionals. Patients have a right to expect the care they receive meets current standards, guidelines and research evidence (Nisselle 2003). One area of concern in some countries is when a conventional professional leaves conventional practice and sets up as a complementary therapist. These practitioners can knowingly or unknowingly mislead patients about the currency/recency of their conventional practice.

Complementary professional associations set standards for education programmes that must be met in order for the practitioner to be accredited, in much the same way as conventional professional associations do. Practitioners successfully qualifying through an accredited education provider delivering an approved programme can apply for full membership of the relevant association. Once membership is gained, continuing professional development and adherence to a code of professional conduct are mandatory, which is the same way conventional associations operate.

In many cases, complementary therapy education courses are validated through organisations such as the UK National Vocational Qualifications and the Australian National Training Authority. Increasingly, courses are offered through universities and are therefore subject to university course accreditation processes. Table 4.1 outlines some of the issues to be considered before undertaking a complementary therapy education programme.

4.9 Responsibilities of Individual Conventional Practitioners Using Complementary Therapies

Health professionals are responsible for the care they provide including:

- being informed about the potential benefits and risks of the therapy;
- considering the traditional basis and research evidence for the therapy for the particular health issue;
- being informed about or know how to access information about complementary and conventional therapies in order to appropriately advise patients;
- obtaining informed consent;
- understanding regulatory considerations and ethical principles:
  - equitable access;
  - standards of quality, safety and efficacy;
  - Quality Use of Medicines including complementary medicines.

Medico-legal considerations

Several inter-related issues affect the 'legal and policy decisions surrounding the integration of complementary and conventional care' (Cohen 2005). Medico-legal issues must be considered at the policy level of any integrative initiative, especially obtaining supportive peer opinion about the integrated model, should

Table 4.1 Some issues to consider before undertaking a complementary therapy course.

1. What complementary therapies are you interested in?
2. How do you want to use the therapy?
3. What courses are available in the complementary therapy? Are they offered by a university or a college?
4. What does the content cover?
   - Does it have sufficient theoretical content and practice aspects to ensure you will have a thorough grounding in the therapy to practice safely?
   - How is the course offered: distance mode, on line, on site, in time blocks such as every weekend for several weeks, mixed mode?
   - If the course is offered online from another country is it recognised in the country in which you hope to practice?
   - How long is the course: can you afford the time and fit it into your usual routines?
   - How much does it cost and are there any hidden costs?
   - Are there any prerequisites you will need to fulfil?
   - Is credit given for any previous relevant learning?
   - Does it articulate with any other courses/degrees?
5. What qualification will be conferred after successful completion of the course? Is the course recognised by any professional body or regulatory authority?
6. What assessment processes will be used: examination, demonstrated competencies, assignments or a combination of these?
7. Where does the clinical practice take place: in a clinical agency or in the classroom?
   - Is it supervised?
   - How is it assessed?
   - Are there agreements in place with clinical agencies or do you have to negotiate on your own behalf?
   - Are you covered by professional indemnity when you are in the clinical areas?
8. Does any professional or regulatory body accredit the course and is the accreditation current?
9. Are the teachers qualified to teach the subjects allocated to them and can they demonstrate recency of practice and evidence of continued professional development?
10. Are there any mentoring or ongoing professional development programme in place for after you complete the course?

a legal issue arise. Legal systems are vastly different around the world and are still largely unknown with respect to complementary therapies and integrated care. Responsibility for practice can be the direct responsibility of the practitioner or the indirect responsibility of an organisation employing or consulting the practitioner (vicarious liability). In employed or consultant situations, the credibility, capacity to provide unsupervised care, scope of practice, and responsibility for overall patient management may need to be defined. These factors apply equally to complementary and conventional practitioners.

Some risk management tips in addition to the portfolio described on page 60 are depicted in Table 4.2 and key safety issues in Table 4.3. The level of complementary therapy practice conventional health professionals undertake depends on their knowledge and competence in the particular therapy. All health professionals can and should ask about, and document, complementary therapy use, and in the case of complementary practitioners, conventional therapy use.

Table 4.2 Risk management tips for safe integrated practice.

Ask patients whether they are using complementary therapies and maintain an up-to-date record of the therapies being used. In some cases it is also important to consider the way the therapy is administered for example aromatherapy see chapter 6. Complementary therapists should maintain records of current conventional medicines and management.

Prescribe complementary and conventional medicines according to the Quality Use of Medicines, current evidence and relevant management guidelines.

Practice within the relevant scope of practice and training and education.

Report adverse events.

Ensure billing is consistent with relevant funding mechanisms.

Consider the ethical issues surrounding the same practitioner prescribing and selling products.

Inform patients about the benefits and risks of management recommendations.

Table 4.3 Key aspects of safety.

Practitioner issues	Product development, advertising and monitoring	Administrative issues
Licences/authority to practice based on appropriate education and credentialing systems. Defined scope of practice according to the professional discipline. Manufacturing acts and regulations. Professional liability insurance and third party reimbursement.	Premarket evaluation of products/medicines prior to approving their approval for supply and use, which includes licensing complementary product manufacturers using processes consistent with international standards. Ensuring random product sampling and adverse event monitoring occurs and public inquiries or concerns are responded to after the product is registered and available on the market. Developing and maintaining systems to monitor products and assessing manufactured products to ensure they meet relevant standards before they are exported to other countries. Monitoring the therapy to produce evidence that it contributes to patient care. This includes having processes in place to accurately report and document the effects, and effective collaboration and referral process.	Defining relevant administrative processes such as cost, purchase, storage and maintenance of equipment. Processes to ensure complementary therapists are knowledgeable and competent, visiting rights for non-staff members are clearly articulated and they carry appropriate professional indemnity and insurance.

Informed consent/refusal of treatment by a patient must be ascertained. Informed consent involves ensuring patients are aware of the benefits and risks of *any* therapy they use. However, this is very difficult when health professionals are treating patients from different cultural backgrounds, which is an area that needs more research and policy guidelines. Methods of obtaining consent vary, and may be verbal, obtained as part of a general standard consent process, or be specific to a therapy so that the risks and benefits can be explained. Patient autonomy plays a critical role in any decision about health care from a legal perspective (Brophy 2003a). However, it has not yet been established whether or when conventional practitioners should provide information about complementary therapies. Although legal systems vary among countries, there are some common principles. Brophy (2003b), citing the case of *Rogers versus Whitaker*, indicated that the judge's decision suggests a doctor's duty, and by extrapolation the duty of other health professionals, consists of more than the obligation to provide a patient with information about material risks. It also encompasses the individual's right to choose to accept or reject the treatment based on the information they receive. In making the decision in *Rogers versus Whitaker*, the judge discussed the types of information that could be given to patients by citing other cases where complementary therapies might offer greater benefit than conventional treatment.

Chapter 3 discussed some of the risks associated with using herbal medicines. Other aspects of risks are described in this chapter. Likewise, should integration occur, some complementary medicine doses need to be adjusted or stopped for varying lengths of time before investigations and surgical procedures are undertaken to reduce risks such as bleeding. Therefore, people need to be adequately advised about such risks to minimise anaesthetic, procedural and metabolic adverse events. These issues are still largely under-recognised and not well defined for people with diabetes but need to be incorporated into patient information sheets. People have a responsibility to disclose important information that could compromise their care, and this includes using complementary therapies, but may not think it is relevant unless they are specifically asked.

Providing information

The NHMRC *Guidelines for Medical Practitioners on Providing Information for Patients* (2004) outline key aspects for communicating with patients. These guidelines support people's right to decide, or at the very least be consulted about, their management. Key information to cover is shown in Table 4.4. One of the main reasons for providing advice is to ensure the person has the appropriate information, oral and written, to help them make an informed decision.

When providing information, it can be difficult to determine exactly how much and what type of information an individual requires. The number and type of questions they ask can provide clues, as can asking relevant questions such as enquiring about the types of therapies the person is interested in (conventional and complementary). Questions can be asked when providing information, when the

Table 4.4   Important information to provide as part of helping patients make decisions about their treatment based on the NHMRC (2004).

---

1. The benefits or outcomes likely to result from using the treatment.
2. The risks involved, which should include information about the general risks and specific risks to the individual associated with combining complementary and conventional therapies. General risks might include the risk of allergy to an herbal medicine and specific risk might be interactions with conventional medicines leading to hypoglycaemia, see chapters 3 and 9.
3. Any potential complications, adverse events and interactions such as physical, mental, social and sexual effects.
4. The side effects of herbal medicines, homeopathic preparations and essential oils.
5. Other possible management options; people often seek other management options when they perceive the risks of their current treatment to be high or unpleasant. If complementary and conventional treatments are integrated, the relative benefits and risk of all the relevant options could be presented.
6. Time they need to allow to use the treatment for each dose/application and how long it will need to be continued (duration).
7. The consequences of not using the therapy.
8. Document the people who were present when the information was provided, whether the person actively sought information, their health status, and the general circumstances operating at the time the information was provided.

---

patients ask, and during assessment, history taking and diagnosis (Brophy 2003b). In fact, questions about complementary therapies should be a standard part of the health history and assessment.

When complementary therapies appear to be indicated and the patient or a relative or guardian is not able to give informed consent, the health professional needs to clarify whether any legislation applies, for example, advanced directives or whether there is an appointed guardian or another suitable decision-maker who is familiar with the patient's views (who may or may not be the next of kin) which is important for patients who come from a culturally different background from the therapist. The information should then be provided to that person.

Recommendations need to be underpinned by evidence where possible or, in the case of some complementary therapies, long, safe traditional practice. However, health professionals should also use their clinical judgement and the outcome of a thorough assessment and history when informing people about treatment options. When a complementary therapy is indicated or recommended, consideration needs to be given to whether the treatment is readily available, reasonable, and whether competent practitioners are available to deliver the treatment (Brophy 2003b).

The recommendation of friends, product advertising in a range of mediums, product labels, and often the Internet, are the primary source of information for people when they self-diagnose and self-treat. Health professionals have little control over these information sources. Where they do, they can help people ascertain the quality of the information. The effect of directly advertising to the public is currently being discussed in several countries. Research indicates that direct advertising promotes the use of medicines rather than 'alternatives', often gives inadequate information, 'medicalises' self-limiting conditions, dramatically affects the demand for prescriptions, increases the number of prescriptions provided, and may reduce the amount of education and quality of the education provided (Hoffman and Wilkes 1999; Galbally 2001; Moynihan *et al.* 2002). Some of these concerns can be addressed by open, non-judgemental attitudes in a therapeutic, caring relationship.

Advertising materials affect decisions (*Complementary Medicines in the Australian Healthcare System* 2003). The National Medicines Policy (1999) states that people have a right to timely access to accurate information about medicines and their use. Advertising in Australia is subject to the *Therapeutic Goods Act* 1991, and the *Therapeutic Goods Advertising Code*, which cover over-the-counter and complementary medicines, and the *Trade Practices Act* 1974 and the Medicines Australia Code of Conduct. Similar systems apply in other countries, for example, the International Pharmaceutical Federation (FMP), which is partly concerned with preventing the use of counterfeit medicines.

Consumer Medicines Information (CMI) must be distributed with all Prescriber Benefits Schedule (PBS) listed medicines in Australia, although the degree to which CMI affects choice is not clear. CMI is information adapted from the prescriber information according to specific guidelines to inform people about their medicines (Sless and Wiseman 1997). At present, CMI is not mandatory for complementary medicines and non-PBS listed medicines. Resources such as *Natural Medicines Instructions for Patients* (2002) may be useful, but have not been evaluated. CMI and product labels can be incorporated into patient education strategies. Quality product labels are another way of informing people about products and medicines. Table 4.5 indicates the main headings of an informative product label.

Table 4.5 Label outline for complementary medicines. The information may differ among countries but should include the basic information outlined below. In some countries specific information is required on labels and more detailed information in package inserts.

Name of the product
Presentation: dose form, strength, flavour if relevant
Indications for use: action
Dose prescribed
How to apply or administer
Contraindications
Warnings and precautions
Potential adverse effects including interactions with other complementary and/or
    conventional therapies
Amount of product in the bottle/tube/pack
Medicine classification (where relevant)
Date of preparation and expiry date
Name and contact details of the manufacturer
Storage conditions

4.10 Evidence-based Care and Clinical Practice Guidelines

Research is the basis of evidence-based care, which is defined as: 'the conscientious, explicit and judicious use of current best practice evidence in making decisions about patients' (Sackett 1996). Evidence-based care reflects the fact that the traditional method of choosing care based on clinical experience and intuition is no longer sufficient and stresses examination of clinical research using formal criteria. However, it does not reflect or replace clinical judgement in individual circumstances. Various methods of rating research studies exist such as Jadad scores and NHMRC levels of evidence.

The Medical Board of Queensland's (2005) policy concerning Alternative and Unconventional Medicine states they endorse editorial comments in the *New England Journal of Medicine* (Angell and Kassirer 1998), which stated:

> There is only medicine that has been adequately tested, and medicine that has not, medicine that works and medicine that may or may not work. Once a treatment has been tested rigorously, it no longer matters whether it was considered alternative at the outset... But assertions, speculation and testimonials do not substitute for evidence.

The editorial reiterates the importance of research evidence but it also demonstrates that complementary practitioners' concerns about their therapies being lost or the 'gems mined' may be well founded. The Queensland policy goes on to state that regulatory authorities are concerned with competence, standards and evidence and points out the difficulty of defining the scope of practice for doctors. Since a great deal of conventional care is not evidence-based but combines art and science, the challenge for integration is to decide how much evidence is required and how much art can be accepted to achieve holistic care.

Conventional practitioners may not be aware that there is a large body of quality complementary therapy research reported in conventional and complementary journals and on the Cochrane and many other databases. For example, the Cochrane Complementary Health Field has been operating since 1996 and lists over 5000 randomised trials, systematic reviews and other trials. Other databases include the University of Maryland website, newsletter and bibliographic database and the COMPMED trials register and the Database of Abstracts of Reviews of Effectiveness (DARE). While these are not exclusive to diabetes, they do contain useful information.

Some complementary therapy professionals have held international meetings to develop research agendas, for example, homeopathy (Meyers 2004). Such initiatives enable complementary practitioners to focus on specific clinical issues and identify the most pressing research gaps. Meyers points out the potential to devalue specific complementary therapies if potentially 'valuable' elements of specific therapies are incorporated into conventional medicine and others are discarded – 'mining the gems from complementary medicine' and indicates research needs to take note of the therapy as a whole (the way it is usually practised). Likewise, Meyers indicates that the responsibility for research belongs with the complementary practitioners. Since many conventional practitioners have the necessary research skills, they could participate in teaching and mentoring complementary therapists, even to the extent of adapting established research methods to address the concept of holism while maintaining rigour in research projects.

Certainly, the concern that there is insufficient good quality evidence to support many complementary therapies is justified, despite the increasing body of well-designed complementary therapy research. Many complementary therapists argue that randomised control trials are difficult to carry out for some complementary therapies and make the case for large-scale rigorous audits and outcome studies to produce clinically relevant and useful evidence (Fluhrer 2002). Basic science researchers may not appreciate the contribution of qualitative, psychological, behavioural, and evaluation research methods, nor be aware of the way rigour is applied in these methods. Importantly, the method should be appropriate to the research questions.

What are clinical practice guidelines?

Guidelines are systematically developed statements that assist health professionals and patients to make decisions about appropriate health care in specific situations (Institute of Medicine 1990). They are designed to support and complement clinical judgement rather than replace it. Guidelines are usually developed considering current quality evidence and are designated as either evidence-based or consensus-based depending on the strength of the evidence that supports the statements made in the guidelines. Four broad levels of evidence are described:

Level 1: evidence derived from systematically reviewed randomised controlled trials.

Level 2: derived from at least one randomised controlled trial.

Level 3: derived from well described non-randomised controlled trials.

Level 4: based on the opinion of respected relevant authorities and derived from their experience, descriptive studies and reports of expert committees (NHMRC 1995).

Current methods of reviewing evidence where randomised controlled trials (RCT) are the most highly valued form of evidence make it difficult to determine how complementary therapies can be justified in some circumstances. However, RCTs may not be the most appropriate method for researching some clinical questions, especially those concerning issues such as patient's beliefs, attitudes and satisfaction, which largely utilise qualitative methods that do not rely on randomisation. Therefore, there may be a need to develop separate levels of evidence for qualitative research methods based on the degree of rigour in the study and the methods used to control bias including researcher bias. One criticism of RCT is that although they enable the results to be generalised outside the study, they often include small samples and subjects who are rigorously selected, and may not truly resemble patients seen in 'the real world'. Both types of studies provide different information and are complementary: RCT demonstrate what is needed; qualitative methods provide important information about how to implement it.

It is vital to consider complementary therapies use as part of the individual's total assessment and management plan. Therefore, current guidelines could incorporate complementary therapies into the decision-making flow chart process, which is often a key part of the guideline. The growing interest in and use of complementary therapies reflect the increasing need to consider the effect of the individual's unconscious and emotional and spiritual make-up on their physical well-being (Watkins 1997) and these aspects are rarely included in current guidelines.

Currently the evidence for many complementary therapies falls into levels 3 and 4. However, the amount of good quality complementary therapy research is increasing and can be included in iterations of the guideline as part of the regular review process.

A wide variety of evidence may need to be considered when developing guidelines for using some complementary therapies. Level 1 and 2 evidence may not be available for all therapies and as some systematic process for evaluating the evidence from long traditional use, case reports and descriptive studies is needed until such evidence becomes available.

Guidelines are largely concerned with setting standards of care from a government and management perspective and cost containment (Jackson and de, Jong 1999). Guidelines are an integral aspect of practice that make provision for continuity of care across different health-care sectors, limit variation in health-care practices, and strengthen the link between research, evidence and clinical practice, and therapy, improving patient outcomes (Grimshaw and Russell 1993). However, guidelines will only be effective if they improve health professional's decision-making.

Interest in clinical standards of care is one reason for the increasing global interest in agreed clinical practice guidelines to reduce variations in the way diseases are managed, to discontinue outmoded practices, and to recommend adopting desirable new pharmacological treatments, products and technology (NHMRC 1995). The rapidly increasing volume of evidence often makes it difficult for clinicians to incorporate new research into practice. In the case of complementary therapies, the amount of level 1 evidence is limited, which means complementary therapies are not considered when many guidelines are developed and complementary therapists are not often numbered among the stakeholders.

Some existing complementary therapy guidelines were identified when writing this chapter (Wafer 1994; Fowler and Wall 1998; NSW Therapeutic Association Group Inc 1999) but their evidence base is limited and the extent to which they have been implemented and evaluated is unknown, see Table 4.6.

The optimal integration of guidelines into clinical practice depends on organisational factors and available resources. These factors are usually the responsibility of the local clinical areas where complementary therapies are used.

Table 4.6 Some existing complementary therapy guidelines.

(a) **Health professional guidelines**
- Australian College of Holistic Nurses, *Policy Guidelines for the Practice of Complementary Therapies by Nurses and Midwives in Australia, 2000.*
- Australian Nursing Federation *Policy Statement Complementary and Alternative Therapies.*
- Health and Safety Commission Sheffield UK *Safety Data Sheets for Substances and Preparations Dangerous for Supply*, 1994.
- *National Occupational Standards for Aromatherapy UK* 2002.
- Nurses Board of Victoria, *Guidelines for the use of Complementary Therapies in Nursing Practice 2005.*
- South East Health, *Complementary Therapies and Nursing Practice 2001.*
- Royal College of Nursing, Australia, *Complementary Therapies in Australian Nursing Practice, 2000.*
- National Centre for Complementary and Alternative Medicine USA *National Guidelines for Use with Complementary Therapies in Supportive and Palliative Care.*
- Medical Board of Queensland *Guidelines on Complementary, Alternative and Unconventional Medicines.*
- Federation of State Medical Boards of the USA Inc 2002 *Model Guidelines for the Use of Complementary and Alternative Therapies in Medical Practice.*
- Watson, K. 2004 Safety guidelines for Chinese herbal dispensing.

(b) **Patient guidelines**
- American Cancer Society 2005 *Guidelines for Using Complementary and Alternative Methods.*
- Pizzorno *et al.* 2002 *Natural Medicine Instructions for Patients.*
- *Sunderland Teaching Primary Care Trust 2002* Complementary Therapies.

As with any change in practice, a process whereby the implementation and outcomes of the guidelines can be overseen and monitored is vital. Incorporating complementary therapy guidelines into the same 'manual' as conventional guidelines enhances the likelihood that complementary therapies will be seen as part of an holistic approach to care rather than as separate and different. There is some evidence that guidelines that operate within the professional–patient consultation and focus on individual patients are more likely to lead to changes in practice (Grimshaw and Russell, 1993).

Complementary therapy guidelines vary in the detail, usefulness and evidence base. In some cases it may be relevant and important to specify the level of education and competence that practitioners providing complementary care need to demonstrate and specify their scope of practice. This might be a basic level of education and demonstrated complementary therapy competency (which may be specific to particular therapies) or autonomous complementary therapy practice with an expanded scope of practice.

Some complementary therapy guidelines already provide a professional context for incorporating complementary therapies into conventional care by describing the educational preparation, selection of therapies and professional considerations such as legislation, professional indemnity, informed consent and documentation needed for safe use, and were designed to be used in conjunction with other relevant professional documents such as code of professional conduct. This practice framework is essentially the same as that for any health professional and is consistent with the duty of care all health professionals have to practise within their level of knowledge and competence. It is based on the premise that practitioners who provide complementary therapies should have undertaken appropriate training including conventional practitioners using complementary therapies. Guidelines need to be broad and flexible enough to effectively guide health care without being unnecessarily prescriptive.

Legal implications of guidelines

Some health professionals are concerned about possible litigation if management is not provided according to clinical practice guidelines (NHMRC 1995). The Australian High Court in Rogers versus Whitaker (1992) indicated that health professionals have a duty to inform patients about the risks associated with the treatment being recommended but a court is likely to make assessments about whether a health professional acted in a reasonable manner according to 'the facts of each case'. In Rogers versus Whitaker, the High Court distinguished between whether the health professional was negligent in a particular form of treatment and whether they were negligent by not providing all the relevant information. Clinical practice guidelines may help professionals and courts make decisions about what is accepted reasonable and relevant practice.

Guideline authors are not considered to be in a relationship with guideline users or those who receive care according to a guideline. However, authors who claim their guidelines are definitive statements of correct management rather than a general guide to clinical decision-making in conjunction with all other relevant information may be at some risk. Therefore, when developing guidelines it is important to take reasonable steps to ensure they are properly prepared, which might include following guidelines for developing guidelines such as those of the NHMRC (1995) or the State Medical Boards of the USA (2002). In addition, guidelines should clearly state they are provided as a general guide, the date of issue and the date when they should be reviewed. A review of the regulation of health professionals is currently underway in Victoria, Australia (Department of Human Services (DHS) 2005). The draft document indicates that people commenting on the consultation draft document indicated that: 'Standards of practice for registrants who incorporate complementary therapies in their practice is best dealt with through guidelines and codes rather than legislation' (DHS 2002). The document went on to note that registration boards should be encouraged to develop suitable guidelines to outline the integration and use of complementary therapies for their registrants. Since most complementary therapy practitioners are not regulated under legislation in Australia (except Chinese medicine in Victoria), one hopes the authors of such guidelines have the relevant knowledge of complementary therapies to develop appropriate guidelines and include relevant complementary therapy practitioners on development panels.

From a health professional's perspective, guidelines can clarify the scope of practice and roles and responsibilities of individual professionals. This may be particularly important when complementary therapies are incorporated into conventional care plans. Although guidelines are not 'legal documents', they are used as evidence of 'best practice' when questions about care arise. Therefore, guidelines may help health professionals identify and avoid foreseeable risks.

Clinicians' responses to guidelines are not always positive and some question their utility in actual or 'real' practice. For example, there are a bewildering number of 'diabetes management guidelines' and there are inconsistencies among them. A survey of Australian general practitioners in 1999 found less than half followed a specific set of guidelines and called for 'only one [diabetes] guideline please!' (Parnell 1999).

A major benefit of guidelines may be their potential to facilitate integrated health care (Jackson and deJong 1999). Integrated care guidelines could make provision for using complementary therapies and enhance continuity of care among complementary and conventional practitioners and practice settings, clarify roles and responsibilities and care timeframes, and communication and referral processes.

4.11 Guidelines for Patients Using Complementary Therapies

A number of guidelines have been developed to help patients make informed decisions about using complementary therapies and then to select specific therapies. Some define complementary therapies, describe the risks of not using conventional treatment, describe the conventional treatment, suggest strategies for discussing complementary therapies with conventional practitioners, outline questions to ask about complementary therapies, give suggestions about how to detect questionable/fraudulent methods, insurance coverage, and list where more information can be obtained.

Others such as Pizzorno *et al.* (2002) provide detailed information about specific disease processes, signs and symptoms, preventative measures, expected outcomes, management options, risk of interactions and adverse events. Some websites describe important information about various therapies and what people can expect to happen (Sunderland Teaching Primary Care Trust 2005). The Sunderland Trust provide a very brief description of the therapy, indicate 'a consultation will form part of the initial session', concisely describe what the treatment involves, and the cost. Very few actually discuss the need to inform patients about what should be on complementary therapy product labels, how to read labels, or point out patients' rights and responsibilities.

4.12 Quality Use of Medicines

Quality Use of Medicines (QUM) is a system that aims to make the best possible use of medicines to improve health outcomes (Commonwealth Department of Health and Ageing 2002). QUM recognises that many people maintain their health without medicines; others require medicines to prevent illness or to manage existing disease processes including diabetes.

Quality Use of Medicines means:

- selecting management options wisely by considering the place of medicines in maintaining health, treating illness and recognising that non-medicine options may lead to better, safer outcomes for example stress management;
- choosing suitable medicines if a medicine is required considering:
  - the findings of the individual assessment;
  - the clinical condition of the patient at the time;
  - risks and benefits of the medicine and other management options;
  - dosage dose intervals and proposed duration of treatment;
  - any co-existing conditions;
  - other therapies being used;
  - the processes for monitoring outcomes;
  - costs to the individual, the community, and the health system as a whole;
  - delivery devices such as insulin, acupuncture.
- using medicines safely and effectively to get the best possible results by monitoring outcomes, minimising misuse, over-use and under-use and improving people's ability to solve medicine-related problems, such as managing multiple medicines, which is usually necessary in diabetes. QUM guidelines can assist practitioners to determine where and how complementary therapies could be incorporated into an individual's care plan as well as demonstrate and collaborative multidisciplinary communication and referral achieved.

4.13 Documentation and communication

An essential aspect of holistic, integrated care is communication between all health professionals involved in an individual's care. Documentation is a key aspect of communication. The appropriate place to document complementary therapy treatments is in the standard care plan, medical record and possibly the medication record in acute settings if pharmacological agents (herbal medicines, essential oils, homeopathy) are used. However, separate processes for referral, complementary care plans and implementation processes are common practice and could contribute to adverse events. A key aspect of the patient's documented management plan should include assessment processes, the management options discussed, investigations and outcomes to be monitored. Documentation should be contemporaneous following each complementary treatment.

4.14   Adverse event reporting

Adverse event reporting is concerned with safety and is an essential aspect of documentation and could be part of management guidelines. If an adverse event occurs, it should be documented on the relevant adverse event reporting form and communicated to the relevant people see chapter 3. Documenting adverse events is as important as documenting their benefits, and contributes to the safety profile of the particular therapy and helps identify trends or problem areas that may need to be addressed by the wider health system. Where an allergy to an herb or essential oil occurs, warnings should be placed in the patient's records to prevent inadvertent prescribing in future situations.

References

American Cancer Society. *Complementary and Alternative Therapies* www.cancer.org/docroot/ETO.com, 2005.

Angell M, Kassirer J. Alternative medicine – the risks of untested and unregulated remedies. *New England Journal of Medicine* 1998; **339**: 839–841.

Australian College of Holistic Nurses. *Policy Guidelines for the Practice of Complementary Therapies by Nurses and Midwives in Australia* Brisbane: Duo Press, 2000.

Australian Government Department of Health and Ageing, Medicare Plus Update, 2004. www.health.gov.au/medicareplus (accessed May 2004).

Bensoussan A, Lewith B. Complementary medicine research in Australia. *Medical Journal of Australia* 2004; **181**(6): 331–333.

Bettiens R. Integrating complementary therapies into mainstream care. *Australian Nursing Journal* 1998; **6**(3): 33.

Brophy E. Does a doctor have a duty of care to provide information and advice about complementary and alternative medicine? *Journal of Law and Medicine* 2003a; **10**(3): 271–284.

Brophy E. Informed consent and CM. *Complementary Medicine*, 2003b; **July–Aug**: 23–28.

Caspi O, Maizes V, Bell I. Integration of clinical practice and medical training with complementary and alternative and evidence based medicine. In: Spencer J, Jacobs J (eds), *Complementary* and Alternative Medicine: An Evidence Based Approach. St Louis Missouri: Mosby, 1999.

Cohen M. CAM practitioners and "regular" doctors: is integration possible? *Medical Journal of Australia* 2004; **180**: 645–646.

Cohen M. Legal issues regarding complementary therapies. 2005. www.camlawblog.com (accessed April 2005).

Cohen M, Ruggie M. Integrating complementary and alternative medical therapies in conventional medical settings: legal quandaries and potential policy models. *University of Cincinnati Law Review* 2003; **72**: 671–729.

Commonwealth Department of Health and Aged Care. *The National Medicines Policy*. Canberra: Commonwealth Department of Health and Aged Care, 1999.

Commonwealth Department of Health and Aged Care. *The National Strategy for Quality Use of Medicines*. Canberra: Commonwealth Department of Health and Aged Care, 2002.

Complementary Medicines in the Australian Health System. Report to the Parliamentary Secretary to the Minister for Health and Ageing, Canberra: Commonwealth of Australia, 2003.

Department of Human Services, Victoria, Australia. *Review of the Regulation of Health Professions in Victoria*, 2005. Available on: http://www.health.vic.gov.au/pracreg/hp-review.htm (accessed April 2005).

Dossey L. Conference on definitions and standards: working on definitions and terms. *Alternative Therapies Health Medicine* 2003; **9** A10–A12.

Elisha R. Make alternative practitioners accountable. *Medical Observer* 2005; **May 6**: 24.

Faas N. *Integrating Complementary Medicine into Health Systems*. Gaithersburg: Aspen Publications, 2001.

Federation of State Medical Boards of the United States Inc *Model Guidelines for the Use of Complementary and Alternative Therapies in Medical Practice*. 2002; **April**: 1–6.

Fluhrer J. Integrative practice overview. *Journal of Complementary Medicine* 2002; **1**(1): 32–35.

Fowler P, Wall M. Aromatherapy, Control of Substances Hazardous to Health (COSHH) and assessment of the chemical risk. *Complementary Therapies in Medicine* 1998; **6**: 85–93.

Fox R, Lau C. Highlights of the International Conference and Exhibition of the Modernisation of Traditional Chinese Medicine Health Products. *Mediscape Rheumatology* 2005; **6**(2): 1–12.

Galbally R. *Review of Drugs, Poisons and Controlled Substances Legislation, Part B*. Canberra: Commonwealth of Australia, 2001.

Grimshaw J, Russell T. Effect of clinical guidelines on medical practice and a systematic review of rigorous evaluations. *Lancet* 1993; **342**: 1317–1322.

Hoffman J, Wilkes M. Direct to consumer advertising of prescription drugs. *British Medical Journal* 1999; **318**: 1301–1302.

Institute of Medicine. Clinical Practice Guidelines: directions for a new program. In: Field, M., Lahr, K. (eds) *Institute of Medicine*. Washington, DC: National Academy Press, 1990.

Jackson C, de Jong I. Clinical practice guidelines and general practice: the sleeping giant in Australian healthcare integration. *Medical Journal of Australia* 1999; **171**: 91–93.

Marshall D, Walizer E, Vernalis M. Optimal healing environments for chronic cardiovascular disease. *Journal of Alternative and Complementary Medicine* 2004; **10**(Suppl)S147–S155.

Meyers S. Finding the whole beyond the parts. *Complementary Medicine* 2004; **3**(2): 55.

Moynihan R, Heath I, Henry D. Selling sickness; the pharmaceutical industry and disease mongering. *British Medical Journal* 2002; **324**: 886–891.

National Centre for Complementary and Alternative Medicine (NCCAM). *Some Guidelines When Considering Complementary Medicine*. Washington, DC: NCCAM Clearinghouse, 2005.

National Health and Medical Research Council (NHMRC). *Guidelines for the Development and Implementation of Clinical Practice Guidelines*. Canberra: NHMRC, 1995.

National Health and Medical Research Council *General Guidelines for Medical Practitioners on Providing Information for Patients*. http://www.health.gov.au/hfs/nhmrc/publications/fullhtml/cpbo.htm. 2004.

National Strategy for the Quality Use of Medicines. Canberra: Commonwealth of Australia, 2002.

New South Wales Health. Discussion paper *Regulation of Complementary Health Practitioners*. www.health.nsw.gov.au/quality/files/compomed_paper, 2002.

Niselle P. Complementary medicine and the law: the medicolegal academic. *Complementary Medicine* 2003; **2**(2): 48–50.

NSW Therapeutic Association Group. *Complementary Medicines in Public Hospitals: A Discussion Paper*, 1999. Available on: http://www.nswtag.org.au (accessed December 2002).

Parnell K. Guidelines falling short of needs *Australian Doctor* 1999; **9 April**, 27.

Phelps K. Our future is integration. *Complementary Medicine* 2004; **4**(1), 9.

Pizzorno L, Pizzorno J, Murray M. *National Medicine Instructions for Patients*. Edinburgh: Churchill Livingstone, 2002.

Prince of Wales Foundation for Integrated Health. *National Guidelines for the Use of in Supportive and Palliative Care*. London: Prince of Wales Foundation; 2003.

Sackett D. Evidence based medicine: what it is and what it isn't. *British Medical Journal*-1996; **312**(7): 419–426.

Schuster J. Holistic care: healing a sick system. *Nursing Management* 1997; **28**(6): 56–59.

Shortall S, Anderson D, Erikson K, Mitchell J. *Remaking Health Care in America*. San Francisco: Jossey Bass, 1996.

Sless D, Wiseman R. *Writing About Medicines for People*. Canberra: Communication Research Institute of Australia, 1997.

Snyderman R, Weil A. Integrative medicine: bringing medicine back to its roots. *Archives of Internal Medicine* 2002; **162**(395): 360–376.

Sunderland Teaching Primary Care Trust Complementary therapies. www.sunderland.nhs.uk (accessed March 2005).

Wafer M. Finding the formula to enhance care: guidelines for the use of complementary therapies in nursing. *Professional Nurse* 1994; **9**(6): 414–417.

Watson K. Safety guidelines for Chinese herbal dispensing. *Journal of the Australian Traditional-Medicine Society* 2004; **10**(3): 101–104.

Whittenmore R. Analysis of integration in nursing science and practice. *Journal of Nursing Scholarship* 2005; **3** 261–267.

Woods K. Standard practice. *Medical Observer* 2005; 13 May: 27–28.

World Health Organization (WHO). *Traditional Medicine Strategy 2002–2005*. Geneva: WHO, 2002.

Case Cited

Rogers v Whitaker, 1992. 75 CLR 479 at 489 per Mason C, Brenman, Dawson & Toohey & McHugh J.

5 Nutritional Therapies

Rocco Di Vincenzo

5.1 Introduction

Nutrition is a very important aspect of managing diabetes. Malnutrition and under nutrition contribute to a number of health-related issues, for example, in older people malnutrition is associated with weight loss, loss of muscle mass, abnormal gait and weakness, and contributes to falls; and falls increase the risk of admission to hospital and death. The International Diabetes Federation and International Obesity Task Force (2006) recommend taking action against the 'obesogenic environment', encouraging physical activity, advocating healthy diets by controlling access to energy-dense foods and drink.

This chapter explores a variety of complementary nutritional medicine (NM) approaches and provides an overview of some commonly used complementary diets: Zone, Atkins/ketogenic, Metabolic Typing and ABO Blood group diets, and discusses the controversial hypoglycaemia-type 2 diabetes link. In addition, the potential role of nutritional supplementation with vitamins, minerals and herbs to optimise health outcomes of people with type 2 diabetes and their risks and benefits are described.

5.2 Nutritional Medicine (NM)

Nutritional medicine (NM) is defined as using diet and nutrient supplements to prevent and manage ill health and disease (University of Surrey 2006). Inadequate diet is a risk factor for illness and diseases such as diabetes, especially type 2 diabetes, and coronary heart disease (Hooper *et al.* 2001; Bazzano *et al.* 2005). NM attributes a greater impact to nutrition in the cause and treatment of a wider range of illnesses and diseases than conventional medicine. Unlike conventional medicine, NM considers reactive hypoglycemia to be a prediabetic condition (Pizzorno and Murray 1998).

Nutritional medicine also considers chromium deficiency could contribute to the development of diabetes. Chromium is a cofactor in all insulin-regulating activities and plays a critical role in glucose tolerance and has been described as the 'glucose-tolerance factor'. Chromium supplementation significantly improves insulin action and insulin sensitivity, reduces fasting glucose, cholesterol and triglyceride levels; and increases high density lipoprotein (HDL), the 'good cholesterol' (Pizzorno and Murray 1998).

Aims of nutritional medicine

The broad aims of NM for people with diabetes are similar to those of conventional nutritional approaches:

1. Identify the presence and extent of specific nutrient deficiencies by undertaking a detailed nutrition history, thoroughly evaluate the digestive capacity including the capacity to absorb and assimilate nutrients, and the functioning of cellular metabolism.
2. Maintain adequate nutrition to achieve optimal growth and development appropriate to age and developmental stage, achieve optimal metabolic functioning, support immune system function, and reduce systematic toxicity to maintain health and sustain life.
3. Improve glucose tolerance to achieve optimal blood glucose, lipids and blood pressure control, see Chapter 1 for metabolic targets.
4. Prevent and manage, where needed, the chronic complications of diabetes including obesity, dyslipidaemia, hypertension, cardiovascular disease and nephropathy.

5.3 Nutritional Medicine Assessment Approaches

Blood and urine tests provide biochemical information about specific nutrient deficiencies, e.g., urine organic acid profile (Young 2004), which is a non-invasive urine test that can help determine whether nutrients are being appropriately absorbed and detects any key nutritional or metabolic deficiencies. It helps practitioners formulate treatment plans for a variety of disorders including diabetes and cardiovascular disease, decide whether supplements are required, and monitor the effectiveness of nutritional interventions.

The urine organic acid profile shows:

- vitamin, mineral and amino acid deficiencies such as carnitine and n-acetyl cysteine. It is the best currently available functional marker of Vitamin B-complex deficiency. It goes some way towards addressing the criticism that NM recommends unnecessary supplementation that produces expensive urine.
- oxidative damage and antioxidant sufficiency markers;
- detoxification sufficiency;
- neurotransmitter metabolites, which can be used to assess central nervous system function;
- methylation sufficiency status;
- lipoeic acid and CoQ 10 sufficiency markers;
- specific dysbiosis marker for bacterial and yeast overgrowth (Bradley and Lord 2004).

Other tests include nail, hair and stool analysis, liver function tests and body composition tests to detect any patterns of symptoms, e.g., calf cramps at night, headaches and a diet deficient in green vegetables such as broccoli and spinach may indicate magnesium deficiency.

Nutritional medicine management strategies

NM treatment consists of a combination of diet and supplementation to achieve the broad aims already outlined by reducing or removing nutrients or foods that cause the illness or disease and/or to increase the nutrients that are deficient. Supplementation is used to correct nutrient deficiencies by complementing and enhancing dietary intake. Even if dietary changes are not required and dietary intake is adequate, supplements are usually recommended.

Supplement types and doses depend on a number of factors including the extent and type of the particular deficiencies present and Recommended Daily Intakes (RDIs) and may be adjusted as dietary changes are implemented. Inadequate diets may require higher doses to achieve a quicker improvement. Once improvement has been achieved, a maintenance supplementation programme is usually recommended. Supplements are discussed in detail later in the chapter.

Hypoglycaemia as a cause of type 2 diabetes

Modern diets are high in refined carbohydrates, saturated and trans fat, animal products, and are low in dietary fibre, which are important contributing factors to type 2 diabetes, obesity, and hypoglycaemia. Insulin is secreted in response to a carbohydrate load as part of the haemostatic mechanisms that maintain blood glucose in the normal range. Often excess amounts of insulin are secreted. Symptoms such as dizziness, headache and irritability can occur as the adrenal glands secrete adrenaline, also part of the normal glucose homeostasis that protects against hypoglycaemia by liberating glucose stores from the liver and muscle.

According to Pizzorno and Murray (1998), if the adrenal glands are repeatedly stressed, they become exhausted and ultimately cannot mount an appropriate response, which contributes to reactive hypoglycaemia. Further stress on the blood glucose homeostatic mechanisms induces insulin resistance and the beta cells become exhausted and insulin production falls, resulting in impaired glucose tolerance and/or type 2 diabetes. Complementary nutritionists may diagnose reactive hypoglycaemia by requesting a five-hour oral glucose tolerance test where serum insulin and glucose are measured half-hourly (Murray and Lyon 2004). This diagnostic method is different from conventional medicine where mixed meal and exercise challenge tests are more likely to be used to provoke hypoglycaemia and insulin and glucose are measured regularly and especially if symptoms occur.

Many experts consider reactive hypoglycemia to be a prediabetic condition. (Barr *et al.* 2002).

Complementary dietary approaches to managing diabetes

There is an ever-increasing amount of information about the complex hormonal effects of diets high in refined carbohydrate on such parameters as blood lipids, glucose, blood pressure, immune response, and inflammation (Cox *et al.* 2001). Managing the macronutrient content of food, carbohydrate, protein and fat is essential to limiting the adverse effects of diet. Other strategies include Zone, Ketogenic diet, Metabolic typing and ABO Blood Type diets.

Complementary therapists use many of the same strategies as conventional practitioners, for example Glycemic Index™.

Glycemic Index™ is well described in many conventional texts and will not be discussed in this chapter, see Jenkins *et al.* 1981; Brand Miller *et al.* 1998; Wolever *et al.* 1991; Opperman *et al.* 2004.

5.4   The Zone Diet

The Zone diet has increased in popularity since it was first introduced in 1995. The Zone diet is essentially a low carbohydrate diet and is based on the rationale that carbohydrates are the cause of many chronic diseases (Sears 1995) although some recent adaptations are quite sophisticated. Major proponents of the Zone diet are celebrities, which no doubt contributes to its popularity with the general public.

The Zone diet addresses hyperinsulinaemia and is essentially a strategy to keep the insulin level in the normal zone or range. Sears (1995) suggested excess insulin creates and sustains obesity and the underlying reason for increasing global obesity is the consumption of too many grains and starches where potatoes, rice, breads and breakfast cereals are all unfavourable carbohydrates because they elevate insulin levels and are stored as fat. He suggested staying slim depends on managing carbohydrate intake. The Zone diet is one of several low carbohydrate eating regimes that, according to Sears, is safe, effective and certainly no trendy, fly-by-night fad. However, any caloric intake in excess of energy expenditure regardless of the source (carbohydrate, protein, or fat) can be stored as fat.

The Zone diet consists of 40 per cent carbohydrate, 30 per cent protein and 30 per cent fat combined in an eating plan where grains and starches are used sparingly. A precise 0.75 protein-to-carbohydrate ratio is promoted for each meal to reduce the insulin-to-glucagon ratio, which purportedly affects eicosanoid metabolism and ultimately produces a cascade of biological events leading to a reduction in chronic disease risk, enhanced immunity, maximal physical and mental performance, increased longevity and permanent weight loss.

The Zone diet recommends eating in accordance with the following 'zones' or proportions: 40 per cent of kilojoules should come from carbohydrate, 30 per cent from protein and 30 per cent from fat, which includes more omega-3 fatty acids/fish oils. Some researchers claim hunter-gatherers ate this way for 100,000 years (Lambert 2004). The Zone diet is usually accompanied by an exercise regimen.

By and large, these recommendations are quite sound but some people find it impractical to adhere to the recommended proportions. While it is good advice to change the proportion of fats in the diet to reduce saturated fats from dairy and meat sources, eat more monounsaturated and polyunsaturated fats from vegetables and, in the case of the omega-3 oils, from fish, it is difficult to fulfil these recommendations using the 40–30–30 Zone diet.

Likewise it is difficult to exercise when the calorie intake is restricted to 1,300 (about 6000 kilojoules) for women and 1,700 (about 9,000 kilojoules) for men. Most people need twice the number of calories the Zone diet recommends to be able to exercise successfully.

The essence of the Zone diet is that refined carbohydrates found in white pasta, rice, bread need to be reduced and good fats such as those found in nuts, seeds, avocado, hummus and fish need to be increased to maintain insulin levels in the appropriate zone. Once this is achieved, hunger is satisfied for the next four to six hours. Anecdotal evidence suggests that people who follow the basic principles of the diet report sustained energy throughout the day and fewer unacceptable highs and lows in blood glucose that are often associated with high carbohydrate diets, and less hunger. Sears (1995) stated:

> You don't have to avoid these carbohydrates completely . . . Treat them like condiments, not as a primary source of your meal. Eat significant amounts of fruits and vegetables at the same time. Balance off with an adequate amount of protein, and you have the guidelines for lifelong weight control. These are all the rules you need to control insulin.

Potential consequences of the Zone diet are:
- People lose weight but it may not be entirely due to the proportion of carbohydrates, proteins and fats because calorie restriction appears to be a component of the plan.
- It may be difficult to adhere to the recommended 40–30–30 major nutrient proportions and some people find it complicated to follow, which can make the diet unsustainable and become yet another fad diet for the individual concerned.
- Due to the caloric restrictions the ability to exercise to the extent needed to promote healthy weight and fat loss may be difficult.
- The social aspects of eating such as going to restaurants or to dinner parties with friends may be difficult if the individual chooses to strictly adhere to the food zones.
- B group vitamin, calcium, magnesium, potassium, and zinc deficiencies can occur if the Zone diet is followed in the long term. Some of these nutrients are often deficient in people with diabetes and the Zone diet may exacerbate existing deficiencies.

There is limited evidence to support Sears' theory of the relationship between diet, endocrinology and eicosanoid metabolism and health outcomes. Some research supports the contention that compensatory hyperinsulinaemia stemming from peripheral insulin resistance is the metabolic disturbance responsible for the cluster of conditions known as the metabolic: hypertension, type 2 diabetes, dyslipidemia, coronary artery disease, obesity, and abnormal glucose tolerance (Cosford 1999; Kelly 2000; Hanson *et al.* 2002; Golden *et al.* 2002; Cordain *et al.* 2003).

The biological plausibility of any diet and health relationship is crucial when deciding whether or not it is worthy of assessment (National Academy of Sciences National Research Council Food and Nutrition Board 1989). While Sears has made a plausible case for a biological link between hyperinsulinaemia and chronic disease, he has not established his broader health claims for the Zone diet in any cross sectional or longitudinal studies. Organisations such as the National Health and Medical Research Council and Diabetes Australia have not officially condemned the Zone diet, but they are not comfortable with the unsubstantiated claims being made. The benefits and risks of the Zone diet for people with diabetes are largely unknown.

5.5 Total Wellbeing Diet

The recently launched Commonwealth Scientific and Industrial Research Organisation (CSIRO) Total Wellbeing diet in Australia, like the Zone diet, is based on increasing protein intake and reducing carbohydrates, although not to the same extent as the Zone diet. The CSIRO recommends at least four servings of red meat per week. Controlled portions of carbohydrates and fresh fruit and vegetables are also permitted. The CSIRO nutritionists claim the diet is a 'scientifically tested and nutritionally balanced plan' that aids weight loss by restricting glucose and therefore reducing hunger (http://www.nutraingredients.com).

The Total Wellbeing diet was based on eight years of research into heart disease and the results of two specific 12-week studies involving 120 obese women who followed the CSIRO diet. Half were placed on a high protein low fat diet; the remainder consumed a high carbohydrate low fat diet. The results indicate that women with high triglycerides lost 25 per cent more weight on the high protein diet than women on the high carbohydrate diet. Much of this extra weight was lost from the abdominal area, indicating improved metabolic health (Noakes *et al.* 2005).

The CSIRO Total Wellbeing Diet caused controversy because it was promoted as being beneficial for everyone when it was only tested on a subpopulation of overweight women with symptoms of metabolic dysfunction. One can assume, however, that it would benefit people with similar issues such as obesity, insulin resistance, diabetes and cardiovascular disease. Sears (1995) indicated the Australian CSIRO indirectly supported his theory when it put its name to a diet plan similar to the Zone diet.

5.6 Ketogenic or Atkins Diet

The ketogenic diet was developed in the 1920s when Atkins noticed an association between fasting and seizure control in people with epilepsy. The ketogenic approach to managing epilepsy was abandoned when effective pharmacological interventions were introduced. The ketogenic diet ultimately resurfaced and was popularised by Atkins for weight loss in the 1970s. The basis of the ketogenic diet is controlling carbohydrates. It relies on finding each individual's tolerance level for carbohydrates that impact blood glucose levels, promoting weight loss and maintaining a healthy weight for life, see Figure 5.1. This involves:

- avoiding processed foods full of sugar and white flour and restricting other high carbohydrate foods;
- eating a wide variety of delicious foods, including protein, 'healthy' fats and nutrient-dense carbohydrates;
- retaining 'good' carbohydrates full of nutrients found in dark green leafy vegetables, nuts and berries.

Ketogenic diets promote weight loss by restricting carbohydrate intake while maintaining or increasing protein and fat intake. It does not mean totally avoiding carbohydrates and only eating steak, bacon and eggs, or eliminating fruit and vegetables. When carbohydrate is restricted, the body depends on fat catabolism for energy production. Glucose becomes less readily available, which slows the Krebs cycle. Body fat becomes the source of fuel and ultimately results in accumulation of acetyl-CoA, the end product of fat metabolism, which is converted to ketone bodies.

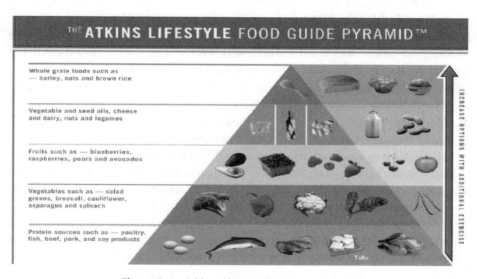

Figure 5.1 Atkins Lifestyle Food Pyramid Guide

Source: Colette Heimowitz, M.Sc. VP, Education, Research Atkins Health and Medical Information Services

The generation of glucose from amino acids (gluconeogenesis) and glycogen breakdown may occur to compensate for reduced carbohydrate in the diet. In the long term, fat synthesis is reduced, secondary to reduced insulin production. According to Atkins, genetics, and the quality and quantity of the carbohydrate consumed determine the individual's insulin response to carbohydrate. Excessive insulin production reduces fat catabolism and increases fat deposition. Other lifestyle factors such as limited physical activity and stress might contribute to development of obesity and insulin resistance, further enhancing the hyperinsulinaemic response to dietary carbohydrate.

Atkins hypothesised in his original book that obese people with insulin resistance are most likely to benefit from the ketogenic diet. It follows that people at high risk for or diagnosed with certain chronic illnesses, including cardiovascular disease, diabetes and hypertension could expect improved clinical parameters if they were encouraged to follow the ketogenic diet.

Four principles of the ketogenic diet

1. *Weight loss*: Both carbohydrate and fat provide fuel for energy. Carbohydrate is the first fuel to be metabolised. When carbohydrates are available they are transformed into energy before other nutrients. Excess carbohydrates are stored as fat. However, when the intake of digestible carbohydrate is sufficiently restricted without caloric restriction, the body converts from the primary metabolic pathway of burning carbohydrate to burning fat as its main energy source, which results in weight loss. Risk factors for heart disease improve when individuals follow a carbohydrate controlled eating plan. For example triglyceride levels reduce by an average of 44 per cent (Abbasi *et al.* 2000).
2. *Weight maintenance*: Each individual has a tightly regulated carbohydrate threshold below which fat burning and weight loss occur. However, if the carbohydrate intake exceeds this threshold, carbohydrate burning predominates, fat accumulates and weight gain occurs. Therefore, each individual has a level of carbohydrate intake at which weight is maintained.
3. *Good health and well-being*: By adhering to a controlled carbohydrate nutritional approach. An individual who chooses to eat nutrient-dense foods including adequate fibre, healthy fats and supplementation as needed is more likely to meet their nutritional needs and maintain good health than they would by following a calorie-restricted, low fat diet. Exercise is also essential to weight control, enhancing energy and maintaining a sense of well-being.
4. *Disease prevention*: By following an individualised controlled carbohydrate nutritional approach that lowers carbohydrate intake resulting in lower insulin production, people at high risk for or diagnosed with certain chronic illnesses, including cardiovascular disease, diabetes and hypertension, can improve their clinical parameters.

These nutritional principles form the core of the four phases of the ketogenic diet:

1. Induction; 2. Ongoing weight loss; 3. Pre-maintenance; and 4. Lifetime maintenance.

Phase 1: Induction

- Limit carbohydrate consumption to 20 g of total carbohydrates per day for a minimum of two weeks. People who need to lose a significant amount of weight can remain in the induction phase longer.
- Satisfy appetite with foods that combine protein and fat, such as fish, poultry, eggs, lamb, pork and beef.
- Consume a balance of healthy natural fats such as monounsaturated, polyunsaturated, and saturated fats. Avoid trans fats from hydrogenated or partially hydrogenated oils.
- Consume carbohydrates in the form of nutrient-dense foods such as leafy green vegetables.
- Drink at least eight 250 ml glasses of water per day.
- Exercise regularly.
- Take nutritional supplements.

Phase 2: Ongoing weight loss

- Slow weight loss commenced in the induction phase by gradually increasing the daily total carbohydrate intake in weekly increments of 5 g. Proceed from 20 g/day of total carbohydrates one week to 25 g/day the next week.
- Increase carbohydrates by five each week until weight loss stops. Choose additional carbohydrates wisely and add nutrient dense foods back into the diet.
- Consume more non-starchy vegetables, such as asparagus and broccoli, berries, e.g. raspberries and strawberries, nuts and seeds, e.g. hazel nuts, almonds, and soft cheeses, e.g. cottage cheese, Stilton, and brie. Once weight loss stops, reduce the daily intake of total carbohydrates by 5 g to continue losing weight slowly. Average 40–60 g of total carbohydrates in this phase. Phase 2 lasts until the individual is within 2–4 kg of their goal weight.

Phase 3: Pre-maintenance

The goal weight is in sight and the individual is 2–4 kg from their goal weight. The last kilos are lost very slowly to ease the individual into a permanently changed way of eating. Each week more grams of total carbohydrates (as much as 10) are added to the daily allowance. As long as weight loss continues, foods such as lentils, melon, starchy vegetables (turnips and carrots) and whole grains can be added. When the goal weight is achieved and maintained for at least a month, the individual has achieved their Atkins Carbohydrate Equilibrium (ACE).

Phase 4: Lifetime maintenance

The aim of Phase 4 is for the individual to maintain their goal weight and ACE. The average grams of total carbohydrates consumed in Phase 4 is 40–120 per day depending on metabolism, age, gender, activity level and or other relevant factors. Regular exercise is encouraged. People who exercise usually have a higher ACE. Changes in activity level, hormonal status or other factors can change the ACE.

Atkins provided specific tips for success in following the four phase plan and especially the maintenance phase. People should do the following:

- Eat at least three meals a day; skipping meals can impede weight loss.
- Not go more than six waking hours without a meal or snack.
- Eat until they are satisfied, but not bloated.
- Drink plenty of water, at least eight 250ml glasses each day.
- Look for hidden carbohydrates in prepared foods.
- Avoid excessive amounts of caffeine, which he suggested can cause hypoglycaemia and promote cravings for sweets.
- Look for reductions in clothing sizes and not rely entirely on the scales.
- Take nutritional supplements.

The carbohydrate ladder

As the ketogenic eating plan progresses through the four phases, carbohydrate foods are reintroduced in the following order:

- salads and leafy vegetables
- hard and soft cheese
- seeds and nuts
- soft fruits such as berries
- beans and pulses
- other fruits such as melon and pineapple
- higher carbohydrate vegetables
- whole grains.

The benefits and risks of the ketogenic diet are shown in Table 5.1. Direct evidence linking the ketogenic dietary approach to improved health outcomes for individuals with or at risk of cardiovascular disease and type 2 diabetes is limited. The relative benefits of high carbohydrate diets compared to low carbohydrate, high protein diets have been discussed and overall appear to support the ketogenic approach. Weight loss is similar in subjects consuming high and low carbohydrate diets, but fasting insulin, the insulin/glucose ratio and triglycerides are lower in subjects on low carbohydrate, high-protein diets (Golay *et al.* 1996) but the ketogenic and Zone diets may not be any more effective than conventional hypocaloric diet with respect to total weight, fat, or lean body mass loss (Landers *et al.* 2002).

Effects of high protein diets on renal function

Changes in renal function including increased kidney size and glomerular filtration rate in people consuming high protein diets have been observed and the opposite in those on high carbohydrate diets. The renal excretion rate and blood pressure do not appear to be affected (Poortmans & Dellalieux 2000; Skov *et al.* 1999).

Table 5.1 Potential risks and benefits of the ketogenic diet.

Benefits	Risks
• Weight loss is achieved • Potential for weight maintenance • Improved health indicators e.g. triglycerides, cholesterol HDL and LDL • Patients have an easy yardstick, providing feedback using Ketostix urine tests. • The high protein content may improve satiety and diet adherence. • Reduced loss of lean body mass. • Probably most useful in obese patients with insulin resistance and pre diabetes. • Better mood regulation. • Increased energy levels. • Increased concentration and alertness. • Increased ability to cope with stress. • Reduced gastrointestinal symptoms. • More energy. • Less preoccupation with food and the need to snack • Les need for caffeine • Less reliance on medicines for some individuals.	• The ketogenic diet is potentially unbalanced and deficient in basic nutrition (yet unproven). • Mostly water weight is lost. Research has consistently demonstrated that weight loss after the first few days on a restricted carbohydrate programme is primarily fat and not water or lean body mass (Young et al. 1971; Sondike et al. 2003). • The ketogenic diet is only effective because calories are restricted. • Adverse effects on the kidneys. • Fat intake is detrimental and will lead to heart disease ketosis is dangerous and causes a variety of medical problems. • Fibre may be lacking in the diet • The ketogenic diet increases the risk of osteoporosis. • Potential for loss of lean body mass. • The ketogenic diet will cause weakness, fatigue and a lack of energy. • Patients do not learn good dietary practices until some weeks after the introduction of ketosis. • Supplementation will be required • Reduced glycogen stores due to less carbohydrate.

The proportions of carbohydrate and protein in the high protein diet were similar to the Zone diet, which are less extreme than the Atkins (ketogenic) diet (Skov et al. 1999). Other researchers have demonstrated an elevated renal acid load and urinary calcium excretion in subjects on high protein, low carbohydrate diets and suggested they could increase the risk of renal calculi and osteoporosis (Reddy et al. 2002).

However, there is little long-term information about the health effects of high protein diets. From the available data it is evident that consuming protein in quantities greater than two to three times the Recommended Daily Allowance (RDI) contributes to urinary calcium loss and may predispose the individual to bone loss in the long term. Therefore, caution using these diets is recommended especially in individuals with a predisposition to nephrolithiasis or kidney disease, and particularly in those with diabetes (Eisenstein et al. 2002).

On the positive side, a small study compared a high protein diet with a high carbohydrate and demonstrated greater weight loss in the high protein diet group. Total cholesterol, triglycerides and LDL cholesterol reduced to a similar extent in both groups (Baba et al. 1999). A more detailed study also published in 1999 revealed greater total weight and fat loss in individuals consuming an *ad libitum* fat reduced, low carbohydrate, high protein diet compared to individuals on a fat-reduced, high carbohydrate diet. Total and HDL cholesterol fell in both diet groups, while triglyceride levels decreased in the high protein diet group but increased in the high carbohydrate diet group. In addition, a two-fold greater intra-abdominal fat loss occurred in the high protein diet group. Total energy intake was lower in the high protein diet group and was attributed to the satiating effects of protein. The researchers suggested low carbohydrate, high protein calorie-controlled diets could be an effective weight-reducing regimen in obese hyperinsulinemic subjects (Baba *et al.* 1999).

Adolescents who followed a low carbohydrate diet lost more weight than those who followed a low fat diet. The low carbohydrate group was able to lose more weight even while consuming more calories – an average of 730kcal more per day than those following the low fat diet (Sondike *et al.* 2003). Similar findings occur in adults (Greene *et al.* 2003). Thus, weight loss is more complex than balancing calories in with calories out. The thermogenic effect of food must be considered and is possibly what the higher protein approach achieves.

Does the ketogenic diet increase risk of cardiovascular disease?

Sharman *et al.* (2002) indicated subjects with a predominance of small LDL particles pattern B demonstrated significantly increased mean and peak LDL particle diameter and more LDL-1 after consuming a ketogenic diet. Sharman *et al.* state: 'The results suggest that a short-term ketogenic diet does not have a deleterious effect on CVD risk profile and may improve the lipid disorders characteristic of atherogenic dyslipidemia.'

Australian research also demonstrates weight loss and improved cardiovascular risk profile (Brinkworth *et al.* 2004); low carbohydrate diets (fewer than 60 g of carbohydrates) are more effective than low fat, calorie-controlled diets in a six-month period and reduce triglycerides without increasing LDL (Noakes and Clifton 2004).

In another study evaluating the effect of a high protein, high monounsaturated fat weight loss diet on glycaemic control and lipid levels in type 2 diabetes, Sondike *et al.* (2003) found both dietary patterns resulted in improvements in the cardiovascular disease (CVD) risk profile as a consequence of weight loss. However, the greater reductions in total and abdominal fat mass in women and greater LDL cholesterol reduction observed in both sexes on the high protein diet suggest that it is a valid diet choice for reducing CVD risk in type 2 diabetes (Parker *et al.* 2002). The low carbohydrate diet appears to be an effective method for short-term weight loss in overweight adolescents and does not harm the lipid profile (Sondike *et al.* 2003).

Dansinger *et al.* (2005) compared the ketogenic, Ornish, Weight Watchers and Zone diets and found each diet modestly reduced body weight and several cardiac risk factors at one year. All diets showed significant reductions in the Framingham

Risk Score (FRS) a measure of 10-year heart disease risk. The four diets promoted weight loss especially in adherent subjects indicating that various strategies can be effective. However, dietary adherence rates to all diets are low. This is important because increased adherence is associated with greater weight loss and reductions in cardiac risk factors with all diets.

The practicalities of the ketogenic diet

Manufacturers recommend a carbohydrate-protein-fat ratio of 20–50–30 for people commencing a ketogenic diet. Although this ratio is not as restrictive as Phase 1 of the Atkins Diet rigorous monitoring and control of ketone levels are essential, especially in type 1 diabetes because of the risk of ketoacidosis. Moderate ketosis may induce insulin secretion in type 2 diabetes secondary to gluconeogenesis from amino acids and fatty acids and might limit fat mobilisation.

Nutrient supplementation is often recommended, particularly antioxidants, magnesium and potassium because Phase 1 of the Atkins Diet is particularly restrictive and eliminates many of the foods that supply ample quantities of these nutrients such as fruit and starchy vegetables. People require pre-diet assessment and regular monitoring of body composition, blood lipids, glucose, and ketones, insulin and serum urate. Ideally, renal urate, oxalate, calcium and magnesium excretion should be assessed pre-diet and monitored throughout the diet period.

Concerns about the ketogenic diet

Effect of the ketogenic diet on renal function

There is no definitive evidence that the protein content of ketogenic diets causes any form of kidney damage but there is some theoretical conjecture. Ornish (2004) stated: 'High total protein intake . . . may accelerate renal function decline.' Likewise, the American Heart Association Nutrition Committee stated: 'Individuals who follow these [high-protein] diets are risk for . . . potential cardiac, renal, bone, and liver abnormalities overall.' (St Jeor *et al*. 2001).

In contrast, Walser (1999) indicated:

> [P]rotein restriction does not prevent decline in renal function with age, and, in fact is the major cause of that decline. A better way to prevent the decline would be to increase protein intake . . . . There is no reason to restrict protein in healthy individuals to protect the kidney

Relative to renal function, healthy kidneys are not damaged by the increased demands of protein consumed in quantities 2–3 times above the RDA. In addition, recent studies suggest, at least in the short term, that the RDA for protein (0.8 gms/kg) does not support normal calcium homeostasis (Kerstetter *et al*. 2000; Manninen 2004). Likewise, there is a positive association between protein intake and bone mineral density (Rapuri *et al.* 2003). Longer and larger studies are required to determine the long-term safety and efficacy of low carbohydrate, high protein, and high fat diets. In the meantime, individuals with normal renal function are at minimal risk of kidney damage or osteoporosis from high protein diets. Individual risks must be assessed and balanced against the real and established risk of obesity (Manninen 2004).

A growing body of evidence demonstrates that a controlled carbohydrate eating plan, if followed correctly, reduces risk factors for heart disease and improves clinical health markers. The body needs fats to survive and fats provide many health benefits. Natural fats increase satiety sooner and keep dieters feeling less hungry for longer. Low carbohydrate diets, in contrast to low fat diets, followed correctly can be more effective than a low fat plan in improving risk factors for heart disease. There is 'A wide body of evidence [that] links the consumption of animal protein protein . . . CVD, cancer, and other chronic clinical illnesses' (Ornish 2004). However, the results are inconsistent. Other research indicates a high intake of protein from animal and vegetables lowers the risk of ischemic heart disease in women and replacing carbohydrates with protein may actually reduce the risk of ischemic heart disease (Hu *et al.* 1999).

Is ketosis dangerous?

The primary fuel in the body is glucose, generated from carbohydrate consumption. When sufficient carbohydrates are not available the body turns to its secondary fuel source – fat. Lipolysis produces ketones (ketosis). Ketosis should not be confused with the abnormal metabolic state ketoacidosis. Ketoacidosis is primarily a concern in insulin-deficient states such as diabetics with hyperglycaemia and alcoholics.

Does the ketogenic diet increase the risk of osteoporosis?

Weight loss due to water loss occurs during the first week of any weight loss programme. Calcium, potassium and magnesium loss accompanies water loss, which is why multivitamin supplementation is important. At this stage calcium is not being leached from the bones. Urinary calcium loss occurs for a few days after which the body adjusts and the calcium urine excretion ceases. No significant changes in calcium balance or intestinal absorption of calcium on high meat diets have been demonstrated in adults in the short or longer term (Spender *et al.* 1983).

However, Ornish (2004) suggested: 'High protein diets may cause loss of calcium and decreased levels of urinary citrate leading to osteoporosis.' Ornish's claim is not supported by other researchers, for example, older people with lower protein intake have increased bone loss compared to those with higher intakes of protein (Hannan *et al.* 2000). Likewise, Dawson-Hughes *et al.* (2004) showed protein supplementation and reductions in carbohydrate intake did not increase urine calcium excretion but did increase IGF-I, a bone growth factor.

Potential loss of lean body mass

Typically, individuals on very low calorie diets can lose muscle mass because they have inadequate intake of protein. The Atkins diet does not restrict calories and the high protein intake offsets any possible loss of lean body mass.

The person becomes weak, fatigued and lacks energy

During the 3–4 days on the Atkins diet people may experience mild fatigue as the body switches metabolic pathways from glucose metabolism to fat metabolism. Reducing caffeine and sugar intake can lead to short-term withdrawal symptoms, which typically resolve within the first week. After the transition, individuals consistently report high energy levels.

A further criticism is that people do not learn good dietary practices until some weeks after the introduction of ketosis, which is not the case with recent versions of the diet. In addition, there are concerns that glycogen stores may be depleted due to the low carbohydrate intake, which could affect response to hypoglycaemia. However, this has not been conclusively demonstrated.

5.7 Metabolic Typing and ABO Blood Type Diets

A useful way to discuss the ABO blood type diet is to compare it with another popular plan, the Eat Right 4 Your Type (D'Adamo 1998). People familiar with the plan often ask whether the Blood Type diet is the same as the Metabolic Typing diet. Wolcott, who developed the Metabolic Typing diet, said blood type is just one of nine different components used in the process of metabolic typing to determine individual nutritional requirements (Wolcott and Fahey 2000). The nine components are:

1. Autonomic Nervous System (ANS), the 'master regulator' of metabolism.
2. Oxidative System or the rate at which nutrients are converted to energy within cells.
3. Catabolic/anabolic and aerobic/anaerobic metabolic states, tissue pH, and selective membrane permeability.
4. Acid/alkaline Balance. There are six different kinds of pH imbalances.
5. Electrolyte stress or insufficiency, which affects blood pressure, circulation, and electric potential.
6. Endocrine type, which determines factors such as the metabolic rate, body type, shape, propensity to gain weight.
7. Constitutional type derived from Ayurveda and Chinese medicine and is concerned with the constitutional qualities of foods relative to the constitutional qualities of individual, see Chapters 10 and 11.
8. Blood type. Food lectins are specific to ABO blood types.
9. Prostaglandin balance, particularly series one, two and three prostaglandin balances. The hypothesis here is that prostaglandin or eicosanoid balance is

essential to inflammation modulation, which in turn may assist to maximise ideal weight control.

The ABO Blood Type diet is concerned with avoiding lectin-containing foods specific to blood type and is discussed in the next section. Wolcott believes the primary energy mechanisms that regulate energy production, maintenance and control such as the ANS, oxidative system and catabolic/anabolic processes, determine the dietary content. These factors are in a constant state of flux, unlike blood type, which is constant.

All foods and nutrients have very specific stimulatory or inhibitory effects on the fundamental homeostatic control systems that regulate every body process at every level of activity, which is the reason nutrition is critical. People have their own unique metabolic type. Proponents of the Metabolic Typing diet believe food and nutrients can have different effects on different metabolic types, exemplified by the old adage, 'one man's meat is another's poison'. Metabolic typing suggests even eating the best organic foods and supplements, and getting plenty of rest and regular exercise may not create health unless the diet suits the individual's metabolic type. Wolcott believes that eating according to individual metabolic type is the only way to ensure food is the medicine God intended it to be, and diets that suit the metabolic type should produce a marked and lasting improvement in mental capacity, emotional well-being, should reduce hunger for several hours, and should maintain energy levels. However, if the individual is still feeling hungry, craving sweets, experiencing a drop in energy level, feeling hyperactive, nervous, angry or irritable or feeling depressed, an hour or so after eating, this might be due to the improper combination of proteins, fats and carbohydrates at the last meal. The diet may be perfect for the person's metabolism, but too much of one type of food in place of another can produce the symptoms listed. This means people can eat high quality nutritious foods and still be unwell (www.healthexcel.com 2000).

Wolcott likens the metabolic typing approach (food is fuel for the body) to selecting petrol for a car. High quality petrol that has been screened carefully to ensure it is free of anything likely to damage the car is more likely to ensure high performance and fuel economy. However, petrol in a diesel-powered engine causes damage, poor performance and is expensive to repair. The fact that the car stopped running does not imply the petrol was poor quality or that the car was defective. It was the wrong type of fuel for the car. Like cars, individual metabolic types require the correct type of fuel in an appropriate blend. According to the metabolic typing theory, the further the diet is from the ideal, the more health problems occur. Wolcott said some of the sickest people he treats were 'designed' to eat high protein foods but are vegetarians. Conversely, carbohydrate metabolic types who eat a high protein diet do have good health.

There are three general metabolic types:

- *Protein types* who do better on low carbohydrate, high protein, and high fat diets. A typical ratio might be 40 per cent protein and 30 per cent each of fats and carbohydrates. However, the proportions depend on individual genetic requirements and might be 50 per cent fats and 10 per cent carbohydrate.

- *Carbohydrate types* who require a high proportion of carbohydrate but the type may vary according to the individual's make-up. Usual requirements are ~60 per cent carbohydrates, 25 per cent protein and 15 per cent fat. However, only 10 per cent fat and 80 per cent carbohydrates in exceptional circumstances. Carbohydrate metabolic types who previously followed a ketogenic diet might improve initially but eventually fail to thrive because they require more carbohydrate. Once a person attains a normal weight and controls insulin-related disorders, they can consume some grains and remain healthy. Carbohydrate types (which account for approximately 15 per cent of the population) actually can do quite well with grains (Wolcott and Fahey 2000).
- *Mixed metabolic types* fall between carbohydrate and protein types and are the most challenging types to manage.

Activity and stress levels affect all metabolic types and affect the quantity of food and the protein/fat/carbohydrate ratio required to achieve and maintain health. Likewise, the circadian rhythm needs to be considered as biochemistry changes throughout the day and influence variables such as hormonal output, pH (acid/alkaline), and waking/sleeping times. Some people need the same proportions of protein, fat and carbohydrates at each meal; others need different proportions at different meals to maintain optimum energy and well-being.

Metabolic typing dietary experts suggest people eat the proportions of proteins, fats and carbohydrates according to their taste and appetite initially. They analyse their reaction to meals to ascertain whether they have selected appropriate right ratios. The ratios should be changed if the response was suboptimal and reactions to the new ratios should be analysed. In this way, the ratio of proteins, fats and carbohydrates can be fine-tuned for each meal.

Wolcott illustrates the importance of ratios and the difference they can make from his own experience. He used to have a salad with some meat for lunch. Several hours later he felt hungry and had strong food cravings. He increased his fat intake to ~40 per cent, and his cravings disappeared. People should not feel hungry an hour after eating. Food cravings may indicate the energy level is low and suggests the individual may not be eating appropriately for their metabolic type.

The Metabolic Typing diet plan is similar to the Zone diet in that it seeks to establish the ideal macronutrient composition for the individual. As yet there are no longitudinal studies that examine the health benefits of the Metabolic Typing diet. It would be very difficult to evaluate because of the number of variables involved. Some critics suggest the Metabolic Typing diet *per se* reveals nothing more than a modern twist on an old food fad.

5.8 ABO Blood Type Diet

Many researchers have reported a relationship between ABO blood group phenotypes and the incidence of certain diseases (Freed 1999). These studies suggest that ABO blood group antigens differentially affect susceptibility to certain diseases and blood group type might suggest the type of diet most likely to optimise health and prevent disease, including diabetes and cardiovascular disease.

- People with blood type A appear to be more prone to heart disease (Whincup *et al.* 1990; Slipko *et al.* 1994).
- People with blood type B are possibly prone to possibly to certain cancers (Su *et al.* 2001).
- People with blood type O may be more susceptible to duodenal peptic ulcer (Shahid *et al.* 1997).

In the 1960s, naturopath James D'Adamo observed that although many patients improved on a low fat/vegetarian diet, others did not respond and sometimes their condition worsened. D'Adamo was familiar with a report prepared by Boyd (1945) that indicated plant-derived lectins could be ABO blood-type specific and that lectins were widely distributed in high nutritional value plants such as cereals, potatoes and beans. D'Adamo (1980) studied patients' ABO blood groups and their response to diet and subsequently published his clinical observations over 20 years in *One Man's Food*. He suggested patients with type A blood reacted adversely to high protein meat diets but improved with vegetable proteins such as soy. He also observed that they produced excess respiratory tract mucus. Dr Peter D'Adamo continued this work and reported some foods are highly beneficial, neutral or undesirable for each blood type and proposed that specific food lectins may enhance biological function and dietary lectin could be manipulated 'to our advantage' according to blood type to prevent illness and treat disease.

The key recommendations for specific blood types are:

- Type 0: Introduce lean red meat 3–4 times per week and eliminate wheat.
- Type A: Replace red meats with fish, chicken and vegetable protein and increase beans and rice.
- Type B: Introduce dairy foods and eliminate chicken.
- Type AB: Increase seafood, tofu, lamb, and turkey and eliminate chicken, corn and most beans.

A number of contemporary studies indicate a variety of disease processes could be initiated, maintained or modulated by cell-surface glycoprotein antigen interactions with endogenous, dietary or microbial lectins. Older studies show many plant-derived lectins are present in food (Nachbar *et al.* 1980), are resistant to cooking and digestive enzymes (Van Damme *et al.* 1998), exert toxic and/or inflammatory reactions (Heneghan *et al.* 1998), and may be absorbed systemically (Wang *et al.* 1998). Plant-derived lectins attach to cell-surface glycoprotein receptors and exert beneficial or detrimental actions on cellular communication, endothelial and mucosal function and immunological activity.

Thus, lectins from plants, microbes and animals (galectins) have been implicated in a wide variety of diseases such as:

- dyspepsia, peptic ulcer, enteritis, bowel flora dysbiosis and 'leaky gut' and coeliac disease (Pustzai *et al.* 1993; Wang *et al.* 1998; Kelly 1998; 1998; Freed *et al.* 1999; Cordain *et al.* 2000);

- autoimmune disease such as rheumatoid arthritis (Cordain *et al.* 2000);
- IgA nephropathy (Coppo *et al.* 1992);
- Graves' disease (D'Adamo and Kelly 2001);
- gastroenteric and systemic infections and response to infection (D'Adamo and Kelly 2001);
- cardiovascular disease, thrombovascular disease (D'Adamo and Kelly 2001);
- insulin resistance and Syndrome X (D'Adamo and Kelly 2001).

The key questions are: to what extent are dietary lectins ABO blood-type specific, and what other factors contribute to lectin-associated disease? D'Adamo suggested ABO blood type grouping offers approximately 90 per cent of the information required to individually tailor people's eating plans (D'Adams and Kelly 2001). However, the individual's blood Lewis antigen status and whether or not they secrete ABH antigen into body fluids, such as mucus, saliva and urine are major confounders (D'Adamo and Kelly 2001).

There is limited evidence for directly adopting the ABO Blood Type diet for people with diabetes or cardiovascular disease. However, it does attempt to individualise diet and nutrient intake according to genetic requirements. In addition, the diet is quite restrictive and needs to be supervised by trained health professionals and tailored to individual needs, to ensure adequate nutrition. Further research could determine whether the ABO Blood Type diet could be a clinically useful way to assess individual physical and biochemical nutrient requirements. The risks and benefits of the ABO Blood Type diet are depicted in Table 5.2 and Table 5.3 outlines some potential clinical guidelines.

Table 5.2 The ABO Blood Type Diet – a risk-benefit approach.

Benefits	Risks
• May offer some simple dietary solutions for people with specific food sensitivities	• Likely to be unnecessarily restrictive and could potentially result in the development of dietary deficiencies
• May be a useful modality adjunct in developing a specific, strategic, goal oriented, individually tailored dietary regimen for people with chronic health problems	• Urgent need for large-scale clinical studies needed to evaluate the efficacy of the Blood Type Diet with regard to a variety of common chronic diseases
• Some significant scientific evidence exists for the link between lectins and biological function	• Difficulty in implementing dietary recommendations in a family consisting of a variety of blood types
• Anecdotal reports of satisfaction in adhering to the blood type diet (90–93 per cent satisfaction) with improvements in digestion, overall sense of energy and well being and weight loss being the most common results reported. (Slipko *et al.* 1994)	• Suspected compliance issues for people living in western environments – requires significant commitment and discipline
	• May offer a false sense of security to those people following it with respect to disease prevention
	• Limited evidence based scientific evidence specifically linking blood type and lectins to biological function

Table 5.3 Clinical Guidelines.

---

1. A modified blood type diet approach is safe and responsible if deemed appropriate between the patient and treating health professional.
2. Individuals without health problems may utilise the diet for preventive purposes and should be advised to consume a varied diet and exercise regularly.
3. Ensure the majority of foods chosen are from the beneficial and neutral lists and not from the 'to avoid' list.
4. From each list, choose predominantly whole foods for their greater nutrient content.
5. Limit refined carbohydrates, hydrogenated/trans fatty acids.
6. Limit time frame to 4–6 weeks to observe health effect. If desired effect is attained, continue with diet, otherwise discontinue and review.
7. Encourage concomitant use of high-quality multivitamin and mineral supplements.
Caution with patients with severe food allergies and for people with blood type O who have kidney disease.

5.9 The USDA Food Guide Pyramid

More than a decade ago, the United States Department of Agriculture (USDA) created a powerful and enduring icon – the Food Guide Pyramid, which illustrates the USDA concept of a healthy diet. The Pyramid was used as a nutrition education tool in schools, appeared in countless media campaigns and nutrition information material, and on countless cereal boxes and food labels. Unfortunately, the information represented in this pyramid has not delivered on its promise to point the way towards evidence-based healthy eating possibly because it was based on old information that does not reflect major advances in understanding the connection between diet and health. The USDA recently replaced the original pyramid with MyPyramid™, a new symbol (the old pyramid turned on its side), and 'interactive food guidance system'. However, there are still flaws in the new system. The USDA Healthy Diet Pyramid is in stark contrast to the Harvard School of Public Health Healthy Diet Pyramid (Figure 5.3) and the Atkins Lifestyle Food Pyramid Guide (Figure 5.1).

MyPyramid

In theory, the USDA pyramid reflects the Dietary Guidelines for Americans that aim to 'provide authoritative advice for people two years and older about how good dietary habits can promote health and reduce risk for major chronic diseases' (USDA 1992). The original pyramid was innovative and successful in conveying a message because the shape suggests some foods are 'good' and should be eaten often, and others are not so good and should only be eaten occasionally. The layers represent major food groups that contribute to the total diet. MyPyramid presents the information in an abstract way and obscures the message, see Figure 5.2.

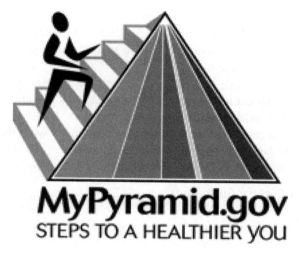

MyPyramid.gov
STEPS TO A HEALTHIER YOU

Figure 5.2 UDSA MyPyramid. Six bands of colour sweep from the apex of MyPyramid to the base: orange for grains, green for vegetables, red for fruits, yellow for oils, blue for milk, and purple for meat and beans. The widths suggest how much food a person should choose from each group. Stairs running up the side of the Pyramid serve as a reminder of the importance of physical activity. It contains no text and was 'designed to be simple'. It encourages consumers to access all the necessary detail they require at MyPyramid.gov.

Harvard School of Public Health Healthy Diet Pyramid

The Harvard School of Public Health developed the Healthy Eating Pyramid as an alternative to the USDA pyramid, see Figure 5.3. The shape resembles the original USDA pyramid but the information more accurately reflect modern research findings. The foundation of the Healthy Eating Pyramid is daily exercise and weight control, which are important considerations when planning diets (Willett 2001). The recommendations suggest including:

- Whole grain foods in most meals to supply energy.
- Plant oils to improve cholesterol levels and supply essential fatty acids.
- Vegetables in abundance and 2–3 pieces of fruit per day to prevent a variety of diseases, reduce insulin resistance, lower blood pressure and cardiovascular risk, and reduce the incidence of macular degeneration, the major cause of vision loss among people over age 65.
- Fish, poultry, and eggs up to twice per day. These are important sources of protein.
- Nuts and legumes 1–3 times per day. Nuts and legumes are excellent sources of protein, fibre, vitamins, and minerals and many types of nuts contain healthy oils.
- Dairy or calcium supplement 1–2 times per day. Calcium, vitamin D, exercise, and a variety of other factors are necessary for bone health.
- Red meat and butter sparingly.

- White rice, white bread, white pasta, potatoes, soft drink and sweets sparingly because they have a high Glycemic Index™and can contribute to a rapid rise in blood glucose levels, which can lead to weight gain, type 2 diabetes, heart disease, and other chronic disorders.
- Multiple vitamins. A daily multivitamin and mineral supplement, but this should not replace healthy eating. Some studies suggest all adults should take vitamin supplements (Fairfield *et al.* 2002).
- Alcohol in moderation. A small amount of alcohol lowers the risk of heart disease but the benefits must be weighed against the risks. For men, a good balance point is 1–2 drinks a day. For women, at most one drink a day.

The New USDA Dietary Guidelines

The new Dietary Guidelines for Americans were released in January, 2005. The new guidelines emphasise the importance of controlling weight and physical activity. The recommendation on dietary fats is a change from considering all fats to be undesirable to emphasising the intake of trans fats should be as low as possible and saturated fat should be limited but no longer require an impractical low fat intake. The potential health benefits of monounsaturated and polyunsaturated

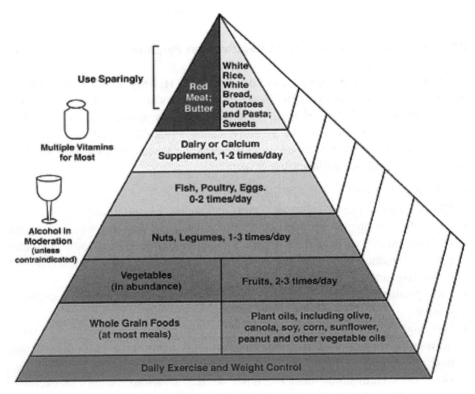

Figure 5.3 Harvard School of Public Health Healthy Diet Pyramid
Source: Willett (2001). © 2001, 2005 by the President and Fellows of Harvard College

fats are recognised. The 2005 Guidelines recommend 20–35 per cent of daily calories should come from fats and high fibre foods. Likewise the new Guidelines recommend limiting sugar and stress the benefits of whole grains instead of emphasising 'complex carbohydrates'.

Proteins in red meat, poultry, and fish, beans and soy proteins are all grouped together and the Guidelines recommend selecting protein foods with a low fat content, which does not take account of the different types of fat present in protein food and overlooks mounting evidence that replacing red meat with a combination of fish, poultry, beans, and nuts offers numerous health benefits. The recommendation to drink three glasses of low fat milk or eat three servings of other dairy products per day to prevent osteoporosis may also be incorrect in light of recent evidence that supports increasing the intake of milk or other dairy products to promote bone mineralisation in children and adolescents (Lanou et al. 2005).

From clinical, observational and anecdotal experience, too much emphasis is placed on reducing fat and protein and treating all carbohydrates as if they are all quickly converted to glucose. Diets in their 'purest' form, Pritikin, Ornish, McDougall, Protein Power, Atkins, The Zone or the Sugar Buster Diets, can all, when followed correctly, eliminate or reduce refined carbohydrates, which the current healthy diet pyramid fails to address. It seems more appropriate to avoid all refined carbohydrates rather than eliminating all carbohydrates.

We seem to have come full circle back to recommendations made by nutritional pioneers 20–30 years ago: eliminate all refined carbohydrates and sugars (processed and not naturally present such as in fruit) because of the potential insulin and nutritional imbalance they can create. The focus should be on eating whole foods (vegetables, fruit, legumes, nuts, grains) whenever possible and following the most basic tenet in CAM, eat unrefined foods as close to possible as their natural state.

5.10 Detoxification Diets

Detoxification is considered to be of paramount importance in complementary medicine and is usually achieved in a liver cleansing programme or more comprehensively a combined bowel and liver detoxification programme. Many naturopaths and integrative medicine practitioners consider the gastrointestinal tract and liver to be primary defence barriers that protect the individual from reactive toxins and infectious organisms. These practitioners believe defective functioning of these organs directly increases the toxic burden, which affects the immune and nervous systems, and produces inflammatory reactions and neurological dysfunction (Alberti et al. 1999).

Many complementary practitioners believe chronic activation of immune and nervous system tissues by the accumulation of toxins could significantly contribute to many of the common chronic degenerative diseases, including diabetes and cardiovascular disease (Baldi et al. 1998). However, there is little direct evidence to support such an assertion. Many complementary practitioners suggest improving and repairing defective gut and liver function may help normalise over-active immune and nervous systems, which could slow and possibly reverse some of the associated degenerative processes (Bland *et al.* 1995; Kilburn *et al.* 1989; Marteau *et al.* 2002; Jenkins *et al.* 2005).

While there is little direct scientific evidence to suggest liver detoxification regimes improve prognostic outcomes for patients with a variety of chronic diseases, there is some evidence that a simple detoxification programme can assist in improving the liver detoxification function, which is consistent with the hypothesis that improved liver detoxification may contribute to well-being.

MacIntosh and Ball (2000) conducted an outcome-focused, non-controlled clinical intervention trial (n = 25). The Metabolic Screening Questionnaire (MSQ) was completed as a subjective assessment of well-being and drug challenge tests (caffeine clearance) were used to assess hepatic detoxification capacity before and after the detoxification programme. There was a statistically significant (47 per cent) reduction in the MSQ scores, which occurred concurrently with a 23 per cent increase in liver detoxification capacity, as reflected by the measure. There was an increase in the urinary sulfate/creatinine ratio after treatment, indicating a trend towards improved liver function.

Some detoxification studies used detoxification programmes for several weeks to months to treat poor health and demonstrated positive results (Kilburn *et al.* 1989; Bland *et al.* 1995; Rea *et al.* 1996) in contrast to MacIntosh and Ball who used a short (seven day) detoxification programme. The MSQ was originally designed as a succinct form of the Cornell Medical Index and concentrated on symptoms that could be related to toxicities (Bland *et al.* 1992) and is a useful measure of multisystem symptomatic level of poor health, regardless of whether a specific diagnosis has been established.

The detoxification programme consisted of consuming a hypoallergenic diet (see Table 5.4), six scoops of a medical food supplement and drinking at least 2 litres of purified water daily. MacIntosh and Ball (2000) demonstrated how a seven-day detoxification programme resulted in a significant reduction in patient symptomatology. The few contemporary clinical studies that have used detoxification to improve poor health have reported successful results (Kilburn *et al.* 1989; Bland *et al.* 1995; Rea *et al.* 1996) and suggest there could be a role for detoxification regimes to improve health and well-being. The more reasonable commercially available detoxification regimes highlight the common adverse effects: headaches, irregular bowel movements, fatigue, skin outbreaks, and flu-like symptoms. No serious adverse events have been documented but people with diabetes would need to consider potential risks such as dehydration and hypoglycaemia.

Most detoxification regimes recommend reasonable diets and advise against their use in pregnancy, breast-feeding and on children younger than 12 years. They also recommend people seek appropriate medical advice before implementing such a regime and to be cautious when undertaking detoxification programmes if they are using medications. This may be particularly important to people with diabetes

Table 5.4 Hypoallergenic diet guidelines.

Ultraclear Program

- For seven days, take 2 scoops Ultraclear mixed in 250ml liquid (e.g. spring or filtered water, or 125ml of water and 125ml of unsweetened juice) 3 times per day.

Foods to eat days 1–3

- No suspected allergens or intolerances, no dairy, no wheat, no concentrated sweets, no caffeine products, no alcohol, no eggs and no oats.
- Any fruits except citrus fruits can be added to Ultraclear or Ultraclear Plus to make a smoothie.
- Any vegetables (best steamed or raw) except potatoes or potatoes.
- Basmati white rice and legumes. Do not eat beans that are difficult to digest; consider peas, lentils and green beans.
- Use nuts and seeds freely – except peanuts.
- Flavourings may include organic butter, olive oil, high-quality sunflower or flaxseed oil for cold uses and herbs and spices except conventional table salt.

Optional foods days 4

- Turkey and fish, other than shellfish, may be added, as well as grains such as buckwheat, millet, amaranth, quinoa and brown rice.

---

on glucose-lowering agents and lipid-lowering agents. It is generally advisable to avoid regimes that are inordinately restrictive.

Given that many detoxification regimes eliminate red meat, dairy products and wheat, they have the potential to cause specific deficiencies such as calcium and iron and it is imperative that fish, legumes and nuts are substituted for the meat, that calcium-fortified soya and rice milks are used to replace dairy foods, and that oats, corn, buckwheat and brown rice are used instead of wheat. Adequate consumption of fruits and vegetables is of paramount importance on detoxification regimens as well as on healthy eating plans.

Adequate calorie, protein and micronutrient intake is important for proper liver functioning and to support detoxification, for example, B group vitamins, magnesium, zinc, vitamin C and glutathione. Supplementation with a good quality probiotic is also recommended (Hawrelak 2005).

The most efficacious detoxification approach considers the presenting symptoms, the particular toxins to which the individual was been exposed, their total toxin burden, and their individual capacity to metabolise and detoxify xenobiotic compounds, which may be largely genetically determined. At present there is limited evidence to support detoxification regimens currently available through health food stores and pharmacies but no serious adverse events have been documented. However, they are best undertaken under the guidance and supervision of a health-care practitioner.

5.11 Nutritional Supplementation

Vitamin deficiency syndromes such as scurvy and beri beri are now uncommon in developed countries, however, suboptimal intake of some vitamins especially antioxidants is common and increases the risk of a number of chronic diseases including cardiovascular disease (Fairfield and Fletcher 2002). Most diets do not contain adequate amounts of vitamins and other micronutrients. Gruner (2005) suggested diet may not be sufficient to correct common nutritional deficiencies and supplementation is required. She suggested the underlying mechanism of NM is based on physiological and biochemical pathways:

> Cells require an optimal level of nutrients to function normally and to fight illness and disease. Chemicals in soil, air and water, as well as stress, mean that we require extra nutrient intake to maintain optimal health, which may not be able to be met by diet alone. Even an organic food-based diet may not be utilised if there is a reduced ability of the gastrointestinal system to absorb nutrients or, if they are absorbed, they may not be efficiently metabolised in the cells.

There is also an extensive and rapidly expanding body of evidence for a wide range of nutrient supplementation in a variety of disease states, including diabetes and cardiovascular disease. For example, herbs such as *Coccinia indica, Panax ginseng, Gymnema sylvestre, Aloe vera, Momordica charantia* and nutrients such as chromium and vanadium improve the blood glucose profile (Yeh *et al.* 2003), see Chapters 9, 10 and 14. There is also increasing evidence for herbal supplements in managing cardiovascular disease especially hawthorn (*Crataegus oxycantha*), garlic (*Allium sativum*), ginger (*Zingiber officinale*), tumeric (*Curcuma longa*), milk thistle (*Silybum marianum*) and nutritional supplements omega 3 fish oils, vitamin E, vitamin C, selenium, coenzyme Q10, and B group vitamins including nicotinic acid (Braun 2004), see Chapter 9. In addition, there is increasing evidence for the role of phytochemicals such as isoflavones, bioflavonoids, carotenoids, glutathione, and alpha lipoic acid in health maintenance. Folic acid supplementation reduces homocysteine, which is linked to cardiovascular disease (Schroecksnadel *et al.* 2004; Yang *et al.* 2005).

Micronutrients

A growing body of evidence demonstrates a link between type 2 diabetes and alterations in the homeostasis of several vitamins, minerals and trace elements such as impaired insulin release, altered insulin action, and glucose intolerance. These states have all been linked to a deficit in the cellular availability of magnesium and minerals and trace elements including chromium zinc, vanadium and selenium in type 2 diabetes.

While there is direct scientific evidence that supplementation with key micronutrients improves blood glucose control in type 2 diabetes (see later), there is little direct evidence that they help prevent, delay or ameliorate many of the associated complications. By association, however, the Diabetes Control and Complications Trial did establish that people with diabetes reduce the likelihood of complications if their blood glucose control is optimised (Turner 1998). This highlights that while there may still be insufficient direct evidence the micronutrients will help prevent, delay or ameliorate many of the associated complications associated with diabetes, there is some research evidence to indicate that a range of micronutrients may be of assistance in optimising blood glucose control in both people with and without diabetes. Definitive conclusions about the efficacy of individual herbs and supplements for diabetes are still to be reached, although they appear to be generally safe.

Some conventional medicines contribute to nutritional deficiencies, especially those that reduce uptake in the gastrointestinal tract or reduce appetite. For example, metformin is associated with reduced uptake of vitamin B12, which can be reversed by calcium supplements (Bauman *et al.* 2000). Medicines that increase gastrointestinal motility and diuretics that increase excretion in the urine also contribute to inadequate micronutrient intake. Only vitamins A, E and B12 are stored in the body, thus a daily intake is essential.

5.12 Vitamins

Vitamin C

Vitamin C plays a major role in the manufacture of collagen, the most abundant protein in the human body. Collagen is an important protein in connective tissue, thus, vitamin C is integral to wound repair, healthy teeth and gums and prevents excessive bruising. People with type 2 diabetes have a relative vitamin C deficiency despite adequate dietary intake, which could be due to inadequate intracellular delivery of vitamin C because vitamin C entry into cells depends on insulin (Cunningham 1991). Chronic vitamin C deficiency in people with type 2 diabetes can lead to a range of problems including increased tendency to bleed, poor wound healing, microvascular disease, increased cholesterol levels, and immunosuppression.

Increased doses of vitamin C have been shown to prevent protein glycosylation and reduce sorbitol accumulation in erythrocytes in type 2 diabetes. Sorbitol accumulation and protein glycosylation are linked to many diabetes complications including eye and nerve diseases. There is some evidence that vitamin C is superior to the Aldose Reductase Inhibitor class of medicines at the reducing sorbitol accumulation in erythrocytes of people with type 2 diabetes at doses as low as 100mg per day (Cunningham *et al.* 1994).

Even though lower levels of vitamin C supplementation can achieve normal erythrocyte sorbitol levels, 2000 mg of vitamin C per day is recommended for its other important effects. While vitamin C supplementation is necessary to achieve this level of intake, patients need to be reminded not to rely exclusively on supplementation but more importantly to integrate dietary measures to maximise vitamin C consumption.

'Nutriceutic' vitamin C and E supplementation (supplementation ~2–10 times the RDI for which a benefit is linked to a mechanism of action) shows some benefits in small trials and is safe and affordable from food or tablet sources. Cunningham (1998) recommended adding 200–600 mg of vitamin C and 100 IU of vitamin E to a healthy diet in type 1 diabetes.

Vitamin B3 (niacin)

Niacin plays a prominent role in energy production, fat, cholesterol and carbohydrate metabolism and production of sex and adrenal hormones. Niacin, like chromium, is an essential component of the glucose tolerance factor (GTF) and is necessary for producing NAD (Nicotinamide Adenine Dinucleotide) in insulin-secreting pancreatic B cells. As a component of the glucose tolerance factor, niacin plays an important role in carbohydrate metabolism. Many refined foods consumed by people who live in Western countries are low in niacin. Grains and other foods that are 'enriched' usually contain added niacinamide, which apparently cannot be converted by the human body into niacin. In addition, many vitamin supplements contain niacinamide, rather than niacin. Although niacinamide is capable of performing most of the functions of vitamin B3, a small amount of niacin seems to be necessary for the synthesis of GTF (Urberg et al. 1987). Both niacin and niacinamide may also be important for blood glucose control through a mechanism unrelated to GTF. As precursors to NAD, which is an important metabolite concerned with intracellular energy production, niacin and niacinamide may prevent the depletion of NAD in pancreatic B cells especially in type 2 diabetes.

Niacin in the form of inositol hexaniacinate can be used to lower lipids in type 2 diabetes. Niacin lowers cholesterol but the dose required, 1–3 gms/day, is often not well tolerated because of side effects such as flushing, stomach irritation, ulcers, liver damage, and fatigue. Inositol hexaniacinate is a better and safer form used successfully in Europe to lower cholesterol and improve blood flow in intermittent claudication. A dose range between 600–1000 mg/3 times per day is usually necessary to achieve an 18 per cent reduction in cholesterol, 1.26 per cent reduction in triglycerides and a 30 per cent increase in HDL (Murray and Pizzorno 1998).

Niacin has been shown to improve blood glucose control in small studies. For example, 500 mg/day supplemental niacinamide was given to four people with type 2 diabetes for one month followed by 250 mg/day for at least 6–12 months thereafter. Blood glucose returned to normal and the two people on glucose-lowering agents were able to discontinue these medicines. All patients experienced diuresis for several months and lost 10–12 kg (Cleary 1990).

It is worth noting that people who do not respond to chromium supplementation may have deficient intake of nicotinic acid (Urberg and Zemel 1987).

Biotin

Biotin is essential to the appropriate processing and utilisation of carbohydrates, fats and protein. Biotin is manufactured normally in the intestines by gut bacteria. The initial step in glucose utilization by the cell is its phosphorylation, mediated by the biotin-dependent enzyme hepatic glucokinase, which is responsible for the first step in glucose utilisation in the liver. Thus, adequate biotin intake is required to initiate intracellular glucose into the cell (No authors listed 1970). Biotin may also play a role in stabilising blood glucose levels through biotin-dependent enzymes acetyl Co A carboxylase and pyruvate carboxylase (Jitrapakdee *et al* 1999).

Vitamin B6

Vitamin B6 supplementation appears to offer significant protection against diabetic neuropathy particularly in vitamin B6-deficine states. Supplementation with ~150 mg/day may relieve the symptoms of peripheral neuropathy. Vitamin B6 may have a role in preventing other diabetes-related complications such as protein glycosylation (Pizzorno and Murray 1998).

Vitamin E

Patients with type 2 diabetes patients appear to require Vitamin E supplements with pharmacologic doses ~ 900IU/day, which appears to reduce oxidative stress, improve insulin action, improve glucose tolerance, and increase total glucose disposal (Paolisso *et al*. 1993).

5.13 Minerals

Magnesium

The RDI for magnesium in Australia is 320 mg for males and 270 mg for females but extra is required in altered physiological states such as pregnancy and lactation where an extra 30 and 70 mg/day respectively is needed. The RDI in the USA is 350 mg for adult males and 300 mg for adult females. People with type 2 diabetes may require double this amount. Adults in the USA require between 143–266 mg magnesium from dietary sources.

The RDI may not be achievable in most western environments particularly in view of the reduced availability of magnesium in many refined foods. Other factors such as illness in this case type 2 diabetes, medications, stress and environmental factors also affect magnesium requirements. Environmental factors affect the magnesium content of the food supply (soils, agriculture, acidic rain, air pollution) and food processing. Many foods contain bioavailable magnesium such as green leafy vegetables, grains, various nuts (almonds, hazelnuts), various fish (bluefish, cod, herring, mackerel), wheat germ, dark chocolate, and tofu, whereas meat, milk, fish and most commonly consumed fruit are low in magnesium.

The daily intake of magnesium is below the RDA for 50 per cent of all males and for 39 per cent of all females tested in a CSIRO study (Baghurst *et al.* 1991). Deficiencies appear to be even more common in the United States where dietary surveys have shown that 80–85 per cent of American women consume less than the RDA for the mineral magnesium (Morgan *et al.* 1975) and in one study, and in another study magnesium intake was only about two-thirds of the RDA (Lakshmanan *et al.* 1984) Although deficiency signs are not common, many chronic pathologies seem to be responsive to magnesium supplementation (Fox *et al.* 2001). Supplemental magnesium may be the best strategy to correct magnesium deficiencies.

Although the National Health and Medical Research Council (NH&MRC) dietary guidelines do not suggest supplemental magnesium level for people with diabetes, it is likely to be beneficial in a bioavailable form (diglycinate, orotate, aspartate), given the tendency to excrete excessive amounts of magnesium in the urine each day.

Magnesium plays an important role in glucose homeostasis by affecting both insulin secretion and action. Significant evidence exists that people with type 2 diabetes are magnesium-deficient and supplements may have a role in preventing retinopathy and heart disease (Pizzorno and Murray 1998). The association between low magnesium and type 2 diabetes was documented in the 1950s (Stutzman 1952) and a significant proportion of those people with type 2 diabetes are magnesium-deficient (25–40 per cent) or at the very least have suboptimal magnesium status (McNair *et al.* 1982).

People with hyperglycaemia often develop polyuria, which might partly explain the higher than normal excretion of magnesium and other minerals. Depending on the dietary and supplemental magnesium intake, the magnesium status may be in negative balance. As a result, less magnesium is available for insulin secretion or action, which could contribute to suboptimal metabolic functioning.

A number of human studies highlight the association between magnesium deficiency and poor metabolic control in diabetes. Magnesium facilitates insulin release and function, once released, it binds to the tyrosine-kinase receptor complex and initiates a cascade of biochemical reactions that results in several physiological and biochemical events involved in carbohydrate, lipid and protein metabolism (Suarez *et al.* 1992; Lefebvre *et al.* 1995). Reduced peripheral glucose uptake is often noted in people with magnesium deficiency. Researchers have shown a relationship between magnesium and insulin resistance in animal studies (Yajnik *et al* 1984; Balon *et al.* 1995) and humans where hypomagnesaemia has been correlated with poor diabetic control and IR in diabetic elderly patients (Tosiello 1996).

Supplemental magnesium (2 g per day) improves insulin sensitivity in insulin resistant individuals. Paolisso *et al.* (1989) compared insulin response and action after chronic magnesium in addition to diet in elderly type 2 diabetes subjects compared to placebo and showed a significant increase in plasma and erythrocyte magnesium levels, an increase in insulin action, increased glucose clearance rate, and a reduction in resting plasma glucose levels.

The researchers concluded that type 2 diabetes subjects may benefit from therapeutic chronic administration of magnesium salts.

In a more recent double blind, randomised, cross-over placebo-controlled trial, Paolisso *et al.* (1992) explored the effects of magnesium supplementation on the ability of elderly insulin resistant people (average age 78) to cope with an intravenous glucose challenge. They administration of 4.5 g (15.8 mmol) magnesium per day for four weeks and reported significant increases in erythrocyte blood cell magnesium levels, enhanced total body and oxidative glucose metabolism, and reduced erythrocyte membrane microviscosity.

Likewise, Nadler *et al.* (1993) showed lean non-diabetic subjects receiving a low dose magnesium liquid diet (< 0.5 mmol/day) experienced a significant reduction in erythrocyte magnesium levels and increased insulin resistance, demonstrated by reduced glucose clearance in response to a intravenous glucose tolerance test. In addition, they also found increased urinary thromboxane levels and enhanced aldosterone-secreting effects of angiotension II. The changes observed in these two parameters may reflect some of the underlying processes that lead to the development of the micro- and macro-vascular complications associated with diabetes.

Kao *et al.* (1999) suggested a magnesium deficiency may be a novel risk factor for impaired glucose tolerance on the basis of; several large observational studies demonstrating strong associations between low serum magnesium levels and type 2 diabetes; *in vitro* studies that demonstrated an effect of magnesium on insulin secretion and peripheral tissue responsiveness to insulin; spontaneous type 2 diabetes in a rat model; and improved short-term insulin response and glucose handling in diabetic individuals.

Previous work suggests several possible mechanisms whereby low intracellular magnesium levels may lead to the development of type 2 diabetes including the fact that magnesium is an essential co-factor in reactions involving phosphorylation; magnesium deficiency could impair the insulin signal transduction pathway; low serum or erythrocyte magnesium levels may affect the interaction between insulin and the insulin receptor by decreasing hormone receptor affinity or by increasing membrane microviscosity; magnesium can also be a limiting factor in carbohydrate metabolism, since many of the enzymes in this process require magnesium as a co-factor during reactions that utilise phosphorus bonds. In summary, it appears that low serum or erythrocyte magnesium levels may be a strong, independent predictor of the development of exponential insulin resistance in type 2 diabetes (Yajnik *et al.* 1984).

Some additional considerations include the fact that electrolyte disturbances are known to affect normal skeletal muscle function. Hypomagnesaemia is related to nocturnal leg muscle cramps, impacting negatively on the quality of life of people with type 2 diabetes by disrupting sleep and causing excessive fatigue. Bachem (1986) showed improvements in 24 patients with type I diabetes suffering frequent nocturnal leg muscle cramps who were given 5 mg/kg/day magnesium aspartate hydrochloride. 20 out of the 24 experienced complete resolution of leg cramps and the remaining noted a marked reduction in the frequency and intensity of their nocturnal leg muscle cramps. Magnesium supplementation should always be considered in people with nocturnal leg muscle cramps, especially if they have type 2 diabetes. Health professionals, however, need to ensure that renal function is not compromised.

Magnesium deficiency can be treated in a number of ways:

1. *Diet*: by encouraging foods rich in magnesium in a way that is nutritionally tailored to the individual. Many magnesium-rich foods are also high calorie and high fat foods, which needs to be taken into consideration.
2. *Nutritional supplements*: Oral magnesium sources are generally available as ionically bound salts such as magnesium chloride (MgCl), magnesium sulphate (MgSO4) and magnesium oxide (MgO). Other forms are the complexed minerals such as magnesium aspartate and magnesium orotate. All of these forms dissociate in solution to release magnesium ions and are known to induce bowel evacuation when taken in therapeutic doses, although magnesium aspartate HCl has also been reported to cause less diarrhoea than many of the other available magnesium supplements. Magnesium aspartate HCl is one of the best bioavailable and absorbed sources (Gums 1987; Mulhbauer *et al*. 1991).

Magnesium supplements are obviously required for patients with low serum and/or red blood cell levels. Many practitioners also routinely recommend magnesium supplements even when serum/red blood cell magnesium levels are within the normal range because the diabetic state encourages magnesium loss.

Potassium

Consuming a potassium rich diet is important for people with type 2 diabetes to improve insulin sensitivity, responsiveness and secretion, and to reduce the risk of heart disease, atherosclerosis and cancer. Potassium is associated with antioxidant, alkaline-rich foods such as fruits and vegetables. Most people with type 2 diabetes should be able to obtain sufficient potassium via diet alone. In cases where requirements are increased, such as use of diuretics, or in the presence of dehydration such as hyperosmolar states (commonly in the elderly), supplementation may be necessary for good health. Care needs to be exercised in the presence of renal disease because potassium may not be excreted and may precipitate cardiac arrhythmias. Kidney function should be regularly monitored in people with diabetes using potassium supplements (Pizzorno and Murray 1998).

Manganese

Manganese is an important co-factor in the many enzyme systems involved in blood glucose control. People with type 2 diabetes have lower levels of manganese than non-diabetics. An adequate daily dose of manganese for a type 2 diabetes patient is 30 mg (Pizzorno and Murray 1998).

Zinc

Adequate zinc intake is essential in people with diabetes because it is involved in all aspects of insulin metabolism. It is essential for the production, storage and secretion of insulin and facilitates the binding of insulin to the insulin receptor. It is required for the normal exocrine and endocrine role of the pancreas and controls gene expression related to glucose and insulin action. Zinc may be involved in the release of insulin from the vesicles within the pancreatic-beta cells (Walsh *et al.* 1994).

People with type 2 diabetes excrete copious amounts of zinc in the urine and supplementation has been shown to help improve insulin sensitivity. Zinc also assists in wound healing in people with diabetes. Good food sources of zinc include whole grains, nuts, legumes, and seeds. The recommended level of supplementation for people with type 2 diabetes is at least 30 mg per day (Pizzorno and Murray 1998).

5.14 Trace Elements

Chromium

A significant amount of experimental and epidemiological evidence exists to indicate that serum trivalent chromium levels are a significant determinant of insulin sensitivity (Offenbacher and Pi-Sunnyer 1980; Riales *et al.* 1981; Levine *et al.* 1968; Anderson 1992). Without chromium, insulin action is compromised and glucose levels are raised (Mooradian *et al.* 1994). Inadequate dietary intake of chromium is implicated in a number of metabolic abnormalities including impaired glucose and lipid metabolism, elevated circulating insulin levels, and reduced numbers of insulin receptors. High intake of simple sugars increases urinary chromium loss (Kozlovsky *et al.* 1986; Davis and Vincent 1997). Kozlovsky stated:

> compared to the reference diets, consumption of high sugar diets increased urinary chromium losses from 10 % to 300 % for 27 of 37 subjects. These data demonstrate that consumption of diets high in simple sugars stimulated chromium losses; this coupled with marginal intake of dietary chromium may lead to marginal chromium deficiency, which is associated with impaired glucose and lipid metabolism.

Chromium is an essential trace nutrient. Deficiency is widespread in the United States (Pizzorno and Murray 1998) and by association, in Australia. Chromium deficiency may be an underlying contributing factor to obesity, hypoglycaemia and type 2 diabetes. Trivalent Chromium (3+) is the only form of chromium that exhibits biological activity and is an integral component of the Glucose Tolerance Factor, which also contains two molecules of nicotinic acid, cysteine, glutamine and glycine.

Supplemental chromium significantly improves glucose tolerance, decreases fasting glucose, cholesterol and triglyceride levels, and increases HDL-cholesterol by improving insulin sensitivity in elderly adults (Offenbacher and Pi-Sunyer 1980; Riales and Albrink 1981; Mooradian et al. 1992; Anderson 1992). Reversing chromium deficiency by supplementing the diet leads to weight reduction while increasing lean muscle mass. In healthy subjects experimentally depleted in chromium, trivalent chromium replacement improved glucose tolerance and reversed abnormal elevations in circulating insulin and glucagon in patients with mild hyperglycaemia (Anderson et al. 1991).

Oral trivalent chromium has also been shown to improve glycaemic control and cholesterol levels in Chinese patients with type 2 diabetes (Anderson et al. 1997). In this study 180 Chinese men and women with type 2 diabetes were given placebo or 200 or 1000 ug of chromium for four months. Dose-related improvements in glycosylated haemoglobin, fasting and two-hour post-prandial glucose, insulin and total cholesterol were demonstrated. A recent case report highlighted the fact that some people with type 2 diabetes self-supplementing with chromium to control their blood glucose become hypoglycaemic (Anderson et al. 1997).

In a double-blind, cross-over placebo-controlled trial whose primary objective was to test the hypothesis that an elevated intake of supplemental chromium is involved in the optimal control of type 2 diabetes, 180 type 2 diabetics were divided randomly into 3 groups and supplemented with: (1) placebo; (2) 100mcg chromium (as chromium picolinate) twice daily; (3) 500mcg chromium (as chromium picolinate) twice daily.

Participants were asked to continue taking their regular medication and instructed not to change their diet and lifestyle. Glycosylated haemoglobin improved significantly after two months in the group receiving 1000 mcg per day and was lower in both chromium groups after two and four months. Two-hour post-prandial glucose tolerance values were also significantly lower in the subjects consuming 1000 mcg of supplemental chromium after both two and four months. Fasting and two-hour post-prandial serum insulin levels decreased significantly in both groups receiving supplemental chromium after two and four months.

Plasma total cholesterol also decreased after four months in the group receiving 1000 mcg chromium. These data demonstrate that supplemental chromium had significant beneficial effects on HbA_{1C}, fasting glucose, insulin and cholesterol variables in subjects with type 2 diabetes. The beneficial effects of chromium in individuals with type 2 diabetes were observed at levels higher than the upper limit of the Estimated Safe and Adequate Daily Dietary Intake (Anderson et al. 1997).

The effect of chromium on glucose metabolism apparently requires its conversion to glucose tolerance factor (GTF), a low-molecular-weight compound that contains chromium, niacin (nicotinic acid), glycine, glutamic acid, and cysteine. GTF has been shown to potentiate the action of insulin at the cellular level (Toepfer et al. 1977; Glinsmann et al. 1966).

Tissue chromium levels were found to decline with age in Americans (Schroeder et al. 1970). In other studies, including one by the US Department of Agriculture, more than 50 per cent of people consumed less than the lower level of chromium recommended by the National Academy of Sciences, Nutritional Research Council (Anderson *et al.* 1985). Chromium aspartate is a well-utilized form of supplemental chromium being solubilized at a wide range of ph. The amounts of chromium used in most clinical trials (150 to 200 µg/day) are apparently inadequate for some patients, even when more efficient chromium compounds are used. Larger amounts of chromium, such as 500 to 1,000 ug/day, have often had a greater benefit (Glinsmann 1966).

These effects may be due to the physiological effect of chromium on insulin responsiveness of skeletal muscle and probably fat cells. This could possibly be mediated by insulin internalisation and the regulation of the synthesis or insertion of insulin receptors into the plasma membrane (Evans and Bowman 1992). Jovanovic-Peterson *et al.* (1996) showed trivalent chromium improves glycosylated haemoglobin, insulin and glucose levels in women with gestational diabetes.

Vanadium

Insulin-like effects of vanadium on glucose metabolism have been demonstrated in animal and human studies but the exact physiological mechanism is not completely understood (French and Jones 1992). Vanadium does not replace insulin action, but appears to improve insulin receptor sensitivity to glucose including in type 2 diabetes (French and Jones 1992; Shechter *et al.* 1995).

Cohen *et al.* (1995) examined the in vivo metabolic effects of Vanadyl sulphate in six people with type 2 diabetes treated with diet and/or sulphonylureas at the end of three consecutive periods: placebo for two weeks, Vanadyl sulphate (100 mg per day) for three weeks and placebo for two weeks. Treatment with Vanadyl sulphate resulted in improved glycosylated haemoglobin and fasting plasma glucose, which were sustained for up to two weeks after Vanadyl was discontinued. Cohen *et al.* suggested Vanadyl sulphate improves hepatic and peripheral insulin sensitivity in insulin resistant humans.

The mechanism of action of vanadium is unclear, however, several studies indicate it is a phosphatase inhibitor and activates serine/threonine kinases distal to the insulin receptor possibly by preventing dephosphorylation by inhibiting phosphatases. These studies suggest vanadium may optimise blood glucose control by mimicking the activity of insulin and increasing tissue sensitivity to insulin (Cohen *et al.* 1995; Halberstam *et al.* 1996; Goldfine *et al.* 2000).

5.15   Essential Fatty Acids; Gamma-Linolenic Acid and Omega 3 Fish Oils

Both omega 3 and omega 6 essential fatty acids (EFAs) have demonstrated benefits in type 2 diabetes. Gamma linolenic acid (18:3n6) has a role in preventing diabetic neuropathy and omega 3 fatty acids protect against atherosclerosis and improve insulin sensitivity in type 2 diabetes. NM recommends increasing the intake of cold water fish such as salmon, tuna, sardines, mackerel, supplementing with ~480mg of GLA/day, and 1–2 tablespoons of flaxseed oil daily (Pizzorno and Murray 1998).

Gamma-linolenic acid (GLA)

Human and experimental studies indicate type 2 diabetes is associated with a disruption in the essential fatty acid (EFA) pathway, which results in microvascular changes that lead to reduced blood flow and neuronal hypoxia (Pizzorno and Murray 1998). Most of the disruption to the EFA pathway is likely to be due to key nutrients deficiencies (zinc, magnesium, Vitamin B6, Vitamin C). The Gamma-Linolenic Acid Multicentre Trial showed that supplementing the diets of people with mild diabetic neuropathy with 480mg Evening Primrose Oil, the equivalent of 12 40mg capsules of GLA/day, for one year markedly improved conduction velocity and amplitude, hot and cold threshold, tendon reflexes and muscle strength.

Omega 3 fish oil (EPA/DHA)

Many studies in type 2 diabetes indicate omega 3 fatty acids lower cholesterol and triglycerides (Pizzorno and Murray 1998). Omega 3 fatty acids can be incorporated into the treatment of cardiovascular diseases such as hypertension as well as non-diabetes-related conditions such as autoimmune disorders such as rheumatoid arthritis and psoriasis.

A three-month study of daily supplementation with docosahexaenoic acid (DHA) produced a clinically significant improvement in insulin sensitivity in overweight individuals (Denkins 2002). In the study, 12 overweight men and women, aged 40–70, consumed 1.8 grams of DHA at breakfast for 12 weeks. None had type 2 diabetes but they all had insulin resistance. Insulin sensitivity improved after 12 weeks of DHA supplementation: 70 per cent showed improvements in insulin-related function, and the change was clinically significant in 50 per cent (Denkins 2002). Denkins (2002) only used DHA. The author does not advocate using isolated fish oils; EPA and DHA should always be taken in a balanced dose. The dose of DHA used in this study was 1.8 g. Most capsules contain 180 mg of EPA and 120 mg of DHA, which equates to 10 regular fish oil capsules/day, which could affect compliance. Fish oil capsules containing 300 mg EPA and 200 mg DHA with vitamin E are available and may be more palatable and increase compliance.

In type 2 diabetes, omega 3 essential fatty acids have been shown to: lower total, LDL cholesterol and triglyceride levels and raise HDL cholesterol; reduce platelet aggregation; reduce endothelial permeability; increase insulin-receptor sensitivity (Popp-Snijders et al. 1987).

It also appears that fish oil has a threshold level of benefit beyond which it begins to exert deleterious effects. Studies indicate that up to 2.5 g of omega 3 fish oil/day, which equates to approximately 450 mg of EPA and 300 DHA, has cardiovascular benefits such as reduced platelet aggregation, systolic blood pressure and triglycerides (Axelrod 1994). However, doses between 4–10 g of omega 3 fish oil/day have deleterious effects such as increased plasma glucose, total and LDL cholesterol and serum apolipoprotein B (Schmidt and Dyerberg 1994). Hence, potential does exist for omega 3 to contribute to a deterioration in glycaemic control and worsening dyslipidaemia. It is difficult to understand these discrepancies. Other nutritional factors such as antioxidants and dosage regimes may play a role.

Although these studies suggest fish oil supplements should be used with caution in people with type 2 diabetes, the deleterious effects might be partially explained by the high levels of lipid peroxides contained in many fish oils preparations (rancid fat), which place undue demand on the individual's antioxidant capacity. A sensible, cautious approach is to do the following:

- Encourage people with type 2 diabetes to consume more deep-sea fish rich in omega 3 fatty acids and/or flaxseed oil, neither of which are associated with deleterious effects in type 2 diabetes.
- Take lower doses, no more than 2–3 g of enteric-coated omega 3 fatty acid fish oils/day, which produce fewer gastrointestinal effects and make use of fish oil supplements containing d-alpha tocopherol or mixed tocopherols between 25–50 IU per capsule to limit the development of lipid peroxides in the capsule in the first place.

Consuming deep-sea fish produces equal or if not superior benefits as fish oil supplementation. Equivalent doses of both lower triglycerides and increase HDL cholesterol levels, but total cholesterol levels remain. Other studies have demonstrated an inverse relationship between fish consumption (mean daily intake of 24.2 g/day), impaired glucose tolerance and type 2 diabetes (Pizzorno and Murray 1998). These, and other epidemiological studies in cultures with a high consumption of deep-sea fish indicate that omega 3 EFAs are beneficial for both type 1 and type 2 diabetes.

Flaxseed oil, which contains alpha-linolenic acid (ALA), is an omega 3 oil that can be converted in the body to EPA (eicosapentaenoic acid) provided the micronutrient status is adequate. In the presence of excessive omega 6 fatty acids, flaxseed oil containing ALA is not as effective at increasing tissue concentrations of EPA or lowering Arachidonic Acid (AA). Hence, practitioners need to consider dietary approaches that discourage excessive omega 6 intake such as excessive grains and omega 6 rich vegetable oils. Flaxseed oil may be the preferred treatment option because many encapsulated fish oils contain lipid peroxides, which deplete body stores of antioxidants and are expensive at therapeutic doses. In addition, flaxseed oil is less expensive. Flaxseed oil should be from cold pressed sources and ideally be kept in opaque glass bottles and stored in the refrigerator for no more than 8–12 weeks.

In essence, people with diabetes are likely to benefit from increased consumption of fish oil, which can easily be achieved by regularly consuming at least 30–40 g per day of deep-sea fish, and/or regularly consuming 1 tablespoon of flaxseed oil, and/or judicious supplementation with 1000 mg/2–3 times/day antioxidant rich fish oil capsules. Many people find it difficult to digest fish oil capsules because they cause regurgitation or cause nausea, which are often related to impaired gall bladder function. In the author's experience, many patients benefit from using a lipase digestive enzyme and/or opt for enterically coated fish oil capsules.

5.16 Other Key Nutrients

Flavonoids

Flavonoids may be useful in type 2 diabetes, for example, quercetin improves insulin secretion and prevents sorbitol accumulation. The nutritional effects of flavanoids include: increased intracellular vitamin C levels, reduced blood vessel permeability and fragility, reduced bruising, and immune support, all of which are desirable in the optimal management of diabetes. In addition to consuming a diet rich in flavanoids, people with diabetes could benefit from an additional 1–2 g of mixed flavanoids per day (Pizzorno and Murray 1998).

Taurine

Nakaya *et al.* (2000) found taurine supplementation significantly improved insulin sensitivity, lowered serum lipids, and reduced abdominal fat accumulation in rats receiving taurine supplements compared to controls. They suggested taurine might improve metabolism by reducing serum cholesterol and triglycerol, possibly by increasing cholesterol secretion into bile acid and reducing cholesterol production through increased nitric oxide production. Taurine has insulin-like action (Kulkowski *et al.* 1984; Franconi 1995).

Lipoeic/thiotic acid

Lipoeic acid improves insulin sensitivity and aids fat loss type 2 diabetes because of its ability to stimulate thermogenesis. In a multicentre, placebo-controlled trial, 74 people with type 2 diabetes received either 600, 1200 or 1800 mg of alpha-lipoeic acid per day or a placebo. After four weeks all treatment groups showed improved glucose disposal compared to placebo. There was no significant difference between the alpha-lipoeic acid doses. The combined results of the treated groups versus the placebo group showed a 27 per cent increase in insulin-stimulated glucose uptake. No serious side effects were noted in any of the treatment groups (Jacob *et al.* 1999). Likewise, intravenous infusions of lipoeic acid increase insulin-mediated glucose disposal (Jacob *et al.* 1996; Evans and Goldfine 2000) and hypoinsulinaemic/hypoglycaemic effects (Becca *et al.* 1999). These studies suggest lipoeic acid could be a safe and effective adjunctive insulin sensitising glucose-lowering agent.

   Alpha-lipoeic acid has also been shown to stimulate basal glucose transport and positively affect insulin-stimulated glucose uptake. The stimulatory effect depends on phosphatidylinositol 3-kinase activity and may be explained by a redistribution of glucose transporters (Glut 4), which suggests it can stimulate glucose transport via the insulin signalling pathway (Estrada *et al.* 1996) and may be particularly valuable in disorders of glucose metabolism such as type 2 diabetes mellitus.

Konrad *et al.* (1999) examined the effect of 1200 mg of supplemental alpha-lipoeic acid/day taken for four weeks on insulin sensitivity, glucose effectiveness, serum pyruvic acid and lactic acid levels after glucose loading in 10 lean and 10 obese controls and 10 lean and 10 obese type 2 diabetics. Fasting pyruvic acid and lactic acid levels were significantly higher in the lean and obese diabetic patients. Alpha-lipoeic acid was associated with increased glucose effectiveness in both lean and obese diabetics and a significantly reduced fasting glucose and improved insulin sensitivity in the lean diabetics. The authors concluded that oral lipoid acid improves intracellular glucose utilisation, possibly by stimulating the pyruvate dehydrogenase complex, and increases insulin-mediated glucose disposal in type 2 diabetes patients.

Increased oxidative stress may be a major factor in the development of diabetic complications, including peripheral neuropathy. Animal studies demonstrate the effects of oxidative stress on the development of diabetic neuropathy and suggest antioxidants could prevent or reverse hyperglycaemia induced nerve dysfunction (Sytze 2002). Antioxidant effects maximise the availability of nutrients in tissues. Antioxidants including alpha-lipoeic acid and vitamin E have been shown to reduce neuropathic symptoms or correct nerve conduction velocity in a limited number of clinical studies. These data are promising and suggest treating symptomatic diabetic polyneuropathy with alpha-lipoeic acid may be beneficial. Additional larger studies with alpha-lipoeic acid are currently being performed. A meta-analysis showed 600 mg/day of intravenous alpha-lipoeic acid taken for three weeks is safe and clinically improves neuropathic symptoms and neuropathic deficits (Konrad *et al.* 1999; Zeigler *et al.* 2004).

5.17 Safe Use of Supplements

It is advisable that nutritional supplementation for people with diabetes is supervised by qualified practitioners and considered as part of the overall management plan including diet and conventional and complementary medicines that can affect absorption, and excretion and therefore actions of supplements and vice versa. Supplements are particularly useful when deficiencies are present or risk factors for deficiencies exist. The RDI should be considered and evidence shown for benefit and risk and doses and dose intervals where possible. Access to trained advice and regular revision of doses and effects is essential.

Adverse events related to supplement

Adverse events related to nutritional supplementation are associated with:

- The supplement itself, which is usually associated with mega doses. Mega doses of the following can cause:

- Hypercarotenaemia.
- Niacin: hyperuricaemia, reduced glucose tolerance, liver toxicity lactic acidosis and prolonged bleeding especially with sustained release preparations.
- Vitamin C: diarrhoea, increased renal oxalate excretion and may be contraindicated in renal disease.
- Omega 3: reduce immunity – supplement with Vitamin E to prevent temporary thrombocytopenia.
- Vitamin E: oily form may increase triglycerides. The water miscible form is recommended for people with diabetes.
- Zinc: reduced immunity, anaemia, neutropenia, leukopenia and copper deficiency.
- Inappropriate use.
- Manufacturing issues such as contamination and adulteration and inadequate labelling, see Chapter 3.
- Interactions with complementary and conventional medicines, which is more likely when people are taking multiple medicines, which is frequently necessary to manage diabetes.
- Presence of liver and kidney disease.

At present, while there seems to be a sufficient evidence to support the role of nutritional supplementation in improving blood glucose control and diabetes health outcomes, there is still insufficient direct evidence to draw definitive conclusions about the efficacy of individual supplements (and herbs) for people with diabetes. However, they appear to be generally safe. The best evidence for efficacy from adequately designed randomised controlled trials is available for chromium, which has been the most widely studied supplement. Nutritional preparations with positive preliminary results include vanadium, lipoeic acid, fish oil and magnesium.

As far as herbal supplements are concerned, the best evidence for efficacy from adequately designed randomised controlled trials is available for herbs such as *Coccinia indica* and American ginseng. Other herbal preparations with positive preliminary results include *Gymnema sylvestre*, *Aloe vera*, *Momordica charantia* and nopal. The available data suggest that these nutritional and herbal supplements may warrant further study (Yeh *et al.* 2003).

References

Abbasi F, McLaughlin T, Lamendola C, Kim HS, Tanaka A, Wang T, Nakajima K, Reaven GM. High carbohydrate diets, triglyceride-rich lipoproteins, and coronary heart disease risk. *American Journal of Cardiology* 2000; **85**(1): 45–48.

Alberti A, Pirrone P, Elia M, Waring RH, Romano C. Sulphation deficit in 'low-functioning' autistic children: a pilot study. *Biological Psychiatry* 1999; **46**(3): 420–424.

Anderson RA. Chromium, glucose tolerance, and diabetes. *Biological Trace Element Research* 1992; **32**: 19–24.

Anderson RA, Cheng N, Bryden NA, Canary J. Supplemental chromium effects on glucose, insulin, glucagon and urinary chromium losses in subjects consuming controlled low-chromium diets. *American Journal of Clinical Nutrition* 1991; **54**: 909–916.

Anderson RA, Cheng N, Bryden NA, Polansky MM, Cheng N *et al*. November Elevated intakes of supplemental chromium improve glucose and insulin variables in individuals with type 2 diabetes. *Diabetes* 1997; **46**(11): 1786–1791.

Anderson RA, Kozlovsky AS. Chromium intake, absorption and excretion of subjects consuming self-selected diets. *American Journal of Clinical Nutrition* 1985; **41**: 1177–1183.

Axelrod L. Effects of a small quantity of omega-3 fatty acids on cardiovascular risk factors in NIDDM. *Diabetes Care* 1994; **17**: 37–45.

Baba NH, Sawaya S, Torbay N, Habbal Z, Azar S, Hashim SA. High protein versus high carbohydrate hypoenergetic diet for the treatment of obese hyperinsulinemic subjects. *International Journal of Obesity Related Metabolic Disorders* 1999; **23**(11): 1202–1206.

Bachem MG. Efficacy of oral magnesium supplementation in type 1 diabetics with nocturnal leg cramps. *Magnesium Bulletin* 1986; **8**: 280–283.

Baghurst KI, Dreosti IE, Syrette JA, Record SJ, Baghurst PA, Buckley RA. January Zinc and magnesium status of Australian adults. *Nutrition Research* 1991; **11**(1): 23–32.

Baldi I, Mohammed-Brahim B, Brochard P, Dartigues JF, Salamon R. Delayed health effects of pesticides: review of current epidemiological knowledge. *Rev Epidémioloque Santé Publique* 1998; **46**(2): 134–142. Review. French.

Balon TW, Gu JL, Tokuyama Y, Jasman AP, Nadler JL. Magnesium supplementation reduces development of diabetes in a rat model of spontaneous NIDDM. *American Journal of Physiology* 1995; **269**(4 Pt 1): E7 45–52.

Barr RG, Nathan DM, Meigs JB, Singer DE. Tests for glycemia for the diagnosis of type 2 diabetes mellitus. *Annals of Internal Medicine* 2002; **137**: 263–272.

Bauman W, Shaw S, Jayatilleke E, Spungen A, Herbert V. Increased intake of calcium reverses vitamin B$_{12}$ malabsorption induced by Metformin. *Diabetes Care* 2000; **23**(9): 1227–1231.

Bazzano LA, Serdula M, Liu S. Prevention of type 2 diabetes by diet and lifestyle modification. *Journal of the American College of Nutrition* 2005; **24**(5): 310–319.

Bland J, Barrager E, Reedy RG, Bland K. A medical food-supplemented detoxification program in the management of chronic health problems. *Alternative Therapies in Health and Medicine* 1995; **1**(5): 62–71.

Bland J, Bralley J. Nutritional upregulation of detoxification enzymes. *Journal of Applied Nutrition* 1992; **44**(3, 4): 2–15.

Bralley, JA Lord RS. New laboratory measures for detection of abnormal microbial growth. *Journal of the Australian College of Nutritional & Environmental Medicine* 2004; **23**(3): 3–7 (www.metametrix.com).

Braun, L. Review of the literature for the evidence for herbs and nutritional supplements in both primary and secondary prevention of cardiovascular disease. *Journal of Complementary Medicine* 2004; **3**(5): 18–26.

Brecca V, Nourooz-Zadeh. A-Lipoid acid decreases oxidative stress even in diabetic patients with poor glycaemic control and albuminuria. *Free Radical Biological Medicine* 1999; **22**(11/22): 1495–1500.

Brehm BJ, Seeley RJ, Daniels SR, D'Alessio DA. Randomized trial comparing a very low carbohydrate diet and a calorie-restricted low fat diet on body weight and cardiovascular risk factors in healthy women. *Journal of Clinical Endocrinology and Metabolism* 2003; **88**(4): 1617–1623.

Brinkworth GD, Noakes M, Keogh JB, Luscombe ND, Wittert GA, Clifton PM. Long-term effects of a high-protein, low-carbohydrate diet on weight control and cardiovascular risk markers in obese hyperinsulinemic subjects. *International Journal of Obesity Related Metabolic Disorders* 2004; **28**(9): 1187.

Cleary J.P. Vitamin B3 in the treatment of diabetes mellitus: case reports and review of literature. *Journal of Nutritional Medicine* 1990; **1**: 217–225.

Cohen MM, Penman S, Pirotta M, Costa CD. The integration of complementary therapies in Australian general practice: results of a national survey. *Journal of Alternative Complementary Medicine* 2005; **11**(6): 995–1004.

Cohen N, Halberstam M, Shlimovich P, Chang CJ, Shamoon H, Rossetti L. Oral vanadyl sulfate improves hepatic and peripheral insulin sensitivity in patients with non-insulin-dependent diabetes mellitus. *Journal of Clinical Investigations* 1995; **95**(6): 2501–2509.

Coppo R, Amore A, Roccatello D. Dietary antigens and primary immunoglobulin A nephropathy. *Journal of the American Society of Nephrology* 1992; **2**(10 Supplement): S173–180.

Cordain L, Toohey L, Smith MJ, Hickey MS. March Modulation of immune function by dietary lectins in rheumatoid arthritis. *British Journal of Nutrition* 2000; **83**(3): 207–217. Review.

Cosford R. April Insulin resistance, obesity and diabetes: the connection. *Journal of the Australian College of Nutritional & Environmental Medicine* 1999; **18**(1): 3–10.

Cox DJ, Gonder-Frederick L, Polonsky W, Schlundt D, Kovatchev B, Clarke W. Blood glucose awareness training (BGAT-2): long-term benefits. *Diabetes Care* 2001; **24**(4): 637–642.

Cunningham JJ. Reduced mononuclear leukocyte ascorbic acid content in adults with IDDM consuming adequate vitamin C. *Metabolism* 1991; **40**: 146–149.

Cunningham JJ. February Micronutrients as nutriceutical interventions in diabetes mellitus. *Journal of the American College of Nutrition* 1998; **17**(1): 7–10.

Cunningham JJ, Mearkle PL, Brown RG. August Vitamin C: an aldose reductase inhibitor that normalizes erythrocyte sorbitol in insulin-dependent diabetes mellitus. *Journal of the American College of Nutrition* 1994; **13**(4): 344–350.

D'Adamo P. *Eat Right 4 Your Type Complete Blood Type Encyclopaedia*. 1998.

D'Adamo PJ, Kelly GS. Metabolic and immunologic consequences of ABH secretor and Lewis subtype status. *Alternative Medicine Review* 2001; **6**(4): 390–405.

D'Adamo P, Whitney C. *The Eat Right Diet*. New York: Century Book Limited, 1998.

Dansinger ML, Gleason JA, Griffith JL, Selker HP, Schaefer EJ. Comparison of the Atkins, Ornish, Weight Watchers, and Zone diets for weight loss and heart disease risk reduction: a randomized trial. *Journal of the American Medical Association* 2005; **293**(1): 43–53.

Davis CM, Vincent JB. Chromium oligopeptide activates insulin receptor tyrosine kinase activity. *Biochemistry* 1997; **36**(15): 4382–4385.

Dawson-Hughes B, Harris SS, Rasmussen H, Song L, Dallal GE. Effect of dietary protein supplements on calcium excretion in healthy older men and women. *Journal of Clinical Endocrinology and Metabolism* 2004; **89**(3): 1169–1173.

Denkins Y. Paper presented at Annual Experimental Biology 2002 Conference, New Orleans, LA, 21 April 2002.

Eisenstein J, Roberts SB, Dallal G, Saltzman E. High-protein weight-loss diets: are they safe and do they work? A review of the experimental and epidemiologic data. *Nutrition Review* 2002; **60**(7 Pt 1): 189–200.

Estrada DE, Ewart HS, Tsakiridis T, Volchuk A, Ramlal T *et al.* Stimulation of glucose uptake by the natural coenzyme alpha-lipoic acid/thioctic acid: participation of elements of the insulin signalling pathway. *Diabetes* 1996; **45**(12): 1798–1804.

Evans GW, Bowman TD. Chromium picolinate increases membrane fluidity and rate of insulin internalization. *Journal of Inorganic Biochemistry* 1992; **46**(4): 243–250.

Evans JL, Goldfine ID. Alpha-lipoic acid: a multifunctional antioxidant that improves insulin sensitivity in patients with type 2 diabetes. *Diabetes Technology and Therapies* 2000; **2**(3): 401–413. Review.

Fairfield MK, Fletcher HR. Vitamins for chronic disease prevention in adults – scientific review. *Journal of the American Medical Association* 2002a; **287**(23): 3116–3126.

Fairfield MK, Fletcher HR. Vitamins for chronic disease prevention in adults – clinical applications. *Journal of the American Medical Association* 2002b; **287**(23): 3127–3129.

Fontvielle AM, Rizkalla SW, Penfornis A, Acosta M, Bornet FR, Slama G. The use of low glycaemic index foods improves metabolic control of diabetic patients over 5 weeks. *Diabetes Medicine* 1992; **9**(5): 444–50.

Fox C, Ramsoomair D, Carter C. Magnesium: its proven and potential clinical significance. *South Medical Journal* 2001; **94**(12): 1195–1201.

Franconi F. Plasma and platelet taurine are reduced in subjects with insulin-dependent diabetes mellitus: effects of taurine supplementation. *American Journal of Clinical Nutrition* 1995; **61**(5): 1115–1119.

Freed DLJ. Do dietary lectins cause disease? *British Medical Journal* 1999; **318**: 1023–1024.

French RJ, Jones PL. Role of vanadium in nutrition: metabolism, essentiality and dietary considerations. *Life Sciences* 1992; **52**: 339–346.

Glinsmann WH, Mertz W. Effect of trivalent chromium on glucose tolerance. *Metabolism* 1996; **15**: 510–502.

Golay A, Eigenheer C, Morel Y, Kujawski P, Lehmann T, de Tonnac N. Weight-loss with low or high carbohydrate diet? *International Journal of Obesity Related Metabolic Disorders* 1996; **20**(12): 1067–1072.

Golden SH, Folsom AR, Coresh J, Sharrett AR, Szklo M, Brancati F. Risk factor groupings related to insulin resistance and their synergistic effects on subclinical atherosclerosis: the atherosclerosis risk in communities study. *Diabetes* 2002; **51**(10): 3069–3076.

Goldfine AB, Patti ME, Zuberi L, Goldstein BJ, LeBlanc R *et al.* Metabolic effects of vanadyl sulfate in humans with non-insulin-dependent diabetes mellitus: in vivo and in vitro studies. *Metabolism* 2000; **49**(3): 400–410.

Greene PJ, Willett W. Pilot 12-week feeding weight-loss comparison: low-fat vs. low-carbohydrate (ketogenic) diets. NAASO meeting 13 October 2003, Obesity Research, September 2003, Oral Abstract #95

Gums JG. Clinical significance of magnesium: a review. *Drug Intelligence Clinical Pharmacology* 1987; **21**: 240–246.

Halberstam M, Cohen N, Shlimovich P, Rossetti L, Shamoon H. Oral vanadyl sulfate improves insulin sensitivity in NIDDM but not in obese non diabetic subjects. *Diabetes* 1996; **45**(9): 1285.

Hannan MT, Tucker KL, Dawson-Hughes B, Cupples LA, Felson DT, Kiel DP. Effect of dietary protein on bone loss in elderly men and women: the Framingham Osteoporosis Study. *Journal Bone Mineral Research* 2000; **15**(12): 2504–2512.

Hanson RL, Imperatore G, Bennett PH, Knowler WC. Components of the 'metabolic syndrome' and incidence of type 2 diabetes. *Diabetes* 2002; **51**(10): 3120–3127.

Hawlerak J. Probiotics for GI disorders. *Journal of Complementary Medicine* 2005; **4**(3): 42–50.

Heneghan MA, Moran AP, Feeley KM, Egan EL, Goulding J *et al.* Effect of host Lewis and ABO blood group antigen expression on Helicobacter pylori colonisation density and the consequent inflammatory response. *FEMS Immunology Medicine and Microbiology* 1998; **20**(4): 257–266.

Hooper L, Griffiths E, Abrahams B, Alexander W, Atkins S *et al.* UK Heart Health and Thoracic Dietitians Specialist Group of the British Dietetic Association. Dietetic guidelines: diet in secondary prevention of cardiovascular disease (first update, June 2003). *Journal Human Nutrition and Dietetics* 2004; **17**(4): 337–349.

Hu FB, Stampfer MJ, Manson JE, Rimm E, Colditz GA, Speizer FE, Hennekens CH, Willett WC. Dietary protein and risk of ischemic heart disease in women. *American Journal of Clinical Nutrition* 1999; **70**(2): 221–227.

International Diabetes Federation. Press release: diabetes and obesity: urgent action needed. available at: www.idf.org, accessed 16 January 2006.

Jacob S, Streeper RS, Fogt DL, Hokama JY, Tritschler HJ, Dietze GJ, Henriksen EJ. The antioxidant alpha-lipoic acid enhances insulin-stimulated glucose metabolism in insulin-resistant rat skeletal muscle. *Diabetes* 1996; **45**(8): 1024–1029.

Jacob S, Ruus P, Hermann R, Tritschler HJ, Maerker E, *et al.* Oral administration of RAC-alpha-lipoic acid modulates insulin sensitivity in patients with type-2 diabetes mellitus: a placebo-controlled pilot trial. *Free Radical Biology Medicine* 1999; **27**(3–4): 309–314.

Jenkins B, Holsten S, Bengmark S, Martindale R. Probiotics: a practical review of their role in specific clinical scenarios. *Nutrition Clinical Practice* 2005; **20**(2): 262–270. Review.

Jenkins DJ, Wolever TM, Kalmusky J, Giudici S, Giordano C *et al.* Low-glycaemic index diet in hyperlipidaemia: use of traditional starchy foods. *American Journal of Clinical Nutrition* 1987; **46**(1): 66–71.

Jitrapakdee S, Wallace JC. Structure, function and regulation of pyruvate carboxylase. *Biochemistry Journal* 1999; **15**: 340 (Part 1):1–16. Review.

Jovanovic-Peterson L, Gutirrez M, Peterson C. Chromium supplementation for gestational diabetic women improves glucose tolerance and decreases hyperinsulinaemia (abstract). *Diabetes Care* 1996; **45** (supplement 2): 337A.

Kao WH, Folsom AR, Nieto FJ, Mo JP, Watson RL, Brancati FL. Serum and dietary magnesium and the risk for type 2 diabetes mellitus: the Atherosclerosis Risk in Communities Study. *Archives Internal Medicine* 1999; **159**(18): 2151–2159.

Kelly GS. The role of glucosamine sulphate and chondroitin sulphates in the treatment of degenerative joint disease. *Alternative Medicine Review* 1998; **3**(1): 27–39.

Kelly GS. Insulin resistance: lifestyle and nutritional interventions. *Alternative Medicine Review* 2000; **5**(2): 109–132.

Kerstetter JE, Svastisalee CM, Caseria DM, Mitnick ME, Insogna KL. A threshold for low-protein-diet-induced elevations in parathyroid hormone. *American Journal of Clinical Nutrition* 2000; **72**(1): 168–173.

Kilburn KH, Warsaw RH, Shields MG. Neurobehavioural dysfunction in firemen exposed to polychlorinated biphenyls (PCBs): possible improvement after detoxification. *Archives of Environmental Health* 1989; **44**: 345–350.

Konrad T, Vicini P, Kusterer K, Hoflich A, Assadkhani A *et al.* Alpha-Lipoic acid treatment decreases serum lactate and pyruvate concentrations and improves glucose effectiveness in lean and obese patients with type 2 diabetes. *Diabetes Care* 1999; **22**(2): 280–287.

Kozlovsky AS, Moser PB, Reiser S, Anderson RA. Effects of diets high in simple sugars on urinary chromium losses. *Metabolism* 1986; **35**(6): 515–518.

Kulakowski EC, Maturo J. Hypoglycemic properties of taurine: not mediated by enhanced insulin release. *Biochemical Pharmacology* 1984; **33**(18): 2835–2838.

Lakshmanan FL, Rao RB, Kim WW, Kelsay JL. Magnesium intakes, balances and blood levels of adults consuming self-selected diets. *American Journal of Clinical Nutrition* 1984; **40**: 1380–1389.

Lambert C. The way we eat now. *Harvard Magazine* 2004; May–June: 50–58, 98–99.

Landers P, Wolfe MM, Glore S, Guild R, Phillips L. Effect of weight loss plans on body composition and diet duration. *Journal of Oklahoma State Medical Association* 2002; **95**(5): 329–331.

Lanou AJ, Berkow SE, Barnard ND. Calcium, dairy products, and bone health in children and young adults: a re-evaluation of the evidence. *Pediatrics* 2005; **115**(3): 736–743.

Lefebvre PJ, Scheen AJ. Improving the action of insulin. *Clinical Investigations in Medicine* 1995; **18**: 340–347.

MacIntosh A, Ball K. The effects of a short program of detoxification in disease-free individuals. *Alternative Therapies* 2000; **6**(4): 70–76.

Manninen AH. High-protein weight loss diets and purported adverse effects: where is the evidence? *Sports Nutrition Review Journal* 2004; **1**(1): 45–51.

Marteau P, Seksik P, Jian R. Probiotics and intestinal health effects: a clinical perspective. *British Journal of Nutrition* 2002; **88**(Supplement 1):S51-7. Review.

Mayer-Davis EJ, Levin S, Marshall JA. Heterogeneity in associations between macronutrient intake and lipoprotein profile in individuals with type 2 diabetes. *Diabetes Care* 1999; **22**(10): 1632–1639.

McNair P, Christensen MS, Christiansen C, Madsbad S, Transbol I. Renal hypomagnesaemia in human diabetes mellitus: its relation to glucose homeostasis. *European Journal Clinical Investigation* 1982; **12**(1): 81–85.

Miller JC. International table of glycemic index and glycemic load values. *American Journal of Clinical Nutrition* 2002; **76**(1): 5–56.

Mooradian AD, Failla M, Hoogwerf B, Maryniuk M, Wylie-Rosett J. Selected vitamins and minerals in diabetes. *Diabetes Care* 1994; **17**(5): 464–479.

Morgan KJ, Stampley GL, Zabik ME, Fischer DR. Magnesium and calcium dietary intakes of the U.S. population. *Journal of the American College of Nutrition* 1985; **4**: 195–206.

Muhlbauer B, Schwenk M, Coram WM, Antonin KH, Etienne P, Bieck PR, Douglas FL. Magnesium-L-aspartate-HCl and magnesium-oxide: bioavailability in healthy volunteers. *European Journal of Clinical Pharmacology* 1991; **40**(4): 437–438.

Murray M, Lyon M. *How to Prevent and Treat Diabetes with Natural Medicine*. New York: Penguin Group (USA), 2004.

Nachbar MS, Oppenheim, JD. Lectins in the United States diet: a survey of lectins in commonly consumed foods and a review of the literature. *American Journal of Clinical Nutrition* 1980; **33**(11): 2338–2345.

Nadler JL, Buchanan T, Natarajan R, Antonipillai I, Bergman R, Rude R. Magnesium deficiency produces insulin resistance and increased thromboxane synthesis. *Hypertension* 1993; **21**(6 Pt 2): 1024–1029.

Nakaya Y, Minami A, Harada N, Sakamoto S, Niwa Y, Ohnaka M. Taurine improves insulin sensitivity in the Otsuka Long-Evans Tokushima Fatty rat, a model of spontaneous type 2 diabetes. *American Journal of Clinical Nutrition* 2000; **71**(1): 54–58.

National Academy of Sciences, National Research Council, Food and Nutrition Board. *Diet and Health: Implications for Reducing Chronic Disease Risk*. Washington, DC: National Academy Press, 1989.

No authors listed. Biotin and glucokinase in the diabetic rat. *Nutrition Reviews* 1970; **28**(9): 242–244. Review.

Noakes M, Clifton P. Weight loss, diet composition and cardiovascular risk. *Current Opinion Lipidology* 2004; **15**(1): 31–35.

Noakes M, Keogh JB, Foster PR, Clifton PM. Effect of an energy-restricted, high-protein, low-fat diet relative to a conventional high-carbohydrate, low-fat diet on weight loss, body composition, nutritional status, and markers of cardiovascular health in obese women. *American Journal of Clinical Nutrition* 2005; **81**(6): 1298–1306.

Offenbacher EG, Pi-Sunyer FX. Beneficial effect of chromium-rich yeast on glucose tolerance and blood lipids in elderly subjects. *Diabetes* 1980; **29**(11): 919–925.

Ornish, D. Was Dr Atkins right? *Journal of the American Dietetics Association* 2004; **104**(4): 537–542.

Paolisso G, D'Amore A, Giugliano D, Ceriello A, Varricchio M, D'Onofrio F. Pharmacologic doses of vitamin E improve insulin action in healthy subjects and non-insulin-dependent diabetic patients. *American Journal of Clinical Nutrition* 1993; **57**(5): 650–656.

Paolisso G, Sgambato S, Gambardella A, Pizza G, Tesauro P, Varricchio M, D'Onofrio F. Daily magnesium supplements improve glucose handling in elderly subjects. *American Journal of Clinical Nutrition* 1992; **55**(6): 1161–1167.

Paolisso G, Sgambato S, Pizza G, Passariello N, Varricchio M, D'Onofrio F. Improved insulin response and action by chronic magnesium administration in aged NIDDM subjects. *Diabetes Care* 1989; **12**(4): 265–269.

Parker B, Noakes M, Luscombe N, Clifton P. Effect of a high-protein, high-monounsaturated fat weight loss diet on glycemic control and lipid levels in type 2 diabetes. *Diabetes Care* 2002; **25**(3): 425–430.

Pizzorno JE, Murray TM. *Encyclopaedia of Natural Medicine*, 2nd edn. Little Brown and Company, 1998.

Poortmans JR, Dellalieux O. Do regular high protein diets have potential health risks on kidney function in athletes? *International Journal of Sport Nutrition and Exercise Metabolism* 2000; **10**(1): 28–38.

Popp-Snijders C, Schouten JA, Heine RJ, van der Meer J, van der Veen EA. Dietary supplementation of omega-3 polyunsaturated fatty acids improves insulin sensitivity in non-insulin-dependent diabetes. *Diabetes Research* 1987; **4**(3): 141–147.

Pusztai A, Ewen SW, Grant G, Brown DS, Stewart JC, Peumans WJ, Van Damme EJ, Bardocz S. Antinutritive effects of wheat-germ agglutinin and other N-acetylglucosamine-specific lectins. *British Journal of Nutrition* 1993; **70**(1): 313–321.

Rapuri PB, Gallagher JC, Haynatzka V. Protein intake: effects on bone mineral density and the rate of bone loss in elderly women. *American Journal of Clinical Nutrition* 2003; **77**: 1517–1525.

Rea WJ, Pan Y, Johnson AR, Ross RG, Suyama H, Fenyves EJ. Reduction of chemical sensitivity by means of heat depuration, physical therapy and nutritional supplementation in a controlled environment. *Journal of Nutritional and Environmental Medicine* 1996; **6**: 141–148.

Reddy ST, Wang CY, Sakhaee K, Brinkley L, Pak CY. Effect of low-carbohydrate high-protein diets on acid-base balance, stone-forming propensity, and calcium metabolism. *American Journal of Kidney Disease* 2002; **40**(2): 265–274.

Riales R, Albrink MJ. Effect of chromium chloride supplementation on glucose tolerance and serum lipids including high-density lipoprotein of adult men. *American Journal of Clinical Nutrition* 1981; **34**(12): 2670–2678.

Rizkalla S, Bellisle F, Slama G. Health benefits of low glycaemic index foods, such as pulses, in diabetic patients and healthy individuals. *British Journal of Nutrition* 2002; **88** (Supplement 3): S255–G2.

Schmidt EB, Dyerberg J. Omega 3 fatty acids: current status In cardiovascular medicine. *Drugs* 1994; **47**: 405–424.

Schroecksnadel K, Frick B, Fuchs D. Homocysteine is an independent risk factor for myocardial infarction, in particular fatal myocardial infarction in middle-aged women. *Circulation* 2004; **110**(4): e37–38.

Schroeder HA, Nason AP, Tipton IH. Chromium deficiency as a factor in atherosclerosis. *Journal of Chronic Disease* 1970; **23**: 123–142.

Sears B. *The Zone.* New York: Harper Collins, 1995.

Shahid A, Zuberi SJ, Siddiqui AA, Waqar MA. Genetic markers and duodenal ulcer. *Journal of Pakistani Medical Association* 1997; **47**(5): 135–137.

Sharman MJ, Kraemer WJ, Love DM, Avery NG, Gomez AL, Scheett TP, Volek JS. A ketogenic diet favourably affects serum biomarkers for cardiovascular disease in normal-weight men. *Journal of Nutrition* 2002; **132**(7): 1879–1885.

Shechter Y, Li J, Meyerovitch J, Gefel D, Bruck R, Elberg G, Miller DS, Shisheva A. Insulin-like actions of vanadate are mediated in an insulin-receptor-independent manner via non-receptor protein tyrosine kinases and protein phosphotyrosine phosphatases. *Molecular Cell Biochemistry* 1995; **153**(1–2): 39–47.

Skov AR, Toubro S, Ronn B, Holm L, Astrup A. Randomized trial on protein vs. carbohydrate in ad libitum fat reduced diet for the treatment of obesity. *International Journal of Obesity Related Metabolic Disorders* 1999; **23**(5): 528–536.

Slipko Z, Latuchowska B, Wojtkowska E. Body structure and ABO and Rh blood groups in patients with advanced coronary heart disease after aorto-coronary by-pass surgery. *Polskie Archiwum Medycyny Wewnetrznej* 1994; **91**(1): 55–60.

Sondike SB, Copperman N, Jacobson MS. Effects of a low-carbohydrate diet on weight loss and cardiovascular risk factor in overweight adolescents. *Journal of Pediatrics* 2003; **142**(3): 253–258.

Spencer H, Kramer L, DeBartolo M, Norris C, Osis D. Further studies of the effect of a high protein diet as meat on calcium metabolism. *American Journal of Clinical Nutrition* 1983; **37**(6): 924–929.

St Jeor ST, Howard BV, Prewitt TE, Bovee V, Bazzarre T, Eckel RH. Nutrition Committee of the Council on Nutrition, Physical Activity, and Metabolism of the American Heart Association. Dietary protein and weight reduction: a statement for healthcare professionals from the Nutrition Committee of the Council on Nutrition, Physical Activity, and Metabolism of the American Heart Association. *Circulation* 2001; **104**(15): 1869–1874.

Stutzman FL, Amatuzio DS. Blood and serum magnesium in portal cirrhosis and diabetes mellitus. *Journal of Laboratory Clinical Medicine* 1952; **41**: 215.

Su M, Lu SM, Tian DP, Zhao H, Li XY, Li DR, Zheng ZC. Relationship between ABO blood groups and carcinoma of oesophagus and cardia in Chaoshan inhabitants of China. *World Journal of Gastroenterology* 2001; **7**(5): 657–661.

Suarez A, Pulido N, Casla A, Casanova B, Arrieta FJ, Romero R, Rouira A. Tyrosine kinase activity in insulin receptors from hypomagnesemic rats (abst.317). *Diabetologia* 1992; **35** (suppl. 1): A82.

Sytze Van Dam P. Oxidative stress and diabetic neuropathy: pathophysiological mechanisms and treatment perspectives. *Diabetes Metabolic Research Review* 2002; **18**(3): 176–184.

Toepfer EW, Mertz W. Polansky MM, Roginski EE, Wolf WR. Preparation of chromium-containing material of glucose tolerance factor activity from brewer's yeast extracts and by synthesis. *Journal of Agriculture Food Chemistry* 1977; **25**: 162–166.

Tosiello L. Hypomagnesaemia and diabetes mellitus: a review of clinical implications. *Archive of Internal Medicine* 1996; **156**: 1143.

Turner R. Tight blood glucose control and risk of macrovascular and microvascular complications in type 2 diabetes: UKPDS 38. UK Prospective Diabetes Study. *British Medical Journal* 1998; **317**: 703–713.

University of Surrey (UK), Department of Food Science Homepage. http://portal/surrey. ac.uk/ugstudy/foodscience (accessed January 10 2006).

Urberg M, Zemel MB. Evidence for synergism between chromium and nicotinic acid in the control of glucose tolerance in elderly humans. *Metabolism* 1987; **36**(9): 896–899.

Van Damme EJM, Peumans WJ, Pusztai A, Bardocz S. *Handbook of Plant Lectins: Properties and Biomedical Applications*. London: John Wiley & Sons, Ltd. 1998; pp. 31–50.

Walser, M. Effects of protein intake on renal function and on the development of renal disease, In: *The Role of Protein and Amino Acids in Sustaining and Enhancing Performance*, Institute of Medicine, Washington, DC: National Academy Press, 1999, pp. 137–154.

Walsh CT, Sandstead HH, Prasad AS, Newberne PM, Fraker PJ. Zinc: health effects and research priorities for the 1990s. *Environmental Health Perspective* 1994; **102** (Suppl 2): 5–46.

Wang Q, Yu L-G, Campbell BJ, Milton J, Rhodes, JM. Identification of intact peanut lectin peripheral venous blood. *Lancet* 1998; **352**: 1831–1832.

Whincup PH, Cook DG, Phillips AN, Shaper AG. ABO blood group and ischaemic heart disease in British men. *British Medical Journal* 1990; **300**(6741): 1679–1682.

Willett W. *Eat, Drink, and Be Healthy: The Harvard Medical School Guide to Healthy Eating*. Fireside, 2001.

Willett W. *World Health News*, Boston. March 29, 2000.

Wolcott W, Fahey T. *The Metabolic Typing Diet*. Broadway Books, 2000.

Wolever TM, Jenkins DJ, Jenkins AL, Josse RG. The glycemic index: methodology and clinical implications. *American Journal of Clinical Nutrition* 1991; **54**(5): 846–854.

Yajnik CS, Smith RF, Hockaday TD, Ward NI. Fasting plasma magnesium concentrations and glucose disposal in diabetes. *British Medical Journal (Clinical Research Edition)* 1984; **288**(6423): 1032–1034.

Yang F, Tan HM, Wang H. Hyperhomocysteinemia and atherosclerosis. *Sheng Li Xue Bao* 2005; **57**(2): 103–114.

Yeh GY, Eisenberg DM, Kaptchuk TJ, Phillips RS. Systematic review of herbs and dietary supplements for glycemic control in diabetes. *Diabetes Care* 2003; **26**(4): 1277–1294.

Young CM, Scanlan SS, Im HS, Lutwak L. Effect of body composition and other parameters in obese young men of carbohydrate level of reduction diet. *American Journal of Clinical Nutrition* 1971; **24**(3): 290–296.

Young, E. http://www.smh.com.au/articles/2004/11/11/1100021915101.html. 2004.

6 Essential Oils (Aromatherapy)

Trish Dunning

6.1 Introduction

Aromatherapy is a specialised form of herbal medicine that uses essential oils. Essential oils are derived from plants but they have a very different chemical composition and therefore effects from the herb from which they are extracted. A number of definitions of 'aromatherapy' exist, but in the context of this chapter aromatherapy refers to the controlled use of essential oils derived from named botanical sources using a variety of application (external) or administration (internal) methods to promote and support health and well-being (Dunning 2005).

In this context, 'controlled' refers to practitioners holding appropriate qualifications, having an accurate diagnosis, selecting appropriate essential oils, practising according to professional and regulatory standards, and monitoring the effects, applying a quality use of medicines approach (Dunning 2005). Essential oils have a long association with health care and are selected for their specific therapeutic properties according to traditional use and evidence where it exists.

Essential oil use is well documented throughout history in perfumery, medicine and religion, often in association with massage, for example, in Ancient Egypt, Rome, Greece, China, India and the Middle East. Chamerland in 1887 and Cadeac and Marnier in 1888 published studies describing the antibacterial properties of essential oils, especially against glandular and yellow fevers. The term 'aromatherapy' means using essential oils derived from plants and is attributed to René Gattefosse, a chemist who burned his hands in a laboratory explosion in 1937. Gattefosse plunged his hands in a vat of lavender essential oil and they healed with little scarring or pain. He subsequently used essential oils in wound care in military hospitals in World War I.

About the same time Couvreur was writing about the medical application of essential oils, and Jean Valnet used essential oils in military hospitals during the Indochina War for their antiseptic properties and continued using them in civilian practice after the war. Penfold in Australia researched tea tree oil and, in Italy,

Gatti and Crayola were publishing their findings about the psychological effects. Maury, another chemist, largely used essential oils in beauty therapy especially in the UK. Her practice of using low doses of essential oils applied in massage had a major effect on aromatherapy practice in many countries. In modern aromatherapy including health care, essential oils are applied in massages, baths, spritzers, skin creams and gels, inhalations and compresses, and administered internally in capsules, pessaries and on inhalant wicks.

6.2 Aromatherapy Care Models

There are three main aromatherapy care models:

1. Medical aromatherapy, also known as aromatology or aromatic medicine, which is largely used in France and involves the internal use of essential oils often in high doses. Internal use is restricted to doctors who undertake specific training beyond their medical degree.
2. Subtle aromatherapy or aromachology is more often used in Germany where odours are used to promote well-being.
3. Topical application and inhalation, most frequently used in the UK and Australia.

The extent of essential oil use by or for people with diabetes is largely unknown although aromatherapy is one of the most widely used complementary therapies in the British National Health Service (Thorgrimsen *et al.* 2005). In Australia, Dunning (2003a) found 16 of 38 diabetes educators used complementary therapies in the management of people with diabetes. Of these, three used aromatherapy. Likewise, Sabo *et al.* (1999) found 63 per cent of 829 diabetes educators in the USA recommended a range of complementary therapies, including massage, to their patients but aromatherapy was not mentioned. Since massage is often combined with essential oils, it is possible patients were exposed to essential oils if they followed the diabetes educator's recommendation.

6.3 Essential Oils

Essential oils are volatile complex chemical compounds containing the odiferous elements of plants extracted by distillation, which produces little change in the oil. Distillation uses the volatility (boiling point) of the components of a mixture to enable them to be separated. Oils extracted using mechanical pressure (expression) and dry distilled oils are also defined as essential oils (International Standards Organisation). Hypercritical carbon dioxide extraction is a relatively recent extraction method and yields very pure oils. Each essential oil contains many chemical compounds that give it its specific pharmacological properties. The essential oil components are formed via secondary metabolism and stored within specialised cells. Only a small percentage of the essential oils produced end up in aromatherapy; the majority are used in the food, perfume and medicine industries (Burfield 2005).

Aromatherapists prefer to use whole unadulterated essential oils rather than isolated individual chemicals or synthetic oils because whole oils have synergistic and quenching properties, some of which have been confirmed by research (Lis-Balchin et al. 1997). Other common extraction methods include solvent extraction, maceration and enfleurage. Most of these methods leave some plant material such as waxes or solvent materials in the oils, which means they are not technically 'pure'. Synthetic and fragrant oils are generally not recommended for use on the body. The major chemical constituents found in essential oils are shown in Table 6.1. Aromatherapists usually blend several essential oils to address the various components of the condition being treated. In addition, pre-formulated proprietary blends (fixed blend) are readily available, for example, analgesic and sedative blends. These may be diluted ready for use or concentrated, in which case they need to be diluted before use.

Carrier substances

In most cases essential oils are not used undiluted. They are applied or administered dispersed in a range of carrier substances, many of which also have therapeutic properties. Carrier substances include a range of cold pressed vegetable oils such as sweet almond, macadamia, olive oil and macerated oils such as calendula and St. John's wort (*Hypericum perforatum*) and hydrosols (the water that remains after essential oils are removed by steam extraction), *Aloe vera*. When used internally, essential oils are contained in incipients such as gel and wax capsules and suppositories.

Essential oil composition standards

Many readily available 'essential oils' are adulterated, or contaminated by other means, which changes their therapeutic effects. At present no agency certifies that essential oils are 'therapeutic grade'. A number of aromatherapy companies have their own internal standards and testing processes but no single agency is responsible for certifying that essential oils meet acceptable chemical composition standards, that is, minimum and maximum percentages of the major components. Current analytical standards include the pharmacopoeias of the UK (BP), Europe, and the USA (USP), material safety data sheets (MSDS) and monographs of individual essential oils such as those produced by: Essential Oil Association Inc (EOA), Scientific Foundation for Herbal Medicinal Products (ESCOP), the German E Commission, and the standards of independent certifying bodies such as: the International Standards Organisation (ISO), the Research Institute for Fragrance Materials (RIFM), the International Fragrance Association (IFRA) and the Association Française de Normalisation (AFNOR).

The ISO and AFNOR standards are often accepted as being the most reliable indicators of quality (but not therapeutic effect) and differentiate between the different grades of essential oils (*Essential Oils Desk Reference 2001*). Generally, if an essential oil contains two or more marker compounds outside the ISO

Table 6.1 Major chemical constituents of essential oils, their reported properties and examples of essential oils that contain high proportions of the particular chemical in their make-up. Reproduced with permission from Australian Scholarly Publishing.

Major chemical constituent	Reported therapeutic properties	Example essential oils
Terpenes Terpenes are hydrocarbons based on the isoprene unit where the compound occurs in chains. Isoprene units join together in groups. **a) monoterpenes** $C^{10}H^{16}$ 10 carbon atoms usually end in 'ene' d-limonene terpinene ocimene pinene myrcene	Highly volatile and evaporate quickly Oxidise readily when they are double bonded Bacteriacidal Antiviral Stimulant Decongestant Antiseptic Analgesic	Almost all essential oils contain some terpenes They are high in most citrus oils, e.g. lemon, lime, mandarin, Orange Angelica Juniper berry Frankincense
b) Sesquiterpenes $C^{15}H^{24}$ 15 carbon atoms e.g. Caryophyllene, Viridiflorene Chamazulene Elemene Bisabolol	Largest group of terpenes in the plant world They make a significant contribution to the oil's odour Only a few are volatile, prone to oxidation Anti-inflammatory Anti-allergenic Antibacterial Antiseptic Calming	Myrrh Cedarwood German chamomile Ginger
c) Diterpenes $C^{20}H^{32}$ camphorene	Not common due to their high molecular weight. Similar properties to sesquiterpenes but have a higher boiling point and lower oxidation rate. Antifungal, antiviral, may be expectorant.	
d) Triterpenes and $C^{30}H^{48}$ **Tetraterpenes** $C^{40}H^{56}$ Also exist in essential oils but are more common in herbs as sterols, steroids and saponins carotenoids		

Alcohols
usually end in 'ol',
e.g. monoterpenols
e.g. geraniol, linalool,
citronellol terpin-4-ol,
menthol Nerol
Isopulegol
There may be different
chemotypes depending on
the growing conditions of
the plant.

Considered most
therapeutically beneficial.
They have a soft, sweet,
herbaceous or woody odour
and are usually safe.
Antibacterial (*E coli, staph
aureus*)
Antifungal (*Candida
albicans*)
Vasoconstrictive
Mild local anaesthetic effect
Stimulant and tonifying to
the immune system Warming

Ho leaf
Rosewood
Tea tree
Palmarosa
Rosa damascena
Sweet marjoram

b) Sesquiterpenols e.g.
farnesol
viridiflorol
patchoulol
alpha-santalol
alpha-bisabolol
Farnesol

General tonic
Anti-inflammatory
May induce vascular
dilatation
Antiviral (*Herpes simplex*)

Jasmine
Niaouli
Patchouli
Vetiver
German chamomile
Rose

Phenols have a benzene ring
in their structure also often
end in 'ol', e.g. thymol,
carvacrol, eugenol.
Some appear as phenolic
ethers and have similar
preoprties to phenols but are
more powerul and may be
neurotoxic in large doses.
Anisole
Antheole
Safrole
Methyl chavicol (estragole)

Phenol (carbolic acid) is a
potent chemical. Not very
volatile. They are the most
reactive agents found in
essential oils and combine
with other positively
charged molecules.
They have a medicinal
odour
More likely to irritate
mucous membranes and
skin. Very stimulating to the
immune system.
Antibacterial (*staph aureus,
pseudomonas, bacilli ceres*)
Antidepressive
Sedative in large doses
May stimulate healing
Similar to phenols.
The odour varies from light
and sweet to pungent and
medicinal often being
similar to liquorice.
If ingested in large
quantities they may be
psychotrophic.
Antispasmodic.
Anti-infectious.
May be neurotoxic at high
oral doses.

Ajowan
West Indian Bay
Cinnamon leaf
Clove bud
Oregano (CT thymol)
Summer savory
Thyme
Basil CT chavicol
Tarragon
Aniseed
Fennel
Star anise
Vanilla
Nutmeg

Table 6.1 (Continued)

Major chemical constituent	Reported therapeutic properties	Example essential oils
Aldehydes often end in 'al', e.g. citral neral geranial cinnamaldehyde cuminaldehyde	Relatively stable volatility. Generally have a sharp lemony, floral odour Readily react with other molecules and oxidise to carboxylic acids, which may cause skin irritation so careful storage is essential. Vasodilator Sedative Anti-inflammatory Antifungal Antipyretic	Lemon verbena Melissa May chang *Eucalyptus citriodora* Citronella Cinnamon bark
Ketones often end in 'one', e.g. menthone camphor thuyone pulgeone pinocamphone Piperitone Verbenone Carvone Jasmone	Ketone essential oils should be diluted. There are a range of odour types from green and oily to fruity, fresh mint and dry. Sedative Mucolytic Analgesic Cell regeneration and wound healing Some ketones are reputed to cause convulsions in large doses if given orally. These oils are not generally used in aromatherapy (wormwood, tansy, pennyroyal, buchu) Some camphor-containing oils are used (Ho leaf, sage, rosemary CT camphor hyssop) and care may be required if there is a possibility of causing seizures e.g. known epilepsy	Aniseed Carraway Dill Hyssop Rue Rosemary CT camphor and CT Everlasting Lavandin Sage
Esters and acids Acids often end in 'ic'. They react with alcohols to form esters. cinnamic acid anisic acid benzoic acid Esters in 'ate' e.g. Many esters in essential oils are formed as reaction	Plant acids are highly soluble in water and high concentrations are found in hydrosols but they are rare in oils. Acids combine with alcohols to form esters, which are very odorous molecules and often have fruity notes. The odour molecules consist of the	Lavandin Lavender Clary sage Roman chamomile Jasmine absolute Myrtle

products during distillation.
linalyl acetate
benzyl benzoate
benzyl acetate
eugenyl acetate
methyl salicylate
neryl acetate
methyl benzoate
linalyl acetate

subgroups amines and imines, which give some essential oils an 'animalistic' odour, e.g. jasmine. They balance perfume blends.
Acids are stimulants
Esters are antispasmodic, anti-inflammatory and immunomodulant.
Effective for skin rashes.

Oxides
often end in 'ole' e.g.
1,8-cineole
methofuran
rose oxide
linalool oxide

Volatile.
Can be skin irritants.
Strongest odourants.
May decompose and thicken over time.
May cause destruction of liver enzymes (cytochrome P450) if taken orally.
Expectorant.
Have a drying effect on skin.
Anti-inflammatory, reduce E2, prostaglandins and leukotrines.
Can irritate the skin.

Eucalyptus
Cardamon
Rosemary CT cineole
Rosa damascena
Geranium
Niaouli
Lavandula latifolia

Lactones
often end in 'in' or 'ine', e.g.
helaniline
nepetalactone

Found in expressed oils and absolutes.
Similar properties to ethers and ketones.
Can be neurotoxic and cause skin allergies.
Big molecules and not found in may oils used in aromatherapy.
Mucolytic.
Expectorant.
Anti-inflammatory.
Antipyretic

Arnica
Catnip
Elecampane
Sweet inule

Coumarins
furocoumarin
*(bergaptene)

Anticoagulant. Use with caution if the person is on anticoagulant therapy.
Sedative.
Potentially carcinogenic in combination with UV radiation on the skin.

Cold pressed citrus oils
Bergamot

Notes: Volatility is an important concept to some aspects of aromatherapy. It refers to the ability of a substance to evaporate, which allows molecules to be present in the air, enter the nose and be detected as an odour. The molecules move from the vaporiser, an area of high concentration, to the air, an area of low concentration by diffusion. Volatile substances readily evaporate.
The method of extraction can influence the terpene content e.g. solvent extracted oils may contain none or very low amounts of terpenes compared to a steam distilled essential oil from the same plant material.
* The recommended safe level of bergaptene is 0.0015 per cent i.e. in 100 gm oil no more than 0.0015 per cent. A typical bergamot contains 0.3 per cent bergaptene and it must be diluted (IFRA).

or AFNOR range, the essential oil does not meet the standard. The Australian Therapeutic Goods Association (TGA) bases essential oil (and herbal preparation) risk on the BP standards and advice of relevant experts for listing purposes (AUSTL).

A range of analytical techniques are used to determine the chemical composition of essential oils and detect additive components (adulteration), including gas chromatography (GC trace), chiral analysis, mass spectrometry, infra-red spectroscopy, optical rotation, specific gravity and refractive index. A number of factors affect the composition of essential oils including storage conditions. Inappropriate storage can cause oxidation, particularly in essential oils containing terpene hydrocarbons and citral rich essential oils such as lemongrass (*Cymbopogon citrates, C flexuosus*), lemon (*Citrus limon*), and orange (*Citrus aurantium*). Oxidation products increase the potential to cause skin irritation (*Essential Oil Desk Reference 2001*; Guba 2004).

Composition standards are an important aspect of the essential oil risk profile and quality control procedures and can help practitioners assess whether essential oils are safe to use. There are a great many 'essential oils' on the market that do not undergo any analytical testing and have no guarantee of purity or quality. Practitioners are advised to buy from and advise patients to buy from reputable sources to ensure essential oils meet the standards for patient safety and for medico-legal reasons. It is important to use essential oils that do the following:

- meet accepted essential oils standards;
- are accompanied by the results of analytical tests and/or a statement from the supplier that guarantees their purity such as Therapeutic Grade Essential Oil (TGEO) or 100 per cent essential oil (PEO);
- are stored and handled appropriately (ISO [standard]/TR 210: 1999);
- are regulated by bodies such as the TGA in Australia where they are listed products and the British Pharmacopoeia (BP) in the UK. Listing arrangements do not necessarily support the benefit or efficacy of essential oils but they indicate the level of risk associated with their use and the quality of the manufacturing standards.

Labels are another aspect of standards. General rules for labelling containers are defined in ISO standard TR 211: 1999. Labels should state the following:

- botanical name and species of the plant the oil was extracted from;
- parts of the plant used;
- country of origin. Growing conditions affect the composition of essential oils;
- extraction method;
- statement of purity such as PEO or TGEO;
- indications for use;
- precautions and/or contraindications;
- batch number;
- expiry date.

Pharmacological effects of essential oils

Essential oils are credited with a wide diversity of therapeutic effects according to their chemical composition, traditional use and some research, see Table 6.2. The main therapeutic effects are:

- *Antibacterial, antiviral, antifungal* against a range of bacteria (*Staphylococci aureus, Escheria coli, Streptococcus, pseudomonas, Bacillus subtilis, Klebsiella, enterococci*); fungi (*Candida trichopophyton*); and viruses (*Herpes simplex*).
- *Mucolytic and expectorant.* Mucolytic oils break down mucous, allowing easier removal and enhance the bacterial effects of essential oils or medications. Mucolytic essential oils may also break down pus and aid wound healing.
- *Anti-inflammatory.* Well-known anti-inflammatory oils are *Lavandula augustifolia*, and chamomile.
- *Wound healing* such as Everlasting and rose hip carrier oil.
- *Antispasmodic* essential oils aid digestion, reduce abdominal pain and flatulence, and relieve smooth muscle spasm, for example, peppermint (*Mentha piperita*).
- *Sedative.* Calm the nervous system.
- A range of *psychological* effects through their action on the limbic system. Odour is encoded in memory along with the associated experience and feelings at the time. Volatile substances can have an effect even when they are not detected, for example, pheromones.
- *Analgesic.* Effects may be due to anti-inflammatory properties, local action on nerves, as well as a psychological component. Well-known examples are clove oil for dental pain, and oil of wintergreen for muscular pain.

Pharmacokinetics and pharmacodynamics of essential oils

Figure 6.1 illustrates the pathways by which essential oils enter and leave the body. Essential oils are absorbed in a similar way to topical medicines depending on the application/administration method.

Inhaled essential oils readily cross the blood–brain barrier and enter the limbic system, cortex and hypothalamus and exert physical and psychological effects. Inhaled essential oils have a fast onset of action in the brain and limbic systems but a slower action on physical systems, see Figure 6.1. It is unrealistic to expect low doses of inhaled essential oil to reach internal organs in any quantity and have high levels of bioavailability. A number of structures respond to odour molecules such as the trigeminal nerve, the spatial nerve and the brain. Some effects occur through intercellular signalling, and by stimulating or inhibiting hormones such as adrenalin and serotonins. There is a wide variation in the threshold at which people detect odours. The study of inhaled essential oils is known as olfaction.

Most studies concerning the pharmacodynamics and pharmacokinetics of essential oils were undertaken on animals. From this research it appears that essential oils take between 72 and 120 hours to be absorbed, metabolised and excreted depending on the size of the animal, the properties of the essential oil, the

Table 6.2 Broad actions of essential oils for each body system and some examples of essential oils that can be used. The list is by no means exhaustive and selection should be based on a thorough assessment, history and examination and consideration given to other factors that may need to be addressed such as stopping smoking, improving diet, relevant precautions for serious disease, and contraindications for specific methods and age. Reproduced with permission from Australian Scholarly Publishing.

Body system	Essential oil action	Essential oil examples	Application methods
Respiratory	Antispasmodic. Antibacterial. Antiviral. Antitussitive Expectorant Febrifuge (reduces fever)	chamomile, cypress, sweet thyme, bergamot, ginger, tea tree, cajeput, rosemary, eucalyptus, sandalwood, hyssop, black pepper	Massage (local or whole body) Inhalation Gargle Bath Nasal wick
Circulatory	Hypotensive Antihypertensive Astringent	lavender, ylang ylang, marjoram, geranium, lemon, clary sage, black pepper, rosemary, sweet thyme, cypress	Massage Bath Ointment, e.g. for haemorrhoids
Digestive	Antispasmodic Stimulate appetite Carminative to reduce nausea and flatulence, Stimulant to relieve constipation Increase flow of bile and liver function	chamomile, fennel, peppermint, bergamot, orange, lemon, cardamom, peppermint, dill, lavender, peppermint, rosemary, lavender, myrrh	Abdominal compress Tea Bath Massage Gargle or mouthwash to treat mouth problems such as ulcers or halitosis Gel applied to sore gums
Muscular	Anti-inflammatory Detoxify Reduce spasm Rubefacient Analgesic	chamomile, lavender, marjoram, black pepper, thyme, cedarwood, lemon, rosemary, juniper, black pepper, ginger, rosemary, sweet birch, oil of wintergreen, hypericum carrier oil	Massage Compresses – cold, hot Ointment
Endocrine	Adrenal stimulant Hypoglycaemic agents Balance thyroid Phytosteroids, phyto-oestrogen	clary sage, basil, rosemary, pine, geranium, juniper berry, frankincense, myrrh	Massage Bath Perfume
Nervous	Sedative and hypnotic Stimulant,	clary sage, marjoram, valerian, hops,	Inhalation Bath

	Boost energy	neroli, German	Perfume
	Rebalance	chamomile, black	Pulse point
	Antidepressive	pepper, coriander,	On pillow
	Analgesia	peppermint,	Compress
		bergamot, geranium,	
		juniper, lavender,	
		patchouli,	
		sandalwood,	
		cedarwood, rosewood,	
		vetiver, rose	
Immune	Antibacterial	tea tree, lemongrass,	Massage such as
	Antiviral	thyme, frankincense,	Lymphatic drainage
	Increase white cell	lavender, rosemary,	
	function	angelica, fennel,	
	Detoxify	juniper berry,	
	Wound healing	eucalyptus, lavender,	
		tea tree, lemon,	
		peppermint, thyme,	
		benzoin, marjoram,	
		rosemary, lavender,	
		chamomile	
Skin	Antiseptic	Lavender, tea tree,	Bath
	Anti-inflammatory	chamomile, geranium,	Pessary
	Cicatrisant	neroli, bergamot,	Powder
	Deodorant	cypress, cedarwood,	Deodorant
	Fungicide	eucalyptus, rosemary,	Poultice
	Parasiticide	lemongrass	Compress
	Local analgesia		Ointment
Reproductive	Antispasmodic	chamomile, clary	Massage
	Emmenagogue	sage, lavender, rose,	Sitz bath
	Galactagogue	fennel, marjoram,	Compress, for
	Hormone balance	lemongrass,	example, to the
	Aphrodisiacs	geranium,	perineum, or breasts
	Analgesic	frankincense, melissa,	Inhalation
	Menopausal	ylang ylang, neroli,	Perfume
	symptoms	rose	

dose and dose interval, application/administration method and the state of health. While animal studies may not directly apply to humans, they do provide important pharmacological information.

There is ample evidence that essential oils are absorbed through the skin, but the absorption rate of the various chemical components in the particular essential oil varies and depends on a number of factors including the size of the individual essential oil molecules. Small molecules penetrate faster than large molecules. Jager *et al.* (1992) detected linalool and linalyl acetate (components of lavender) in the blood 5 minutes after a 10-minute abdominal massage using 2 per cent *Lavandula angustifolia* in peanut oil. Carvone was detected in the blood 10 minutes after massage (Jager *et al.* 2001) and salicylate in the subcutaneous tissue within

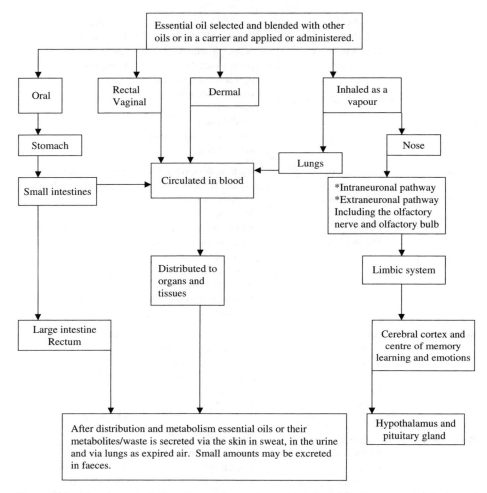

Figure 6.1 Flowchart depicting the pathways by which essential oils enter the body and their metabolic and waste products leave the body. *Intraneuronal pathway takes hours to days for substances to different areas of the brain and involves axonal transport. The extraneuronal pathway most probably involves transport through the perineural channels that deliver substances directly brain tissue, cerebrospinal fluid or both and through which substances reach the central nervous system within minutes (Frey 2002).

30 minutes for up to 60 minutes after 20 per cent methyl salicylate was applied to the forearm (Cross *et al.* 1997). Larger molecules such as coumarin take up to an hour to penetrate (Ford *et al.* 2001). In addition, covering the area after the oils are applied increases the absorption rate to 70 per cent of the dose compared to only 4 per cent in uncovered skin (Bronaugh 1999). However, if the skin is broken, or the stratum corneum damaged or thin due to trauma, burns, age or some forms of dermatitis, up to 100 per cent of the applied dose may be absorbed (Guba 2000).

This information is important when selecting essential oils for specific purposes, for example, when fast pain relief is required. An essential oil that takes 10 minutes to penetrate may be a better choice than one that takes an hour. Combining an essential oil with a fast onset of action with one that acts more slowly may produce more sustained relief and require fewer reapplications.

Research has been underway for some time to determine whether essential oils can enhance absorption of topically applied conventional medicines. Components such as D-limonene, 1,8-cineole and nerolidol have been shown to enhance penetration of both hydrophilic and lipophilic substances (Cornwall *et al.* 1994). Such research suggests topical application of essential oils may be contraindicated or caution required if topical conventional medicines such as antianginal agents and hormones are used at the same time, or dose adjustments might be needed. It also suggests they could be used together for a faster onset of action in some circumstances such as angina.

6.4 Essential Oils and Diabetes Education and Management

Essential oils can complement diabetes education and management provided they are selected and applied/administered appropriately. The effects of the essential oils should not be assessed in isolation from the application/administration method. There is good traditional evidence for using essential oils in some aspects of diabetes management and some limited research evidence. Potential benefits include:

- achieving emotional and physical balance, which improves metabolic control, and reduces complication and infection risk;
- managing the symptoms associated with long-term complications such as pain, skin itch, peripheral neuropathy, foot ulcers, stress and anxiety, muscle tension, poor circulation, sleep disorders, nausea and reduced bowel motility in gastroparesis;
- enhancing memory and recall in diabetes education sessions;
- improving appetite and nutritional status;
- providing prevention, for example, boosting immunity as a preventative measure or during prolonged stress;
- maintaining skin integrity and skin condition in foot care and vascular insufficiency in the legs where ulceration is a risk, and in end stage renal disease;
- reducing isolation and improving the independence of visually impaired people by acting as location cues, and in pet care if they have a guide dog;
- enhancing counselling sessions.

In some cases essential oils might complement the effects of conventional medicines such as oral glucose-lowering agents and enable lower doses to be used. For example, reducing stress may reduce insulin resistance and improve glucose uptake.

People with diabetes usually require several conventional medicines to achieve metabolic targets and actual and potential medicine/essential oil interactions need to be considered, bearing in mind that information about such interactions is limited. Possible adverse events include bruising if the patient is using anticoagulants and massage is used to apply the essential oils. Essential oils with a high eugenol content, or oil of wintergreen and white birch may be contraindicated in these circumstances. Citral rich essential oils may be contraindicated for internal use and in the presence of glaucoma. Massage should be very gentle, see Chapter 13. Eucalyptus may enhance the effects of glucose-lowering agents and predispose the person to hypoglycaemia (Springhouse 2001).

Therefore, a number of factors need to be considered when selecting essential oils, assuming the treatment is provided by or under the direction of a qualified aromatherapist. These factors include:

- holistic patient assessment to determine their physical, psychological and spiritual status and whether essential oils are indicated;
- conventional management regimen. It is imperative that essential oils be considered as part of the overall management plan rather than 'added on', to achieve integrated continuity of care;
- the relationship between the practitioner and the client;
- pharmacological actions and safety of particular essential and carrier substances, contraindications, and interactions with conventional or other complementary medicines the individual may be taking (Quality Use of Essential Oils (QUEO) (Dunning 2005));
- the application method, for example, some people may dislike being touched, massage may cause bruising. Inhaling essential oils is likely with most external application methods. It is difficult to predict the effects of odour on individuals. In addition, volatile substances can have an effect without the person necessarily being aware of an odour, for example, pheromones, which influence sexual behaviour, are odourless. Therefore, the effects of essential oils on other people in the vicinity, including the therapist need to be considered. Taking an 'odour history' is an important part of an aromatherapy assessment;
- the evidence base, which might be traditional use or research.

The actual process of selecting essential oils is the same as the process for selecting conventional medicines or procedures but different terms might be used, for example, 'terrain': 'Terrain is the potential makeup of the genetic elements which have modelled the organism in a certain structured neuro-endocrinal state, and a particular functional structure which is the result of these genetic elements' (Lapraz 1995).

Some nurse aromatherapists undertake assessments according to Gordon's Functional Health Patterns (Buckle 1997). Dossey *et al.* (1995) described an holistic assessment process that makes provision for continual assessment, identifying opportunities to enhance health through health education, self-care, and establishing appropriate attitudes and behaviours, which is an important aspect of diabetes management. The application/administration method that will be used to deliver the essential oils must also be considered.

Using essential oils in diabetes management

Price (1993) and Worwood (1996) list a range of essential oils as being 'good for diabetes' for example:

- *Eucalyptus species*
- *Thymus vulgaris* (thyme)
- *Pinus sylvestrus* (pine)
- *Aabies siberica* (pine)
- *Foeniculum vulgare* (fennel)
- *Anthemis nobilis* (Roman chamomile)
- *Citrus limon* (lemon)
- *Coriandrum sativum* (coriander)
- *Salvia sclarea* (clary sage)
- *Rosmarinus officinalis* (rosemary), however, one study in rabbits found rosemary, chemotype not known, caused hyperglycaemia.
- *Vetiver zizanoides* (vetivert).

However, Price and Worwood do not define 'good for diabetes' or indicate the mechanism of action of any of these essential oils with respect to diabetes. Other authors state that aromatherapy is contraindicated in diabetes and provide a list of specific essential oils to avoid without indicating why they are contraindicated. For example, Lawless (2001: 29) states angelica should be 'avoided in all cases of diabetes', Sellar (1992: 5) is less dogmatic, merely stating 'some say diabetes'. However, with an appropriate assessment and application method, and in appropriate doses, angelica may have mental health benefits, aid transitions, and relieve the abdominal discomfort of gastroparesis when applied in abdominal compresses.

Hypoglycaemic effects of essential oils

There is limited evidence to support a direct hypoglycaemic effect of specific essential oils although it is possible some orally administered essential oils could stimulate insulin production or glucose uptake. Worwood (1996: 110) lists geranium (*Pelargonium graveolens*) and juniper berry (*Juniperus communis*) as 'hypoglycaemics: for helping to balance blood sugar levels' but does not indicate the mechanism of action or doses. Reducing stress reduces stress hormones levels that contribute to hyperglycaemia, therefore, improved blood glucose control may be a secondary benefit of reduced stress. However, research is needed to determine whether essential oils have direct hypoglycaemic properties and their mechanism of action, and if they do, the most effective application/administration method, doses and dose intervals.

Essential oil effects on blood lipids

Hyperlipidaemia often accompanies hyperglycaemia. In diabetes, high cholesterol, high triglycerides and low HDL are common. Although normalising blood glucose helps control blood lipids, lipid lowering agents are frequently necessary. At present there is insufficient evidence of a lipid-lowering effect of essential oils. However, essential oils such as lavender, peppermint and rosemary are cholagogues (stimulate bile), which may play a role in fat metabolism. It is likely they would need to be taken internally to achieve large enough doses to have direct lipid-lowering effects but external use may have secondary lipid-lowering effects by reducing blood glucose through reducing stress.

Effects on hypertension and cardiovascular disease

The cardiovascular system plays an important role in the distribution of essential oils within the body, thus changes in the cardiovascular system may affect their distribution and therapeutic effects, and thus the choice of essential oils, doses and dose intervals. Hypertension is a common complication of diabetes and plays a large role in the development of retinopathy, cardiovascular disease and renal disease. Unpleasant, trigeminally stimulating odours cause an increase in blood pressure (Allen 1988). Stress may play a role in short-term elevation of blood pressure (pain, acute illness). Thus stress reduction may be important in these settings.

Some authors suggest essential oils dilate the peripheral blood vessels, reduce oedema, and lower blood pressure, for example, (*Cananga odorata*) ylang ylang, (*Lavandula angustifolia*) lavender, and (*Origanum marjorana*) sweet marjoram in a cold pressed carrier oil and applied as a massage (Battaglia 1995). Rekieten and Rekieten (1957) demonstrated 1-menthol dilated systemic blood vessels and reduced blood pressure in laboratory settings, but the clinical applicability of their findings is not known. Frazer and Kerr (1993) recorded 'improved' systolic blood pressure before and after back massage in seven elderly residents in an aged care setting but there are methodological limitations to this study. Massage alone reduces muscle tension and lowers blood pressure, see Chapter 13, but it is not known whether the combination of massage and essential oils is more effective than either treatment alone. Battaglia (1995) states (*Hyssopus officinalis*) hyssop, (*Rosmarinus officinalis*) rosemary, (*Salvia officinalis*) sage and (*Thymus vulgaris*) thyme are contraindicated in people with hypertension but does not say why, and there does not appear to be any evidence to support the contraindication (Guba 2000).

Cardiac investigations and surgery

Stevenson (1994) randomised 100 post-cardiac surgery patients into four groups who received (1) 20-minute aromatherapy foot massage with essential oils; (2) 20-minute foot massage with an inactive carrier; (3) counselling; and (4) no intervention. Heart rate, respiratory rate and blood pressure were measured and a modified Spielberger questionnaire (STAI) was used to assess psychological parameters, pain, anxiety, tension, calm, rest and relaxation, before and after the massage on five occasions. The physiological changes were not significant but the psychological effects were statistically and clinically significant and persisted at the two-hour follow-up. STAI scores improved by eight points compared to 0.7 in the control group and 1.32 in the counselling groups. Managing psychological stress using essential oils is reported to reduce fear during acute coronary events (George 1997).

Borromeo (1995: 135) assessed the effects of inhaled lavender from cotton balls on anxiety using the State Trait Anxiety Scale and a repeated measures design in 25 coronary care patients, and sleep quality using a visual analogue scale. The effects were assessed 60 minutes after inhalation commenced and again the next day. Borromeo concluded that passively diffused lavender did not significantly affect anxiety or sleep. Peppermint has been shown to reduce nausea following cardiac surgical procedures such as stenting (Anderson and Gross 2004).

Precautions in people with cardiac disease

Applying essential oils in the same area as topical conventional medicines such as nitroglycerin is contraindicated because the essential oils can enhance the absorption and affect the efficacy of topical medicines. The pressure of massage should be light in patients on aspirin or anticoagulants especially if essential oils with anticoagulant properties are used to reduce the risk of bruising and bleeding. Mentholated products such as cigarettes and confectionery have caused cardiac fibrillation in patients on quinidine, which suggests concomitant use of essential oils rich in menthol should be used with caution in patients taking quinidine-containing medicines (Thomas 1962). The safety aspects of using essential oils around electrical equipment and medical gases such as oxygen must be taken into consideration.

Urinary system

The urinary system plays a key role in:

- eliminating medicines, essential oils and waste products, particularly urea, creatinine, phosphates and sulphates;
- regulating fluid balance and blood pressure and plays a role in the production of red blood cells by releasing erythropoietin when the oxygen tension in the renal blood flow is reduced;
- converting inactive vitamin D to its active form (1, 25 hydroxycholecalciferol), which is necessary to maintain calcium balance;
- producing prostaglandin E (PGE) and prostaglandin I (PGI), which have vasodilatory effects and play a role in maintaining renal blood flow.

Herbal medicines are implicated in renal damage (Combest *et al.* 2005) but it is not clear whether essential oils also cause renal damage. Nephropathy is a well-known long-term complication of diabetes and caution is required when using any pharmacological substance especially when renal function is compromised. The renal status should be assessed before using essential oils internally in people with diabetes but topical and inhaled applications are likely to be safe. Like conventional medicines, some essential oils may be contraindicated or dose or dose frequency adjustments may be required.

Anecdotally, essential oils may be used to do the following:

- stimulate the circulatory and lymphatic systems, which assists in removing excess fluid and waste products and relieving oedema;
- manage pain;
- relieve skin irritation/itch and maintain skin condition in patients with end stage renal disease and those on dialysis;
- stimulate appetite in patients on dialysis;
- reduce nausea;
- improve sleep;
- manage anxiety, emotional distress and depression, which often accompany end stage renal disease;
- provide spiritual care in end stage renal disease.

Casey and Kerr (2003) established an aromatherapy clinic in the Renal Unit at Westmead Hospital in Sydney. Their project involved educating staff and offering aromatherapy treatments to patients. Treatments consisted of hand, foot, neck and shoulder massages, foot and hand baths, compresses and inhalations depending on the individual's needs and desires, but primarily for emotional support. Most treatments averaged 20 minutes.

Casey and Kerr initially evaluated the effectiveness of the service using a ten-point rating scale administered before and after each treatment. Variables measured were physical comfort, emotional comfort, pain, and fatigue. Improvement occurred on all these parameters after the treatment. A range of essential oils was used to treat dry, itchy skin, muscular aches and pain, and emotional factors including fear. Although the study has a number of limitations, the findings are clinically relevant and could be transferred to other settings. Certainly, the potential of the blend developed to manage skin itch associated with renal disease shows great promise and is supported by other researchers.

Ro et al. (2002) used a control group (n = 16) and a treatment group (n = 13) to determine whether aromatherapy reduced pruritus in patients undergoing haemodialysis in Seoul, Korea. The treatment group received an aromatherapy arm massage three times a week for four weeks. Pruritus score, skin pH, skin hydration and pruritus-related biochemical markers were measured before and after each treatment. Hydration significantly improved in the treatment group and the itch reduced.

Likewise, Itai et al. (2000) investigated the effects of inhaled lavender and hila oils and a control substance in 14 women undergoing chronic haemodialysis to estimate the psychological effects using the Hamilton Rating Scales for Depression (HAMD) and Anxiety (HAMA). No changes were detected under control conditions but hila oil significantly reduced the mean scores of both the HAMD and HAMA, and lavender reduced HAMA scores after the treatment. It is difficult to interpret these findings based on one pre-treatment depression score taken out of context, but the results suggest some essential oils can contribute to the mental well-being of individuals with end stage renal disease (ESRD).

6.5 Precautions to Consider When Assessing the Suitability of Essential Oils in Patients with Renal Disease

Medicines and essential oils are largely excreted via the kidneys. They need to be water-soluble in order to be reabsorbed in the kidney tubules. The liver is largely responsible for making lipid-soluble substances water-soluble for excretion. Some components of essential oils are more water-soluble than others, for example, terpenoid alcohols, aldehydes and esters (Tisserand and Balacs 1995, p. 63). It is not clear whether essential oil compounds are reabsorbed in the kidney tubules in the same way as some conventional medicines, although lipid soluble terpenes and terpenoid ketones may be reabsorbed in this way.

Peak plasma concentrations of substances present in the blood reach normally functioning kidneys, hence they are vulnerable to damage. Essential oils do not appear to cause damage to healthy kidneys if they are used in traditional aromatherapy doses and application methods. However, oral dosing is known to cause kidney damage. When renal disease is present, the potential for damage increases and lower doses are recommended, especially for internal use.

Many aromatherapy texts state that juniper oil (*Juniperus communis*) is a 'kidney irritant', contraindicated in kidney disease because it is high in terpenes, which are metabolised in the kidneys. The statements may be based on dog studies where the urine became cloudy after high, doses of juniper oil. However, the clouding appears to be due to juniper metabolites rather than kidney damage (Guba 2000). Tisserand and Balacs (1995, p 64) indicate there is 'nothing in the composition of juniper oil, which would seem to give cause for concern'. Laboratory studies in rats have implicated *d*-limonene and methyl salicylate in kidney damage but the doses used in these studies were high and there is no indication the findings apply to humans. Methyl salicylate is a common component of conventional analgesic medicine especially for muscular pain and is found in some essential oils.

However, it is important to consider the possibility that excretion of essential oil components may be reduced in people with renal disease and cumulative effects can occur with continual use even if lower doses are used. In addition, skin-sensitising essential oils may not be the best choice because end stage renal disease is associated with itch, which causes distress and reduced quality of life as well as representing a portal for infection if the person breaks the skin while scratching.

6.6 Essential Oil Use

Gastrointestinal system

Some essential oils have antispasmodic, carminative or stimulating effects on the gastrointestinal tract and may have a role in managing constipation, diarrhoea and nausea. Constipation is common and is associated with lack of dietary fibre and fluid, many disease processes, and some medicines and can cause haemorrhoids, flatulence, bloating, indigestion and halitosis. Identifying and treating the underlying cause are important.

Essential oils of black pepper (*Piper nigrum*), fennel (*Foeniculum vulgare*), peppermint (*Mentha piperata*) or the citrus oils such as orange (*Citrus aurantium*) in an abdominal massage or combined with acupressure or reflexology to stimulate the appropriate points might relieve autonomic neuropathic discomfort by reducing spasm, dyspepsia and flatulence. Peppermint and ginger (*Zingiber officinalis*) are traditional antinausea essential oils. The herbs from which the essential oils are extracted are often used in herbal teas to relieve nausea and dyspepsia associated with gastrointestinal disease, surgical and investigative procedures and pregnancy (Parker 1999).

Foot care

People with diabetes need to take particular care of their feet, especially if they have peripheral neuropathy and vascular disease and reduced sensation because of the high risk of undetected injury, infection and consequent amputation. Neuropathy can compromise sleep, quality of life, and relationships and predispose the individual to depression due to chronic pain. Pain management is discussed in Chapter 15.

Essential oils can be incorporated into foot self-care as well as managing active foot problems. Essential oils such as *Mentha piperata* and *Lavandula angustifolia*, can be used in massage blends, in creams and lotions to maintain moisture and prevent cracks that can be a portal for infection, as well as treating *Tinea pedis*, for example, tea tree. If used with a foot massage or reflexology, the circulation, tissue oxygenation and nourishment can be improved. *Gentle* exfoliation using a pumice bar or foot gels with added *fine* abrasive agents, for example, finely ground almonds or oatmeal and essential oils can help remove old skin and prevent callous formation. Great care needs to be taken especially if the sensation is reduced to ensure the skin is not abraded.

Fungal foot infections such as *Tinea pedis* and onychomycosis are relatively common in people with diabetes. Combinations of essential oil constituents camphor (*Cinnamomum camphora*), menthol (*mentha piperita*) and thymol (*Thymus vulgaris*) and eucalyptus (*Eucalyptus globulus*) are effective against most organisms that cause onychomycosis (Ramsewak *et al.* 2003), *Melaleuca alternifiolia* is effective against *Candida spp* and *Malassezia*, (Hammer *et al.* 2002) and *Tinea pedis* (Hammer *et al.* 1998). While these studies may not have included people with diabetes, there is no reason to suspect the results would be any different.

Essential oils in clean water, or hydrosols can also be used to cleanse wounds and reduce initial pain, swelling and inflammation while waiting for professional advice. Minor cuts and abrasions can be managed using anti-inflammatory essential oils such as (*Lavandula angustifolia*) lavender, (*Styrax benzoin*), (*Chamaemelum nobile*) Roman chamomile, (*Comiphora myrrha*) myrrh, benzoin helichrysum

(*Helichrysm italicum*), and rosewood (*Aniba rosaeodora*) diluted in a carrier. A range of foot massage techniques and exercises can strengthen foot muscles and ligaments and assist in preventing pain and rigidity. People can be taught basic foot self-massage or their relatives can be shown the techniques if the individual cannot reach their feet.

Excessive perspiration, poor circulation, and inadequate foot hygiene contribute to foot odour. Essential oils such as cypress (*Cupressus sempervirens*), *Mentha piperata* and rosemary (*Rosmarinus officinalis*) in short foot baths or in fine white clay or powder can help reduce foot odour. Foot soaks can reduce swelling and are psychologically relaxing (Sacki 2000). However, long foot soaks can cause tissue maceration and infection risk.

Skin and wound care

Modern principles of wound healing involve maintaining a constant temperature and moisture in the wound, debriding necrotic tissue to allow healing to take place from the base of the wound upwards, protecting the surrounding skin, preventing infection, and applying standard infection control procedures especially where pus or exudate is present, and appropriate waste disposal. Accurate foot assessment and appropriate referral are mandatory and conventional management should not be delayed. Essential oils can be used to do the following:

- cleanse the wound using a hydrosol or low dose essential oil solution;
- reverse the inflammatory process using wet dressings such as a hydrosol or anti-inflammatory essential oil compress *Lavandula angustigolia* or chamomile for acute hot, red, swollen and oozing wounds. Alternatively ointments, creams emulsions or pastes containing *Aloe vera* or MediHoney for dry, scaly wounds;
- relieve local pain and irritation;
- protect the surrounding tissue;
- encourage self-care.

Wounds should be assessed regularly to ensure healing is taking place and the management modified as needed. Essential oils can be applied as a dressing, diluted in an emulsifier in a medicated bath, in powder or clay to absorb moisture and prevent skin surfaces rubbing together or rubbing on clothing, or in sprays or aerosols depending on the ongoing assessment and the goals of therapy. Referral for conventional assessment and care should not be delayed. Essential oils on a secondary dressing may reduce unpleasant odours, which can be distressing for the individual.

A number of studies support using essential oils in wound care. Hartman and Coetzee (2002) used a 6 per cent solution of *Lavandula angustifolia* and *Matricaria recutita* in grapeseed oil directly onto wounds and surrounding tissue twice a day on Grade II chronic ulcers that had been present for at least three months and had not responded to conventional care. Patients aged between 50 and 83 years were randomly allocated to the treatment (n = 5) or conventional care control group (n = 3). One person had two wounds: one wound was treated with the essential oils and the other with conventional care. The wounds were assessed using a standard wound classification scale. Wound healing was faster in the essential oil group. After 56 days the control wound in the patient with two wounds was treated with essential oils at the patient's request, because of the faster healing rate in the other wound. None of the wounds became infected during the trial, but exudate and erythema increased in the essential oil group before healing commenced.

Kerr (2002) developed a wound care formula, which was applied daily in a trial of seven patients with skin tears in an aged care facility. A rating scale was used to assess healing. Other factors assessed included general condition, skin integrity, level of mobility and medication use. Healing occurred but staff noted the formula did not deslough wounds and secondary dressings were needed to retain moisture. The formula was subsequently modified and the essential oil concentration increased to 9 per cent and subsequently 12 per cent in a third iteration. Kerr reported no adverse events at these essential oil concentrations. In fact, local redness and irritation decreased and the analgesic effect increased. Kerr's findings suggest that the current essential oil dose recommendations for topical applications may be too low, but more research is needed to determine effective doses and dose intervals.

Neither Hartman and Coetzee nor Kerr's studies involved people with diabetes but there is no reason to assume similar results would not occur. Supporting wound care with appropriate nutrition, rest, and other appropriate care such as antiembolic stockings, not smoking, relieving pressure, managing pain, reducing odour and considering the psychological and quality of life issues are also necessary.

6.7 Mental Health and Psychological Care

The effect of odour on behaviour and emotions is often referred to as psychoaromatherapy. Similar fields in conventional nursing are psychoneuroendo-crinology and psychoneuroimmunology. The increasing interest in these specialities attests to the interconnectedness of the physical and psychological aspects of an individual (mind–body connection) and underscores why holistic patient care is essential.

Psychological effects of odour

Odours can affect mood and emotion on a deep, unconscious level. Physical effects such as motor, autonomic and EEG changes have been demonstrated in the presence of a range of essential oils (Torri 1988; McCoy 2002; Moss *et al.* 2003). These and other researchers have identified a range of essential oils that have antidepressive, stimulating, sedative, calming and adaptogenic (balancing) effects. Odour-invoked mood changes may be small, but essential oils can be used to improve psychological well-being in a preventative health-care plan. Essential oils can enhance the effects of other mental health care activities such as meditation, colour therapy and massage and conventional medicines.

Diabetes is associated with increased anxiety, fear and depression, which can lead to lowered self-esteem and physical functioning, inadequate self-care, and more frequent presentations to health-care services (Ciechanowski *et al.* 2000). Therefore, preventative, holistic care that includes stress management and mental and spiritual health is imperative. Essential oils, especially combined with massage, counselling and meditation, may represent the greatest application of essential oils in diabetes care, bearing in mind the fact that the individual's expectations of the therapy affects its effectiveness (Brougham 2005).

Research into the psychological effects of essential oils using standardised measurements such as electromagnetic activity, heart rate, task performance, and subject self-reports has been undertaken in Japan, the USA and Europe (Jellinek 1998/1999). Proposed mechanisms of action include:

- *Quasipharmacological.* Small doses entering the blood from inhaled or topically applied essential oils.
- *Semantic.* Effects that reflect how the odour is experienced in the context of the individual's specific situation.
- *Feelings of pleasure or displeasure* (hedonic states), which influence a wide range of mental responses and emotional states, and which can be influenced positively or negatively by pleasant or unpleasant odours. Links between olfaction, emotion and cognition means odours and emotions are closely associated during memory encoding (Brougham 2005). Thus ambient odours can be contextual reminders and used as cues for behaviour change and to enhance learning (Herz 1997). More research is required to determine whether these findings apply to people with diabetes.

The effects of odours are very subjective. Responses to odours may have been stored in memory along with the event they are associated with, years before. Subsequent exposure to the odour can evoke memories of the smell, the incident and the feelings that occurred at the time, for example, happiness, sadness or anger. Asking people about their odour preferences is an important part of the health history, akin to asking about allergies, especially when cognition is impaired.

Depression, mood and cognitive functioning

Many studies of varying quality have been undertaken into the effects of a range of essential oils on mood and cognitive functioning over the years. A recent study (Moss *et al.* 2003) set out to determine the effect of *Lavandula angustifolia* and *Rosmarinus officinalis* on mood and cognitive performance in 144 healthy volunteers. Subjects were randomly assigned to one of three groups and performed a standardised computerised cognitive battery of nine tasks that represent six factors involved in cognitive functioning. The tests were conducted in cubicles containing either lavender, rosemary, or no fragrance. Visual analogue mood scales were completed before and after exposure to the odour and after completing the cognitive tests.

Lavender caused a significant reduction in working memory, reaction time for the memory and attention-based tasks compared with controls. Rosemary significantly enhanced performance overall (quality of memory) but reduced memory speed compared with controls. Both the control and lavender oil groups were significantly less alert than the rosemary group and the control group was significantly less content than either of the essential oil groups. The study demonstrates essential oils do affect mood and performance and supports the traditional uses of the two essential oils tested. The results could be translated into a number of health-care settings including patient and health professionals' education. Despite Moss *et al.*'s findings, studies of the effects of lavender on behaviour, cognition and mood produce mixed, often contradictory results. Lack of standardisation between the tests and different population groups may account for some of the differences.

Komori *et al.* (1995) compared the effects of citrus fragrances on neuroendocrine hormone levels and immune function in 20 depressed male hospital inpatients treated with antidepressant medicines using the Hamilton Rating Scale. Scores improved after citrus fragrances were vapourised at a fixed rate. Symptom remission took between four and eleven weeks. There were no differences between the essential oil and antidepressant medicine groups except lower doses of antidepressants were needed in the essential oil group. Since there is a high incidence of depression in people with diabetes, essential oils may mean lower doses of medicines could be used, but more research is needed.

Many animal studies indicate physical and psychological effects of essential oils or their components on the nervous system such as reduced agitation, sedation and a reduced number of epileptic seizures. The effects may be due to a range of actions such as altering cell membrane functions and/or inhibiting or enhancing receptor binding. Kirk-Smith (2003) pointed out the difficulties encountered when conducting psychological research and indicated that, although an effect of an odour may be found, it is difficult to determine how the effect was produced. In addition, there are ethical issues involved in studying some vulnerable populations such as people with psychiatric illnesses, which need to be considered.

Individual factors and expectations, perhaps more than other factors, affect an individual's psychological response to odours. Therefore, taking a very careful aroma history is essential. Doses and dose intervals also need to be considered. Factors affecting psychological responses include:

- cultural experiences;
- 'expectation effect': the effects the individual expects to occur;
- emotions and circumstance surrounding previous exposure to the odour;
- state of mind at the time the odour was first smelled;
- degree of physical and mental wellness on original exposure and at the current time;
- hedonistic factors;
- smell adaptation or odour suppression.

6.8 Essential Oil Application/Administration Methods

External administration

Table 6.3 depicts commonly used external application methods and traditionally recommended doses.

Table 6.3 Recommended essential oil doses for the various application methods. These doses are based on the traditional use and the recommendations of experts. They are not derived from dose-finding trials. The dose interval also needs to be considered. Reproduced with permission from Australian Scholarly Publishing.

Application method	Number of drops of essential oil based on standard essential oil dropper top, for adults. Note: age and health status need to be considered.
Massage	**Adults** In general, the recommended dose does not exceed 3.5 per cent–5 per cent of a blend. There are, however, documented and anecdotal instances where higher percentages of essential oils have been used safely. **Children** Children over 7 years and the elderly 1–1.5 per cent Children 2–7 years 0.5 per cent **Babies** 0–1 year no essential oils Approximately 25–30 ml of a carrier substance is required for an adult full body massage depending on skin condition and amount of body hair.
Bath	4–7
Vaporiser	4–7
Tissue, cotton ball, clothing	1–2
Inhalation over hot water or nebuliser (thick oils and carriers will clog nebulisers)	2–3 in a bowl of steaming water
Unscented lotions and creams	4–5 drops in 60 mls
Gargle	2–3 drops in 30 mls of water
Room sprays	4 drops/280 ml
Poultice	2–3 drops in $\frac{1}{2}$ cup of medium e.g. clay, oatmeal, chopped comfrey
Compress	2–3
Undiluted on the skin (tea tree, lavender)	1

Internal administration

Appropriate training and competence are necessary before using essential oils internally: orally, vaginally or rectally or as drops or on a wick into the nose or ear. Most undiluted essential oils are irritating to mucous membranes and the eyes and need to be administered in low doses and in appropriate low irritant gels, creams or liquids. Steam-distilled essential oils are preferred for internal use. Essential oils are components of many conventional and complementary medicines for example, peppermint oil capsules, gripe water, throat lozenges and gargles and cold and flu remedies.

Inhalation

Steam inhalations provide moisture and protect the mucous membranes of the respiratory tract. Low doses of essential oils are recommended. High doses change mucociliary function and may reduce fluid secretions and cause dryness and irritation (Harris and Harris 2003). Inhalations can be used to administer essential oils so they quickly reach the systemic circulation to manage a range of conditions such as stress, depression and for their local anti-inflammatory and anti-infectious properties. However, high doses can irritate the eyes and mucous membranes and trigger an asthma-like attack. The traditional method is to place drops of the essential oils into hot water and inhale the steam after covering the head with a towel. This method is no longer used in conventional medicine and is contraindicated for children and carries a risk of burns.

A number of inhalation administration devices are available. The extent to which they are used in health care settings is unknown, but some offer safety advantages over some traditional methods.

Recommended doses

When deciding on an appropriate dose and dose interval, the person's health status, age, pregnancy or lactation, concomitant medications and any previous essential oil-related adverse events, need to be ascertained. In general, frail elderly people, babies and children, and people with alcohol or drug addictions require lower doses because these factors affect the pharmacodynamics and pharmacokinetics of essential oils, as well as herbal and conventional medicines, see Chapter 3.

Experts disagree about the relative toxicity of various essential oils and there may be differences between various chemotypes of some essential oils. The question of whether the whole oil is less toxic than isolated chemical constituents is also unresolved. A strong tradition in aromatherapy is that the synergistic and quenching effects of the various components in an essential oil reduce the potential toxic effects of other components. These effects make it difficult to isolate the contribution and specific toxic effects of any one chemical component of an

Table 6.4 Potential toxicity of essential oil application/administration methods relevant to the amount of essential oil absorbed and the dose delivered (Franchomme and Penoel 1990). The greater the number of + signs the greater the toxicity risk. Reproduced with permission from Australian Scholarly Publishing.

Application/administration method	Potential toxicity rating
Oral	+++++
Vaginal	++
Rectal	+
Topical	+
Inhalation	0

essential oil. Quenching refers to the ability of some chemical components of an essential oil to reduce or eliminate unwanted side effects caused by the other components. Quenching is well known in aromatherapy and perfumery where essential oil chemicals are deliberately combined to reduce the irritant effects of some essential oils.

In addition, it is not always easy to interpret the meaning of LD_{50} doses because results vary among laboratories, the LD should not be considered in isolation, and dose ranges, dose intervals and dose response curves are not established for most essential oils. Generally, LD_{50} dose $< 1\,g/kg$ indicates high risk, and doses $> 5\,g/kg$ represents low risk (Burfield 2000). Franchomme and Peonoel (1990) developed a system to indicate the relative toxicity risk associated with each application/administration method taking into account the amount of essential oil absorbed and typical doses, see Table 6.4.

6.9 Essential Oil Safety Issues

Risk profiles for essential oils can be determined using information from the individual patient assessment and information obtained from:

- material safety data sheets (MSDS) which can be obtained from essential oil suppliers who are required to supply MDS to customers. However, these sheets may not be compiled by a chemist and may contain mistakes so the information should be checked.
- essential oil monographs;
- internet databases;
- quality publications;
- aromatherapy professional organisations.

Recently the American National Standards Committee adopted a 16-section format developed by the Chemical Manufacturers' Association that includes toxicological information (Burfield 2000). Practitioners are advised to have safety information available and in some countries this is an occupational health and safety regulation.

The Research Institute for Fragrance Materials (RIFM) is independent of manufacturing interests and publishes data on fragrance products including essential oils and makes risk assessments and recommendations for use of individual substances based on skin testing, oral and dermal LD_{50} tests, phototoxicity, and photosensitisation and sensitisation. This information is considered by the International Fragrance Association (IFRA), which produces guidelines for the fragrance industry. RIFM has tested more than 1300 substances, some of which are banned and the amounts of others that can be added to products is limited or specific criteria must be fulfilled before they can be used. Essential oils fit into both of these categories. Some of the data is now out-of- date and in addition, does not address the way essential oils are used in aromatherapy.

Reputable manufacturers adhere to the IFRA guidelines as a self-regulatory process. A range of other bodies also exists and some collaborate, for example, the European Flavours and Fragrance Association, the British Essence Manufacturers Association. Others are more directly associated with essential oils such as the International Federation of Essential Oil Aroma Trades and in some countries medicines regulatory authorities.

Various statements have been made about the toxicity of inhaled essential oils but the data are inconclusive and maximum exposure limits for most essential oils and application method are unknown. Although some data from industry are available, it seems likely only small doses reach the systemic circulation after inhalation as used in aromatherapy practice. Contact allergy from inhalation does occur (Schlatter and Korting 1993). However, the sensitising properties of some of the components are modified by others (quenching), and individual susceptibility, which makes it difficult to predict sensitising capacity.

Most of these issues apply generally. However, the potential neurotoxic effect of some essential oils may mean they need to be used with caution in the presence of neuropathy, although there is no data to support this suggestion. Many essential oils have a direct effect on the central nervous system and children and the elderly are particularly at risk of adverse events (Day *et al.* 1997).

General safety precautions when using essential oils

- Generally, essential oils should not be applied on the skin undiluted, except by a competent aromatherapist.
- Sensitivity can develop to any essential oil in susceptible individuals such as those with a history of allergies and eczema.
- Internal administration carries a higher risk of serious adverse events and should only be undertaken by or at the direction of a qualified practitioner.
- Prolonged massage could contribute to hypoglycaemia if meals are delayed or carbohydrate intake is reduced. The individual should be given appropriate advice when scheduling an appointment. Likewise hypotension is possible especially if the person has autonomic neuropathy or is elderly.
- Some essential oils are more likely to cause allergic reactions than others and patch testing before using essential oils for the first time may be indicated, especially in atopic individuals. Low molecular weight allergens (haptens) are present in some essential oils and are capable of causing an inflammatory response.

- The same essential oils should not be used for long periods of time because some have a cumulative effect or cause sensitivity after a period of time.
- Traditional recommendations about essential oils precautions and contraindications should be followed, for example, during pregnancy and lactation, epilepsy, asthma, and doses in certain age groups and conditions. However, the evidence to support many essential oils recommendations is limited. The dose interval and the total dose over a day and the findings of the history and assessment and potential cumulative effect also need to be considered.
- Contraindications to specific essential oils must be considered especially treating the frail elderly, people with alcohol or addictions, children and pregnant women.
- It is possible to extrapolate dose intervals from available data, for example, monoterpenes are volatile and have a short duration of action while heavier molecules such as lactones and coumarins have a slower absorption rate and a longer duration of action.
- The correct essential oil dose and dose interval likely to produce the desired outcome (effective dose) should be known. Many aromatherapists believe 'less is more', which means essential oils are powerful agents and large doses are unnecessary. This concept is consistent with the QUM principle to use the lowest possible dose to achieve the desired effect, see Chapter 4, but effective therapeutic doses and dose ranges for specific situations are unclear. Appropriately monitoring the individual's response can help establish the effective dose for the individual.
- Some essential oils are not used in aromatherapy, for example, wormwood, pennyroyal, rue, camphor, bitter almond and sassafras, because of their known toxicity. Some aromatherapists include oil of wintergreen on the exclusion list; however, if it is used appropriately, it is an effective analgesic for muscular aches and arthritic pain in a massage blend and the odour is more acceptable than synthetic menthol in salicylate-based conventional medicines.
- Essential oils must be appropriately stored to preserve their therapeutic effects. They must be kept out of the reach of children and cognitively impaired or suicidal patients to avoid inadvertent or deliberate overdose. This includes having vaporisers out of reach rather than on coffee tables.
- Care around fire and where people smoke, or other flammable substances are in use, is essential. Essential oils are highly flammable. Likewise, empty bottles, unused portions of oils and other products must be disposed of appropriately to reduce the fire risk. Candle vaporisers are a common cause of fires and other safer alternatives are recommended.
- Educating patients who self-apply essential oils is an important aspect of safe use because most of the adverse events associated with essential oils occur because of misuse by the public.

6.10   Essential Oil – Conventional Medicine Interactions

There is limited information about essential oil and conventional medicines interactions but they need to be considered, especially with internal use, and whenever conventional and herbal medicines are used concomitantly. Reports of unexpected bleeding during surgery have been attributed to interactions between anticoagulant herbs and conventional medicines and supplements, therefore surgery and investigations may be times when caution needs to be used for essential oils.

Grapefruit juice affects particular enzyme systems and may reduce the effects of cyclosporin and some calcium channel blockers, but this information does not apply to topical or inhaled grapefruit essential oils. Orally administered bitter orange essential oil may have similar effects to grapefruit juice, however lemon, lime, sweet orange and mandarin do not (Guba 2004).

There are reports of photosensitization from topical lime juice and sun exposure, and from a combination of lime juice and sun filter occurring where the sun filter was applied (Rogers 2002). This is an interesting finding since lime juice is not extracted from the peel and suggests lime juice may have similar photosensitising effects to lime essential oil or that the reaction was idiosyncratic. In the latter report one product may have potentiated the effect of the other or the lime juice may have reduced the effectiveness of the sun filter. Citrus essential oils are known UV sensitisers. Rogers' report suggests the effectiveness of some sun filter products *might* be reduced if they are applied after a massage containing lime essential oil. However, no such reports were identified and the components in the lime juice may not be the same as the UV sensitising component of the essential oil.

Topically applied conventional antifungal products can interact with Warfarin and lead to bleeding and bruising by potentiating the effect of the Warfarin by inhibiting its metabolism through the cytochrome $P4_{50}$ system. Although only small doses of topically applied antifungal medicines reach the systemic circulation, they may be sufficient to have an effect. Again, it is not clear whether this interaction applies to anticoagulant essential oils, but the possibility should be considered. Essential oils with known anticoagulant effects are *Gaultheria procumbens* (wintergreen) and white birch, which contain significant amounts of methyl salicylate and may cause haemorrhage or bruising.

Concomitant use of valerian and barbiturates and other central nervous system depressants leads to prolonged sleep, drowsiness and falls risk (O'Mathu'na 2003). Again, it is not clear whether topically applied or inhaled essential oils carry the same risk but increased surveillance is recommended.

The potential adverse event profile of vegetable oils (carrier oils) also needs to be considered. For example, ingested *Aloe vera* gel can interact with diuretics and cause confusion, weakness and irregular heartbeats due to potassium depletion. *Aloe vera* is used as a carrier medium for essential oils but probably would not enter the body in significant amounts after topical application and is unlikely to represent the same risk as internal use. Internally administered evening primrose oil can reduce levels of phenothiazine and anaesthetic agents and lower the seizure threshold, which increases the risk of seizures but is unlikely to have the same effect when used as a carrier for topically applied essential oils.

References

Allen W. Effect of various inhaled vapours on respiration and blood pressure in anaesthetised and unanaesthetised subjects. *American Journal of Physiology* 1988; 620–632.

Anderson L, Gross J. Aromatherapy with peppermint, isopropyl alcohol, or placebo is equally effective in relieving postoperative nausea. *Journal of Perianaesthesia Nursing* 2004; **19**(1): 29–35.

Battaglia S. *The Complete Guide to Aromatherapy*. Virginia, Qld: The Perfect Potion, 1995.

Borromeo A. The effects of aromatherapy on patient outcomes of anxiety and sleep quality in coronary care patients. Unpublished PhD thesis, Texas Women's University, 1995.

Bowles J. *Basic Chemistry of Aromatherapeutic Essential Oils*. Sydney: Allen & Unwin, 2003.

Bronough D. In vivo percutaneous absorption of fragrance materials in rhesus monkeys and humans. *Food Chemical Toxicology* 1990; **28**(5): 369–373.

Brougham C. Effects of essential oils on mental performance. *Chemo Sense* 2002; 4(**2**): 7–11.

Buckle J. *Clinical Aromatherapy in Nursing*. New York: RJ Buckle Associates, 1997.

Burfield T. Safety of essential oils. *International Journal of Aromatherapy* 2000; **10**(1/2): 16–29.

Burfield T. Odour perception of essential oils. *Aromatherapy Today* 2003; **25**: 33–37.

Burfield T. The adulteration of essential oils and the consequences to aromatherapy and natural perfumery. http://www.naha.org/original/articles/adulteration_1.htm (accessed November 2005).

Casey M, Kerr J. An aromatherapy clinic in a public hospital ward. *Simply Essential* 2003; **48**: 12–14.

Catty S. *Hydrosols: The Next Aromatherapy*. Vermont: Healing Arts Press, 2001.

Ciechanowski P, Katon W, Russo W. Impact of depressive symptoms on adherence, function and costs. *Archives of Internal Medicine* 2000; **160**: 3278–3285.

Clarke S. *Essential Chemistry for Safe Aromatherapy*. Edinburgh: Churchill Livingstone, 2002.

Combest W, Newton M, Combest A, Kosier J. Effects of herbal supplements on the kidney. *Urology Nursing* 2005; **25**(5): 381–386.

Cornwell P, Barry B, Stoddart C, Bouwstra J. Wide-angle X-ray diffraction of human stratum corneum: effects of hydration and terpene enhancer treatment. *Journal of Pharmacy & Pharmacology* 1994; **46**(12): 938–950.

Cross S, Anderson C, Thompson M, Roberts M. Is there tissue penetration after application of topical salicylate formulations? *Lancet* 1997; **350**: (9078): 636.

Day I, Ozanne-Smith J, Parsons B, Dobbin M, Tibballs J. Eucalyptus oil poisoning among young children: mechanisms of access and the potential for prevention. *Australian and New Zealand Journal of Public Health* 1997; **21**(3): 297–302.

Dossey B, Keegan L, Guzzetta C, Kolkmeier L. *Holistic Nursing*. Aspen: Aspen Publishers, 1995.

Dunning T. *Care of People with Diabetes: A Manual of Nursing Practice*. Oxford: Blackwell Publishing, 2003a.

Dunning T. Complementary therapies and diabetes. *Complementary Therapies in Nursing and Midwifery* 2003b; **9**: 74–80.

Dunning T. Applying a quality use of medicines framework to using essential oils in nursing. *Complementary Therapies in Clinical Practice* 2005; **11**: 172–181.

Essential Oil Desk Reference 2001 Essential Oil Publishing, USA. (no author cited)

Ford R, Hawkins D, Mayo B, Api M. The in vivo dermal absorption and metabolism of [4-^{14}C] coumarin by rats and by human volunteers under simulated conditions of use in fragrances. *Food and Chemical Toxicology* 2001; **39**: 153–162.

Franchomme P, Penoel D. *L'Aromathérapie Exactement*. Limoges: Roger Jollios, 1990.

Frazer J, Kerr J. Psychological effects of back massage on elderly institutionalised patients. *Journal of Advanced Nursing* 1993; **18**(2): 238–245.

Frey W. Intranasal delivery: bypassing the blood brain barrier to deliver therapeutic agents to the brain and spinal cord. *Drug Delivery Technology* 2002; **2**(5): 46–49.

George M. Complementary therapies in a high-tech healthcare environment: a pleasing and powerful partnership. In: McCabe P (ed.), *Complementary Therapies in Nursing and Midwifery: From Vision to Practice*. Melbourne: Ausmed Publications, 2001; pp. 235–265.

Guba R. Toxicity myths—the actual risks of essential oil use. *International Journal of Aromatherapy* 2000; **10**(1/2): 37–49.

Guba R. Quality matters: 'natural variation'. *Essential News* 2004; **15**, March 3–4.

Hammer K, Carson C, Riley T. In vitro activity of *Melaleuca alternifolia* (tea tree) oil against dermatophytes and other filamentous fungi. *Journal of Antimicrobial Chemotherapy* 2002; **50**: 195–2000.

Hartman D, Coetzee V. Two US practitioners' experience using essential oils for wound care. *Journal of Wound Care* 2002; **11**(8): 317–320.

Harris R, Harris B. Aromatic medicine: the interfaces of absorption. Course notes from seminar presented in Melbourne, 2003.

Itai T, Amayasu H, Kuribayashi M, Kawamura N, Okada M *et al*. Psychological effects of aromatherapy on chronic haemodialysis patients. *Psychiatry and Clinical Neurosciences* 2000; **54**(4): 393–397.

Jager W, Buchbauer G, Jirovetz L, Fritzer M. Percutaneous absorption of lavender oil form a massage. *Journal Society of Chemists* 1992; **43**: 49–54.

Jellinek D. Odours and mental states. *International Journal of Aromatherapy* 1998; **9**(3): 115–120.

Kerr J. Research project – using essential oils in wound care for the elderly. *Aromatherapy Today* 2002; **23**: 14–19.

Kirk-Smith M. The psychological effects of lavender 11: scientific and clinical evidence. *International Journal of Aromatherapy* 2003; **13**(2/3): 82–89.

Komori T, Fujiwara R, Tanid M, Nomurn J, Yokoyama M. Effects of citrus fragrance on immune function and depressive states. *Neuroimmunomodulation* 1995; **5**: 174–180.

Lawless J. *Essential Oils: An Illustrated Guide*. London: HarperCollins, 2001.

Lis-Bulchin M, Deans S, Hart S. A study of the changes in the bioactivity of essential oils use singly and as mixtures in aromatherapy. *Journal of Alternative and Complementary Medicine* 1997; **3**(3): 249–256.

McCoy N. Pheromonal influences on sociosexual behaviour in young women. *Physiology and Behaviour* 2002; **75**(3): 367–375.

Moss M, Cook J, Wesnes K, Duckett P. Aromas of rosemary and lavender essential oils differentially affect cognition and mood in healthy adults. *International Journal of Neuroscience* 2003; **113**(1): 15–38.

O'Mathu'na D. Herb–drug interactions. *Alternative Medicine Alerk* 2003; **6**(4): 37–44.

Parker L. A guide to the use of aromatherapy in irritable bowel syndrome. *Aromatherapy World* 1999; **Summer**: 18–19.

Price S. *Aromatherapy Workbook*. London: Thorsons, 1993.

Ramsewak R, Nair M, Stommel M. In vitro antagonist activity of monoterpenes and their mixtures against 'toe nail fungus' pathogens. *Phytotherapy Research* 2003; **17**(4): 376–379.

Rekieten N, Rekieten M. The effect of L-menthol on the systemic blood pressure. *Journal of the American Pharmaceutical Association* 1957; **46**(2): 82–84.

Ro Y, Ha H, Kim C, Yeom H. The effects of aromatherapy on pruritis in patients undergoing haemodialysis. *Dermatology Nursing* 2002; **14**(4): 231–234.

Rogers T. Contact dermatitis. *Australian Doctor*. 2002; **Nov** 29: 33.

Sabo C, Michael S, Temple L. The use of alternative therapies by diabetes educators. *The Diabetes Educator* 1999; **25**(6): 945–954.

Sacki Y. The effect of foot bath with or without essential oil of lavender on the autonomic nervous system: a randomised trial. *Complementary Therapies in Medicine* 2000; **8**(1): 2–7.

Satchell A, Saurajen A, Bell C. Treatment of interdigital *Tinea pedis* with 25 per cent and 50 per cent tea tree oil solution: a randomised, placebo controlled, blinded study. *Australasian Journal of Dermatology* 2002; **43**(3): 175–178.

Sellar W. *The Directory of Essential Oils*. Saffron Waldren: CV Daniel Company, 1992.

Shaller M, Korting H. Airborne contact dermatitis from essential oils used in aromatherapy. *Clinical and Experimental Dermatology* 1993; **20**: 143–145.

Springfield Corporation. *Herbal Medicine Handbook*. Springfield, PA: Springfield Corporation, 2001.

Stevenson C. The psychophysiological effects of aromatherapy massage following cardiac surgery. *Complementary Therapies in Medicine* 1994; **2**(1): 27–35.

Thomas J. Peppermint fibrillation. *Lancet* 1962; 27 Jan, 222.

Thorgrimsen L, Spector A, Wiles A, Orrell M. Aromatherapy for dementia. Cochrane Library (Oxford) (Id # CD 003150), 2005.

Tisserand R, Balacs T. *Essential Oil Safety: A Guide for Health Professionals*. Edinburgh: Churchill Livingstone, 1995.

Torii W. Contingent negative variation and the psychological effects of odour. *Perfumery: The Psychology and Biology of Fragrance*. London: Chapman & Hall, 1998; pp 107–120.

Worwood V. *The Fragrant Mind: Aromatherapy for Personality, Mood and Emotion*. London: Transworld Publishers, 1995.

7 Counselling and Relaxation Therapies

Sue Cradock *and* Chas Skinner

7.1 Introduction

Before discussing counselling and relaxation therapies in detail it may be useful to reflect on how these approaches could be integrated into conventional health care and why people might seek these approaches. Stress is acknowledged to be a factor in modern life and makes it difficult for people to cope generally, and specifically to take care of themselves. Additionally stress can have a very direct effect on blood glucose levels in people with diabetes. However, very little time or attention seems to have been paid to exploring potential stressors with people with diabetes and how they could monitor and manage stress in practical terms. In contrast, great attention is paid to other aspects of managing diabetes such as healthy eating, physical activity, monitoring blood glucose levels, taking medication, and attending health checks. One could ask whether stress is not addressed because diabetes clinicians do not have the time, or the knowledge or skills, or because they do not think it is important enough or part of their role to explore how stress management could enhance diabetes self-management.

It may also be useful to reflect on why people seek complementary or alternative therapies and approaches (CAM). Is it because the therapeutic approaches they are offered in conventional diabetes care are not enough to help them satisfactorily manage their diabetes? Are CAM therapists seen as having more time to explore their client's anxieties and have appropriate environments in which they can listen to and explore other ways of understanding the individual's situation in order to access self-resourcefulness? Or is it simply that people do not like medication and want a more natural answer? These issues are explored in more detail in Chapter 2. Counselling and other therapies help people process their experiences or understand their internal conflict as well as help them recognise the creativity of the imagination, take appropriate responsibility, enable forgiveness and moving on.

This chapter explores why people with diabetes might seek counselling and relaxation therapies in order to reduce the negative emotional and physical effects of diabetes. It also outlines the range of therapies that may be recommended or personally sought and the evidence for their use.

7.2 The Body and the Mind

While it is common to think of body function being altered only by external agents such as medications or surgery, or by physical activities such as exercise or massage, we each have the capacity to regulate our physiology to a far greater extent than is generally known. It is now well accepted that people's thoughts, beliefs and feelings about what is happening to them affects their experience of serious illnesses/events such as cancer or recovery from surgery and that these factors may have a greater impact on their response than the physical impact of the condition itself. This recognition has led to a growing interest in the development of a range of 'psychological therapies' as part of mainstream health care but also in other health systems. While some of these appear to be new therapies, they can often be linked to traditional eastern approaches and philosophies.

These approaches are gaining interest and an evidence base as a result of research into the effect of stress on the mind – body system, and the benefits of reducing that stress as well as the power of the placebo effect (Benson 1996). The underlying contribution of maladaptive stress responses to vascular disease is now accepted and while the links have been made between high stress situations and worse vascular events/outcomes, the recognition that stress reduction approaches can have significant effects on lowering blood pressure, lipids and blood glucose has not resulted in their use in mainstream healthcare. Surwit et $al.$ (2002) suggested that stress management could be a meaningful addition to a comprehensive treatment programme for patients with type 2 diabetes. Surwit et $al.$'s study on the benefits of stress reduction programmes showed significant improvement in HbA_{1c} but, similar to many educational programmes, the effect appeared to diminish over time.

The power of the placebo effect is well known in health care and is considered to be one of the earliest medicinal therapies that invoked the mind – body connection (Grattan 2004). The belief that something or someone can improve an individual's physical state has a dramatic effect on survival rates in some cases and sometimes improves well-being. The link between the mind and the body may also highlight the power of the relationship between a patient and their care provider, which is now often referred to as a 'therapeutic relationship' that requires a great deal of knowledge and skill to enhance its effect.

The placebo effect yields beneficial clinical results in 60–90 per cent of diseases including angina pectoris, bronchial asthma, herpes simplex, and duodenal ulcer. Because of the heavily negative connotations of the words 'placebo effect' the term should be replaced by 'remembered wellness'. Remembered wellness has been one of medicine's most potent assets and it should not be belittled or ridiculed. Unlike most other treatments, it is safe and inexpensive and has withstood the test of time (Benson 1996). Three components bring forth the placebo effect:

1. Positive beliefs and expectations on the part of the individual.
2. Positive beliefs and expectations on the part of the physician or health-care professional.
3. A good relationship between the two parties.

7.3 Diabetes and the Psyche

Living with diabetes presents countless challenges ranging from the mundane to the monumental, from finding time to check the blood glucose in the middle of a busy day, to learning to live with the reality of a major diabetes complication. People have to live with diabetes 24 hours a day, 365 days a year. Since the treatment regimen for diabetes affects essentially everything the person does, good diabetes care involves significant changes in lifestyle for most people. Few people would choose to eat as carefully and stay as active as people with diabetes are supposed to, and nobody would choose to follow the regimen of medication taking, blood glucose monitoring, and medical follow-up recommended for most people with diabetes. People often find meeting these demands especially challenging because their efforts are not guaranteed to produce positive results – or they may have been given that impression. Hard work increases the chances for good outcomes but it does not guarantee them; people frequently report daily fluctuations in their blood glucose levels even when they follow the same regimen every day. Managing diabetes is hard work for those who live with it.

Diabetes-related distress

Diabetes is a family disease because it affects everyone who loves, lives with, or cares for a person who has diabetes. The way all these people respond affects how the person with diabetes feels and how they take care of their diabetes. People who feel unsupported or hassled say it is a major source of distress. Feeling unsupported or hassled by family and friends is yet another source of distress. Some people feel that family and friends tempt them to ignore their diabetes or do not support their efforts to manage the disease for example 'Eat a little cake; a bite won't hurt you,' or, 'Why do we always have to wait for dinner until after you test your blood?' Others feel their family (and friends) go to the opposite extreme, monitoring and criticising every action that could affect blood glucose levels for example 'You know that cookie is not on your diet; are you trying to kill yourself?' or, 'You haven't walked in weeks. You'll never control your diabetes that way.'

Some people report that their family and friends fluctuate between providing too little support and harassing them. Both lack of support and criticism add stress to the life of a person who has diabetes, often generating feelings of isolation, frustration, anger, and guilt. This distress is a problem in its own right, and these feelings can compromise self-care, physical well-being, and the quality of a person's most important relationships. Stress can also be experienced as a result of health-care provision when people feel they have to achieve what the doctor, nurse or dietitian expects of them. They often struggle to fulfil these expectations especially when they are set unrealistic or unspecified goals, which is frequently the case. Health-care professionals often do not recognise the impact of their words or the struggle involved in achieving the tasks they 'set', for example, 'Lose two stone in weight'; 'You must lose weight'; 'You need to get better control.' People with diabetes often express concerns about not having enough time to talk about the daily struggle of living with diabetes and indicate their health-care providers appear not to want to listen to them (Rubin and Peyrot 2001).

Research on diabetes-related emotional distress indicates 'Worrying about the future and the possibility of serious complications' is consistently rated as most distressful by people with type 1 as well as type 2 diabetes, followed by 'Feelings of guilt and anxiety when you get off track with your diabetes management.' The complications people might have to face later in the disease requires renewed adaptation and the re-establishment of emotional equilibrium (Rubin and Peyrot 2001; Taylor *et al.* 2005). Some people do not see diabetes as a serious threat to their health, which might be associated with the fact type 2 diabetes is often asymptomatic in the early stages. However, a significant number of people with diabetes appear to overestimate the seriousness of diabetes and its consequences. For instance, in one study patients were asked to estimate their 10-year risk of developing heart disease and stroke and 40 per cent of over-estimated their risk by at least 20 per cent (Frijling *et al.* 2004). Such optimism may be beneficial when perception of vulnerability to illness and efficacy of therapy motivate people to become actively involved in self-management of diabetes. However, if individuals do believe in the efficacy of treatment strategies, yet feel unable to implement them, high levels of fear that cause feelings of helplessness and denial are likely to develop.

Fear of complications is a major concern for many people and may result in avoidance and neglect of diabetes care by some people and in extreme concern and over-reaction to diabetes in others. Hypoglycaemia is also associated with distress. The acute effects of hypoglycaemia range from transient discomfort, to embarrassment when neuroglycopenia affects behaviour, to emergencies when hypoglycaemia is profound or it occurs when a person is driving. Some people greatly fear hypoglycaemia and a few purposefully keep their blood glucose levels high enough to make low glucose levels highly unlikely. However, the higher levels dramatically increase the risk of diabetes complications (Rubin 2002; Irvine *et al.* 2002).

Therefore, given the profound and varied psychological factors associated with diabetes, it is no great surprise that there is a great deal of research attempting to establish whether people with diabetes have more emotional problems than people with other chronic illnesses and or the general population. Much of the research is couched as clinical mental health problems.

Depression and diabetes

Most of the diabetes 'mental health' research concerns depression in people with diabetes. Much of this literature does not differentiate between the different types of diabetes. Researchers adopting this approach generally conclude that the prevalence of depression is 2–3 times higher in people with diabetes than in the general population and that depression is associated with poorer glycaemic control, macrovascular and microvascular complications, increased health-care costs, and higher mortality rates (Lustman *et al.* 2000; de Groot *et al.* 2001; Anderson *et al.* 2001). The mechanisms behind these associations are unclear at present but could be:

- *Behavioural* – when you are depressed you to eat and drink more and be less active.
- *Physiological* – changes in blood glucose regulation affect neurotransmitter and endocrine levels.
- *Bi-directional* – being more active reduces depression, and changes in neurotransmitter and hormone levels affect blood glucose regulation.

However, it is becoming increasingly clear that health professionals need to consider the relationship between depression and diabetes as being different for type 1 and type 2 diabetes. For example, a recent systematic review of the literature on depression in type 1 diabetes found no evidence of increased rates of depression in people with type 1 diabetes (Barnard in press) whereas the data in type 2 diabetes clearly show higher rates of depression. Furthermore, evidence is beginning to accumulate that depression is in fact a risk factor for the development of type 2 diabetes (Eaton *et al.* 1996) and that depression rates may only be elevated in individuals with co-morbid conditions and or complications (Pouwer *et al.* 2003).

Researchers often focus on other clinical conditions, however, a systematic review of the literature showed generalised anxiety disorder (GAD), the most prevalent of the anxiety disorders, occurs more frequently among people with diabetes, 14 per cent as opposed to 3–4 per cent observed in US community studies (Anderson *et al.* 2002). Furthermore, anxiety disorders only appear to be associated with hyperglycaemia when the association is established through a diagnostic interview, but not when anxiety is self-reported. While there is little evidence about the long-term effect of stress on diabetes outcomes, clinicians recognise that short-term stress can affect blood glucose levels and the actual effects vary between and within individuals.

People with diabetes are at higher risk of developing cardiovascular disease, therefore, the evidence suggesting stressful situations such as high job stress, anger, and hostility are a stronger predictor of coronary heart disease than hyperlipidaemia and smoking is of interest (Rosengren *et al.* 2004). Interestingly, recent research suggests work stress doubles the risk of developing the metabolic syndrome even after controlling for physiological risk factors such as obesity (Chandola *et al.* 2006).

Interestingly, Ernst *et al.* (1998) reported depression is one of the most common reasons people use complementary and alternative therapies, see Chapter 2. However, the amount of rigorous scientific data to support the efficacy of complementary therapies in the treatment of depression is extremely limited. Most evidence for beneficial effects concern exercise, herbal medicines (*Hypericum perforatum*) and to a lesser extent, acupuncture and relaxation therapies, which highlights the need for further research involving randomised controlled trials into the efficacy of complementary and alternative therapies in the treatment of depression (Ernst *et al.* 1998).

Needle anxiety

Health professionals caring for people with diabetes frequently raise the issue of needle phobia. Likewise, people with diabetes often talk about their fears about injecting and may even describe themselves as having a needle phobia. However, it is important to recognise that genuine phobia or long-lasting fear of self-injecting and self-testing is relatively rare in insulin-treated individuals; where it does occur it is usually accompanied by serious psychological comorbidity, which indicates it may be a different manifestation of an underlying problem (Mollema *et al.* 2001). Nevertheless, injecting or drawing blood on a daily basis is not usual human behaviour.

It is important that health professionals acknowledge people's reluctance to use insulin and monitor their blood glucose and support people with diabetes to work through these issues. Where there is a genuine and specific needle phobia, appropriate treatment with systematic desensitisation should be effective. Most people report their fears about injecting resolve after they inject or test their blood glucose for the first time, which suggests needle anxiety is a very normal response that can be reduced by a competent health-care professional. The fact that individuals often raise it may signal a need to be 'emotionally' heard.

Eating patterns

The effective management of both type 1 and type 2 diabetes requires individuals to be more focused on their food choices and the implications for diabetes control. Young females are usually already conscious of their body shape and perceived cultural norms. The increased attention can affect their body image and self-concept and lead to disordered eating habits and/or insulin omission to manage their weight. The focus on food might partially explain an increase in the rate of the clinical condition known as Eating Disorders Not Otherwise Specified (EDNOS) seen in young females with type 1 diabetes (Nash and Skinner 2006). The pressure to lose weight and substantially change food choices and eating habits can be stressful for people with type 2 diabetes and lead to a deepening sense of failure, guilt and frustration, especially if they do not have appropriate support from professionals. Given that obesity is associated with depression, and food is frequently used as a source of comfort in our society, it is clear that diet is an emotive issue that many people with diabetes struggle with.

7.4   Overview of General Concepts and Approaches

The body – mind connection has created increased interest in the Western world outside of and within medical care. Traditional eastern psychological models have been used and developed as well as a range of other approaches, which are becoming part of mainstream Western life and, in some cases, mainstream health care. The core aim of all these approaches is to reduce the harmful effects of stress on the mind – body system by promoting well-being. The range of therapies probably represents the range of interests of the human race. One approach does not suit everybody, nor will one approach work best all the time. Health-care professionals have a responsibility to be aware of the range of approaches that may benefit their patients. Knowledge of only one approach limits the potential to appropriately advise everybody.

While most approaches are seen as 'complementary' to conventional medical interventions, some are now being used as first line therapy in some areas of conventional medicine, for example meditation in the treatment of hypertension. Some approaches are based on a self-help approach and others on the 'therapeutic' interaction with a trained professional, which provides individuals with a further range of options. A recent meta-analysis of the effect of psychological interventions in people with type 2 diabetes (counselling, cognitive behaviour therapy, or psychodynamic therapy) showed improvements in long-term glycaemic control and reduced psychological distress (Ismail *et al.* 2004).

Traditional Western psychological models

Psychodynamic therapies is a general name for therapeutic approaches that try to help the individual bring to the surface their true feelings so that they can experience and understand them. It is based on a philosophy that, if a person can first unravel the subconscious thoughts and feelings that were repressed over years because they are too painful to acknowledge, yet have caused harm in the form of depression and anxiety, they are easier to resolve. Being able to see subconscious feelings for what they really are reduces the pain the individual associates with them, which results in reduced anxiety and depression.

Behavioural therapies aim solely at changing what people do; they are not really interested in thoughts and feelings. These therapies focus on providing rewards for alternative behaviours. Behavioural 'treatments' can emphasise the importance of structured activity, helping the patient learn that they can gain some control over their environment.

Cognitive therapies work from a philosophy that long-term cognitions or thoughts have resulted in a set of behaviours through learning and conditioning. They emphasise the important role thinking plays in how people feel and act. Therefore, if people are experiencing unwanted feelings and behaviours, it is important to identify the thinking that is causing those feelings/behaviours and learn how to replace this thinking with thoughts that lead to more desirable reactions. Examples are Cognitive Therapy, Cognitive Behavioural Therapy, and Cognitive Analytical Therapy.

Traditional Eastern models

Meditation is described as a group of mental practices performed to achieve spiritual, psychological and physical goals. It was developed over 3000 years ago from Hinduism and Buddhism. One form, transcendental meditation, became popular after the Second World War and is described as a form of concentrative meditation where the individual repeats a mantra over and over while sitting in a comfortable position. Concentrating on the mantra prevents any distracting thoughts from arising. Professor Benson from Harvard University studied transcendental meditation in the 1970s and engendered further interest in the technique when he released the results of a study that examined the effect of meditation on a group of monks, which described the 'relaxation response'.

Mindfulness meditation, on the other hand, encourages the individual to notice everything going on around them but not to think about them. The goal is a clearer, calmer, non-reactive state of mind. Meditation was found to be one of the therapies most commonly used by people with diabetes in a study of the prevalence and pattern of complementary therapy use by people with diabetes in the USA, although the type of meditation was not defined (Egede *et al.* 2002). This study also identified diabetes as an independent predictor of use of complementary therapies.

Studying and evaluating meditation research

Caspi in a critique of the literature surrounding meditation research highlighted:

> Like other complex, multifaceted interventions in medicine, meditation represents a mixture of specific and not-so-specific elements of therapy. However, meditation is somewhat unique in that it is difficult to standardize, quantify, and authenticate for a given sample of research subjects. Thus, it is often challenging to discern its specific effects in order to satisfy the scientific method of causal inferences that underlies evidence-based medicine. Therefore, it is important to consider the key methodological challenges that affect both the design and analysis of meditation research. Among the challenges are the mismatches between questions and designs, the variability in meditation types, problems associated with meditation implementation, individual differences across meditators, and the impossibility of double-blind, placebo-controlled meditation studies. Among the design solutions offered are aptitude x treatment interaction (ATI) research, mixed quantitative-qualitative methods, and practical (pragmatic) clinical trials. Similar issues and solutions can be applied more generally to the entire domain of mind – body therapies.

> (Caspi and Burleson 2005)

The challenges outlined in Caspi's comment apply to many stress management and interpersonal therapies. Therefore the next section outlines some commonly used complementary counselling approaches and provides some indication of the evidence available to support their use.

Yoga

The word 'yoga' from the Sanskrit word *yuj* meaning to yoke or bind and is often interpreted as 'union' or a method of discipline. Unlike stretching or fitness, yoga is more than just physical postures. It is a system of exercises, which help the individual gain control of their body and mind. Jayasinghe (2004) suggested that yoga improves breathing and focuses the alignment of the body. Yoga, when used as a form of complementary medicine, is a combination of breathing exercises, physical postures, and meditation, that has been practised for over 5,000 years in alternative medical systems such as Ayurveda, see Chapter 10.

Khalsa *et al.* (2004) conducted a bibliometric analysis on the biomedical journal literature involving research on the clinical application of yoga and revealed an increase in publication frequency over the past three decades and a substantial and growing use of randomised controlled trials. The types of medical conditions studied include psychopathological such as depression and anxiety, cardiovascular diseases such as hypertension and heart disease, respiratory diseases, for example, asthma, diabetes and a variety of others. The majority of the available research was conducted by Indian investigators and published in Indian journals, particularly yoga specialty journals, although recent trends indicate increasing contributions from investigators in the US and England (Khalsa 2004).

Bijlani *et al.* (2005) studied 98 people in a heterogeneous group of patients with hypertension, coronary artery disease, diabetes mellitus, and a variety of other illnesses. The intervention consisted of asanas (postures), pranayama (breathing exercises), relaxation techniques, group support, individualised advice, lectures and films on the philosophy of yoga and the place of yoga in daily life, meditation, stress management, nutrition, and knowledge about the illness. The researchers reported that the intervention led to favourable metabolic effects, but only within a period of nine days.

In contrast, Kerr *et al.* (2002) in the UK found no improvements in a study that examined the influence of yoga on 37 people with poorly controlled diabetes. Patients were randomised to a traditional intensive education programme and simple exercises, or a 16-week (32 session) Hatha yoga plan. Participation in regular yoga sessions did not improve glycaemic control but insulin requirements remained stable in the yoga group and increased in the control group. Although quality of life was not altered, all but one subject in the yoga group opted to continue yoga in the long term after completion of the study.

Studies into the direct effect of yoga techniques on physiology have demonstrated that people with type 2 diabetes practising yoga asanas and pranayama can achieve better glycaemic control and pulmonary function. The exact mechanism by which these postures and controlled breathing, interact with somato-neuro-endocrine mechanisms affecting metabolic and pulmonary functions has not been determined (Malhotra *et al.* 2002a). Yoga asanas appear to have a beneficial effect on glycaemic control and improve nerve function in mild to moderate type 2 diabetes with sub-clinical neuropathy (Malhotra *et al.* 2002b).

7.5 Stress Management Techniques

There is a range of stress management approaches and techniques to help people reduce tension and induce a state of relaxation. The most common techniques used in the western world are biofeedback, guided visual imagery, progressive muscle relaxation and transcendental meditation. Biofeedback involves an individual being connected to a device that monitors some biological measure such as muscle tension, heart rate, galvanic skin response, and EEG. Thereafter, the individual is asked to experiment with thoughts and or bodily states, for example, muscle tension to determine which activities reduce tension, which is evident on the relevant monitor (biological feedback device). Thus, the individuals learn their own technique for tension reduction and therefore relaxation, which with time and practice they can perform without being connected to the biofeedback machine.

Guided visual imagery attempts to help people enter into a relaxed state by trying to mentally place themselves in a different situation. A tape is used to guide the individual through the process, by prompting them to imagine they are somewhere pleasant and relaxing (typically a walk in the countryside), and encouraging the individual to place themselves in the different place with increasing accuracy by reminding them of the sounds, sights, smells and feelings that go with chosen location. Like biofeedback, with time and practice, the individual will not need to use the guidance provided on the tape or CD. Guided imagery is a widely used technique and used in the Chronic Disease Self-Management Program (Lorig *et al.* 2004) to help individuals develop their self-management skills. Participants in the Chronic Disease Self-Management Programme are encouraged to make their own tape or CD to use.

Where guided visual imagery is predominantly a mental approach to relaxation, progressive muscle relaxation is primarily a physical relaxation programme. Progressive muscle relaxation is a technique where individuals are asked to focus their attention on a particular muscle or group of muscles, they are then asked to tense the muscle/group of muscles and after holding the tension for a short while to release the tension and thereby relax the muscle. Often the instructions are provided on tape or CD. The process is repeated for each muscle group in the body. Over time the person learns to do the exercise without needing the tape or CD.

How can these techniques help people with diabetes?

Stress management techniques are used in diabetes on the hypothesis that stress and tension stimulate hepatic glucose release and increase insulin resistance due to the stress hormones that are released in stressful situations. In addition, when people are stressed, they tend to use compensatory behaviours such as smoking more, drinking more, and reducing activity, which also increases blood glucose levels. Although these effects are thought to occur in everybody, there is substantial variability in how people respond to stress. Therefore, these approaches may be of most significant benefit to the subset of people who are physiologically stress reactive, about 20 per cent of population. In addition, stress management programmes do not just teach people stress management techniques, they invariably contain some psycho-educational component, predominantly based on Cognitive Behaviour Therapy, and benefits can be expected from this approach as well.

Surwit et al. (2004) evaluated the efficacy and feasibility of a cost-effective outpatient group programme for stress management training in a randomised, controlled trial. Individuals with type 2 diabetes (n = 108; not on insulin; mean age 57.3 ± 10.7 years; mean HbA_{1C} 7.9 ± 1.8 per cent) were randomised to either a control group (n = 48) receiving five weekly group sessions of diabetes education, or the experimental group (n = 60), attending five sessions of stress management training, involving progressive muscle relaxation (PMR), instruction in stress-reducing cognitive and behavioural skills (identifying stressors, guided imagery, thought stopping), and education about the health consequences of stress. Participants practised PMR between sessions using audiotapes. Over six months, HbA_{1C} results improved equally in both groups. At the 12-month follow up, improvements were only sustained in the stress management group and resulted in a significant 0.5 per cent reduction in HbA_{1C}. The intervention did not have any effect on perceived stress, anxiety, and general psychological health. Researchers did not find evidence to support the hypothesis that stress management is of greater benefit to subjects with higher levels of anxiety.

In an earlier small, controlled study on stress management training for groups of people with type 2 diabetes (n = 22; mean age 61.0 ± 10.2 years; mean HbA_{1C} 11.0 ± 1.9 per cent), participants were randomised to relaxation training or routine medical care (Aikens et al. 1997). Sessions were conducted weekly for six weeks and lasted one hour. During the sessions participants undertook PMR, imagery, and group discussion of stressful life events. At the four-month follow-up, the training did not have any effect on glycaemic control, generalised distress, anxiety, or daily hassles. Higher levels of anxiety and distress at baseline were associated with less improvement in glucose tolerance in the intervention group. These short-term interventions aimed at reducing physiological arousal in older people were not successful in modifying the psychological variables related to stress and had mixed effects on glycaemic control. These findings suggest that highly anxious individuals might respond better to individually administered interventions.

The impact of a stress management and relaxation programme on glycaemic control and mood was evaluated in a randomised, wait-list controlled study (Stenstrom *et al.* 2003). Participants were people with type 1 diabetes who perceived themselves as having stress-related difficulties in their daily life and in the management of their diabetes (n = 36; mean age 40.8 ± 12.4 years; mean HbA_{1C} 7.3 ± 1.4 per cent; mean duration of diabetes 10.5 years; 61 per cent female). The programme consisted of 14 two-hour group meetings, in which instruction in stress and stress management, muscle relaxation, mental imaging, and mental goal setting were practised. Improvements in relaxation and tension were greatest for those with poorest scores at baseline. No improvements in mood or HbA_{1c} were reported, probably due to already neutral to positive mood states and satisfactory glycaemic control at the start of the study.

One issue that should be considered when evaluating the research and clinical utilisation of stress management programmes, is that not everyone is stress re-active. Some individuals seem to show marked elevations in blood glucose levels in relation to stress. However, not everybody shows these effects. Some individuals show no obvious association between blood glucose levels and stress levels (Yasar *et al.* 1994; Clarke *et al.* 1997). These studies also suggest people with diabetes are fairly good at identifying whether they are stress re-active in terms of their blood glucose levels. Polonsky (1999) suggested a relatively simple method for establishing stress re-activity. Although the relative proportions of stress re-active individuals is unknown, current data suggest only a minority of individuals with diabetes are stress re-active. However, large population data are not yet available to inform this issue.

Mindfulness-Based Stress Reduction Therapy (MBSR)

MBSR is a structured 8–10 week, group programme with patients from diverse problems with groups usually consist of between 10 and 40 participants. Single weekly sessions are typically 2.5 hours long, and there is an additional single all-day session per course on a weekend day. Each session covers particular exercises and topics that are examined within the context of mindfulness. These include different forms of mindfulness meditation practice, mindful awareness during yoga postures, and mindfulness during stressful situations and social interactions. Because development of mindfulness is predicated upon regular and repeated practice, participants enter upon enrolling into a commitment to carry out daily 45-min. Homework assignments primarily in the form of meditation practice, mindful yoga and applying mindfulness to situations in everyday life.

As for the other relaxation/stress management approaches it would be expected that those individuals who are physiologically highly stress re-active would experience benefits in terms of blood glucose regulation. In addition, the programme is expected to help people keep their focus on the present moment, and so help alleviate general anxiety and possibly more diabetes-specific anxieties. The programme also may facilitate individuals becoming more proactive in managing their health.

There are two published meta-analyses showing that, for a diverse range of individuals with chronic illness, people attending an MBSR programme report substantially reduced psychological distress, fewer symptoms, and lower blood pressure, and studies indicate that over 90 per cent of individuals continue to use some form of mindfulness practice several years after completing the programme (Baer 2003; Grossman *et al.* 2004). Group MBSR holds particular promise for individuals with comorbid anxiety problems and people with chronic pain. Although no studies have reported data on diabetes patients, one would expect that the MBSR approach would be particularly beneficial for individuals with diabetic painful peripheral neuropathy.

Autogenic Therapy (AT)

Autogenic Therapy (AT) is a powerful and comprehensive therapeutic system encompassing both mind and body. AT teaches skills that enable people to utilise their own capacity for self-healing and self-development (http://www.autogenic-therapy.org.uk/). AT consists of a training course during which clients learn a series of simple exercises in body awareness and relaxation designed to switch off the stress-related 'fight and flight' system of the body and switch on the 'rest, relaxation and recreation' system. During training the individual has the opportunity to learn and experience *passive concentration*, a state of alert but detached awareness, which enables the trainee to break the vicious circle of excessive stress, whatever its origins.

McGrady and Horner (1999) undertook a controlled study to determine the effect of mood state, specifically depression, anxiety, and daily hassles on the outcome of biofeedback-assisted relaxation in type 1 diabetes. Eighteen subjects completed the study, nine in the biofeedback-assisted relaxation group and nine in the control group. There were no significant group differences in blood glucose between those receiving biofeedback-assisted relaxation and the subjects continuing usual care. Five of the nine experimental subjects and one of the nine control subjects were identified as succeeders according to an arbitrary criterion. Treatment failures were more depressed, more anxious, and took longer to complete the protocol than succeeders.

Statistically significant correlations were found between high scores on inventories measuring depression, anxiety, and hassles intensity and higher blood glucose levels and smaller changes in blood glucose as a result of treatment. The findings suggest mood has an important impact on the response to biofeedback-assisted relaxation. Further research is necessary to determine whether assessing anxiety and depression followed by appropriate treatment where necessary should precede biofeedback-assisted relaxation in people with type 1 diabetes.

Kostic found that selected type 2 diabetes patients, especially those who are most responsive to stress would benefit from AT and achieve better glucose control and lipid metabolism, which are not always achieved using conventional treatment.

Hypnosis

Hypnosis is defined as a process where a person induces an altered state of attention or degree of awareness in another person by suggesting the subject experiences changes in sensations, perceptions, thoughts and behaviour (Allen 2002). There is widespread use but limited evidence of any beneficial effects of hypnosis in managing diabetes and vascular disease. Ratner studied the effect of hypnosis in a group of adolescents with type 1 diabetes (n = 7 aged 11–19 years). Patients were managed in the diabetes clinic and received their usual care. All seven had long-term poor control, which did not improve in the six months immediately prior to the study. To ensure that each patient would serve as his or her own control, no management changes were made other than the addition of hypnosis. Six of the seven patients were followed for more than six months. No changes were made to prescribed insulin regimens, diet, or exercise. Post-treatment, the average HbA_{1C} dropped from 13.2 per cent to 9.7 per cent, and the average fasting blood glucose from 426 mg/dl to 149 mg/dl.

Prayer

Intercessory prayer has been shown to have no significant effect on medical outcomes after hospitalisation in a coronary care unit (Aviles *et al.* 2001). However, Yeh *et al.* (2002) attempted to characterise the use of complementary and alternative medicine (CAM) among people with diabetes mellitus residing in the United States. The study included, 2055 people and was undertaken between 1997 and1998. Ninety-five (95) respondents reported having diabetes, of these 57 per cent reported using CAM in the past year; fewer respondents (35 per cent) reported using CAM specifically for diabetes.

Therapies used for diabetes included solitary prayer/spiritual practices (28 per cent), herbal remedies (7 per cent), commercial diets (6 per cent), and folk remedies (3 per cent). Excluding solitary prayer, only 20 per cent of respondents used CAM to treat diabetes. They concluded that the prevalence of CAM therapy use among people with diabetes is comparable to that among the general population. Use of CAM therapies specifically to treat diabetes, however, is much less common (Yeh *et al.* 2002).

Cognitive Behavioural Therapy (CBT)

Cognitive behaviour therapy (CBT) is based on the fact that people's feelings are largely determined by how they think and their behaviour. Therefore, CBT focuses on two broad strategies to facilitate emotional well-being. The first is to consider the activities an individual engages in and how they serve to reinforce the current mood states. For example, depressed people tend to withdraw from social contact and meaningful activities, which feed thoughts about being unwanted, not valued and not pleasant to be with. Through activity scheduling, the individual is gently encouraged to engage in activities designed to improve their self-perceptions.

People suffering from anxiety often avoid the object or situation that drives their anxiety, and in so doing, the individual feeds their negative beliefs and the anxiety. The individuals' anxiety can be partly alleviated by gently encouraging people to face their anxieties through activity scheduling.

The cognitive component of CBT therapies focuses on helping people come to terms with the automatic negative thoughts that drive their emotions. Once individuals are helped to identify these thoughts and the typical cognitive distortions they apply, they can be supported to challenge these thoughts and reduce their impact and frequency. However, CBT is more a family of therapies, including such therapies as Rational Emotive Therapy, Dialectical Behaviour Therapy, and Mindfulness Based Cognitive Therapy, rather than one specific therapy. Different versions emphasise different aspects of the process.

In a recent pilot study, the utility of short, structured, well-described group interventions based on principles of cognitive behavioural therapy was tested in people with type 1 diabetes in long-term poor glycaemic control (Snoek et al. 2001). The feasibility and efficacy of the CBGT programme were also tested. The programme aimed to assist patients to overcome negative beliefs and attitudes toward diabetes and achieve better glycaemic control without compromising emotional well-being. Twenty-four patients participated in a four-week programme. Each session lasted 1.5 hours and was delivered by a diabetes nurse specialist and a psychologist in small groups of 6–8 patients. Each session addressed a different topic:

- the cognitive behavioural model of diabetes;
- stress and diabetes;
- living with the future (worries about complications);
- social relationships.

Training focused on cognitive restructuring, stress management techniques, and behavioural strategies such as cueing and self-monitoring. CBGT proved feasible in this selected group and was well appreciated. The results showed a substantial drop in HbA_{1C} at the six-month follow-up and emotional well-being was preserved.

The effectiveness of an extended (six-week) version of the programme was evaluated in a randomised, controlled trial. Participants were selected on the basis of long-standing high HbA_{1c}, high levels of self-reported psychological distress and depressive symptoms, and relatively low self-efficacy. The results show that CBGT was successful in improving self-efficacy, diabetes-related distress and mood at the three-months follow-up, but glycaemic control did not improve (van der Ven et al. 2005).

Weinger et al. (2002) randomised people with type 1 diabetes to either an eight-week psychologist-led CBGT intervention similar to van der Ven et al's eight-week programme, or cholesterol education classes, to control for attention. The programme used cognitive restructuring and relaxation techniques to help participants achieve better glycaemic control. At the six-month follow-up, adherence and HbA_{1c} were improved in both groups. There were no differences in HbA_{1c} between the groups at post test, although the CBGT participants achieved modest a improvement from pre- to post test. Quality of life was improved in the experimental group only. The small studies suggest that overall, short, structured CBGT interventions are relatively effective in improving psychological well-being.

Cognitive Analytic Therapy (CAT)

CAT is a form of psychotherapy that involves a therapist and an individual working together, by looking at the issues that hindered changes in the past, in order to understand better how to move forward in the present. Questions such as, 'Why do I always end up feeling like this?' become more answerable. www.rcpsych.ac.uk/info/glosTreats.htm.

Fosbury *et al.* (1997) compared the effect of individual outpatient CAT in a randomised controlled trial consisting of 26 chronically poorly controlled people with type 1 diabetes (10 CAT, 16 education). CAT consisted of time-limited psychotherapy sessions delivered by a psychotherapist. A diabetes nurse specialist provided the individual diabetes education. Of the 26 patients, 18 were female, mean age was 31 years (range 19–52 years), and baseline HbA_{1c} was 11.9 ± 1.7 per cent. Interestingly, glycaemic control improved significantly in the control group at the three-months follow-up, with a mean fall of 1.3 per cent in HbA_{1c} by the nine-month follow-up the HbA_{1c} had reduced further to 0.9 per cent. Three months after completing CAT, mean HbA_{1c} had dropped 1.5 per cent and had reduced by 2 per cent at the nine-month follow-up. Although not statistically different from education, glycaemic improvement showed a prolonged effect in CAT.

Solution-Based Therapy

Solution-focused brief therapy is an approach to psychotherapy based on solution building rather than problem-solving. It explores current resources and future hopes rather than present problems and past causes (http://apt.rcpsych.org). In a non-randomised controlled pilot study, a group intervention based on motivational solution focused therapy was delivered to adolescents (11–17 years) to help them improve their poor glycaemic control ($HbA_{1c} > 8.5$). The intervention was based on motivational interviewing and solution-focused therapy, including elements of CBT. Participants attended six sessions held weekly. Control subjects were randomly selected from those refusing to participate. The intervention proved effective in improving HbA_{1c} at the six-months follow-up (10.2 per cent to 8.7 per cent, $p < 0.05$; controls 9.8 per cent). These findings should, however, be interpreted cautiously: the reach of the intervention seems low with only 21 of 126 (17 per cent) eligible patients willing to participate. Using patients who refused the intervention as controls also seems problematic. Therefore, it remains unclear whether the improvements can be attributed to the intervention or simply to motivation to change (Viner *et al.* 2003).

Motivational Interviewing (MI)

Motivational Interviewing (MI) has been described as a directive, counselling style for eliciting behaviour change by helping people explore and resolve ambivalence. MI has been implemented in a variety of health-care settings within adult populations. The results from two systematic reviews show impressive effect sizes (> 0.33) for studies delivering MI in substance misuse. The results are less conclusive for other lifestyle areas. Most of the published research with teenagers and MI has been in the substance misuse field where some pilot studies demonstrate positive results in the diabetes field (Dunn et al. 2001).

The preliminary benefits of MI theory demonstrated in pilot studies were recently tested in a randomised controlled trial of MI with adolescents (Skinner et al. 2005). To address the criticism of MI, that scientific evaluation of the methods is lacking, and issues relating to interventionist training, supervision, and quality monitoring, Skinner et al. used direct clinical supervision. Furthermore, to provide a more rigorous test of the MI, individuals randomised to the control group received supportive counselling from a diabetes nurse specialist. Long-term follow-up data showed those receiving MI had significantly lower HbA_{1c}, particularly those individuals entering the study with poor control.

Combination therapeutic approaches

A number of US institutions offer mind–body programmes, which combine some of the methods described in the preceding sections, as well as professional training in these therapies. For example, the Center for Mind – Body Medicine in Washington, DC. (http://www.cmbm.org/) provides a programme that combines guided imagery, several types of meditation, autogenic training (self-hypnosis), biofeedback, breath work, movement, journal writing and drawing, self-awareness, exercise, and nutrition. As yet there are no published studies that demonstrate the effectiveness of this total approach. The Harvard Mind/Body Medical Institute led by Professor Benson (http://www.mbmi.org/research/published.asp#Review) focuses on the impact of stress reduction techniques and undertakes research into the effects of stress on anxiety, hypertension, and other conditions but not specifically in diabetes. Researchers at the Harvard Mind – Body Institute state: 'To the extent that one's medical condition and/or symptoms are caused or made worse by stress, we can help.'

Elder, in a review of the English language literature related to Ayurveda and diabetes care encompassing herbs, diet, yoga, and meditation as modalities that are accessible and acceptable to Western clinicians and patients found a considerable amount of data from both animal and human trials suggesting the efficacy of Ayurvedic interventions in managing diabetes, see Chapter 10. However, the reported human trials generally fall short of contemporary methodological standards and yet again highlighted the need for more research in the area of Ayurvedic treatment of diabetes, assessing both whole practice and individual modalities (Elder 2004). Likewise, essential oils are often used for their psychological effects in vaporisers during counselling, in massage for a range of reasons including stress management as well as self-care, see Chapter 6.

7.6 Summary

This chapter explored some of the reasons people with diabetes might seek complementary and conventional counselling and relaxation therapies in their journey with diabetes. It also attempted to consider the evidence so far available regarding some of the more common techniques. Common themes emerging in the literature are:

1. Taking time to work through each individual's issues and barriers to self-care with a therapist who typifies the characteristics of acceptance, respect, curiosity and honesty (ARCH) is important. The focus should be on helping the individual realise their goals and aspirations, not necessarily improving blood glucose results.
2. For individuals, putting time into everyday life enables them to bring themselves back to a state of equilibrium, harmony or centredness.
3. While the goal of these interventions is not primarily improved metabolic outcomes, it appears that there is improvement in these as a result of improved emotional well being.

One of the challenges of the increasing interest in mind – body links is that professionals will seek to develop new interventions, which will be prescribed across whole populations and may help some people and not others, rather than recognising that, possibly, the value of the various therapies outlined in this chapter is that they assist the individual to strengthen their own resources. Requirements of individuals vary – so how do health professionals introduce the range of therapies to the people with diabetes we care for and assist them to seek therapies likely to help? It appears that the focus should be on helping people know themselves more, rather than health professionals continuing to assume they know what is best. Such a change will involve many health professionals using consultation skills that assist personal exploration of diabetes and life, as well as providing people with signposts to therapies that they may not have otherwise be aware of.

In addition, there is recognised need for great openness and explicitness regarding the shared responsibility among health-care and complementary care providers and patients (Kainz 2003). However, an unintended consequence of modern therapies that focus on mind – body interaction is the risk that people with diabetes will experience guilt and self-blame for contracting a disease such as cancer and/or for failing to heal themselves. If these therapies are 'prescribed' within the current 'acute care' paradigm, their impact may not be as expected.

Penultimately, this chapter focused on people with established disease, Grattan (2004) highlights that, while many people seek CAM to help with the emotional strains of life and diabetes, others use CAM as a preventative approach. For example, 18.9 per cent of adults in the US sought out 'mind – body' therapies such as meditation, yoga and imagery as an alternative to the lack of effect of statins in preventing cardiac illness (Grattan 2004). Grattan suggested that, while studies show the 'tremendous effect of statin therapy in reducing cardiovascular event reduction', they remind us that this represents a 70 per cent failure rate and that 'scores of patients' have realised this and are seeking alternatives to reduce their risk of deteriorating cardiovascular disease. He postulated that this finding is likely to be an increasing phenomenon as people access more information via the Internet, interpret it and take responsibility for their own health promotion and may be particularly true in countries where direct health costs are escalating.

The last word goes to an editorial written by Frank Snoek (2001):

Clearly, the mind matters in diabetes. Man is not simply a machine, as Descartes suggested more than 300 years ago. It seems we have come full circle in our beliefs about the mind body relationship. Body and mind clearly interact and in complex ways that we do not yet fully understand. To me, taking the mind into consideration is anything but 'alternative' and is certainly congruent with a holistic approach to caring for people with diabetes.

References

Aikens J, Kiolbasa T, Sobel R. Psychological predictors of glycemic change with relaxation training in non-insulin-dependent diabetes mellitus. *Psychotherapy and Psychosomatics* 1997; **66**: 302–306.

Allen R. Hypnosis. *Complementary Medicine* 2002; **Sept/Oct**: 32–36.

Anderson R, Freedland K, Clouse R, Lustman P. The prevalence of comorbid depression in adults with diabetes: a meta-analysis. *Diabetes Care* 2001; **24**: 1069–1078.

Anderson R, Grigsby A, Freedland K, de Groot M, McGill J, Clouse R *et al*. Anxiety and poor glycemic control: a meta-analytic review of the literature. *International Journal of Psychiatry in Medicine* 2002; **32**: 235–247.

Aviles J, Whelan S, Hernke D, Williams B, Kenny K, O'Fallon W *et al*. Intercessory prayer and cardiovascular disease progression in a coronary care unit population: a randomized controlled trial. *Mayo Clinic Proceedings* 2001; **76**(12): 1192–1198.

Baer R. Mindfulness training as a clinical intervention: a conceptual and empirical review. *Clinical Psychology* 2003; **10**: 125–143.

Benson H. Harnessing the power of the placebo effect and renaming it 'remembered wellness'. *Annual Review of Medicine* 1996; **47**: 193–9.

Bijlani R, Vempati R, Yadav R, Ray B, Gupta V, Sharma R *et al*. A brief but comprehensive lifestyle education program based on yoga reduces risk factors for cardiovascular disease and diabetes mellitus. *Journal of Alternative and Complementary Medicine* 2005; **11**(2): 267–274.

Caspi O, Burleson KO. Methodological challenges in meditation research. *Advances in Mind-Body Medicine* 2005; **21**: 4–11.

Chandola T. Brunner E. Chronic stress at work and the metabolic syndrome: prospective study. *British Medical Journal Online First* 2006; (accessed February 2006).

Clarke W, Cox D, Gonder-Frederick L, Julian D, Schlundt D, Polonsky W. The relationship between nonroutine use of insulin, food, and exercise and the occurrence of hypoglycemia in adults with IDDM and varying degrees of hypoglycemic awareness and metabolic control. *Diabetes Educator*, 1997; **23**: 55–58.

de Groot M, Anderson R, Freedland K, Clouse R, Lustman P. Association of depression and diabetes complications: a meta-analysis. *Psychosomatic Medicine* 2001; **63**: 619–630.

Dunn C, Deroo L, Rivara F. The use of brief interventions adapted from motivational interviewing across behavioral domains: a systematic review. *Addiction* 2001; **96**: 1725–1742.

Eaton W, Armenian H, Gallo J, Pratt L, Ford D. Depression and risk for onset of type II diabetes: a prospective population-based study. *Diabetes Care* 1996; **19**: 1097–1102.

Egede L, Ye X, Zheng D, Silverstein M. The prevalence and pattern of complementary and alternative medicine use in individuals with diabetes. *Diabetes Care* 2002; **25**(2): 324–329.

Elder C. Ayurveda for diabetes mellitus: a review of the biomedical literature. [Review] *Alternative Therapies in Health and Medicine* 2004; **10**(1): 44–50.

Ernst E, Rand J, Stevinson C. Complementary therapies for depression: an overview. *Archives of General Psychiatry* 1988; **55**: 1026–1032.

Fosbury J, Bosley C, Ryle A, Sonksen P, Judd S. A trial of cognitive analytic therapy in poorly controlled type I patients. *Diabetes Care* 1997; **20**: 959–964.

Frijling B, Lobo C, Keus I, Jenks K. Patient perception of CHD risk. *Patient Education and Counselling* 2004; **52**: 47–53.

Grattan J. Mind body approach to cardiac illness. In Frishman WH, Weintraub MI, Micozzi MS, (eds) *Complementary and Integrative Therapies for Cardiovascular Disease*, St Louis, Mo: Mosby, 2004, pp. 108–126.

Grossman P, Niemann L, Schmidt S, Walach H. Mindfulness-based stress reduction and health benefits: a meta-analysis. *Journal of Psychosomatic Research* 2004; **57**: 35–43.

Irvine A, Cox D, Gonder-Frederick L. Fear of hypogylcaemia: relationship to physical and psychological symptoms of patients with insulin-dependent diabetes mellitus. *Health Psychology* 2002; **11**: 135–138.

Ismail K, Winkley K, Rabe-Hesketh S. Systematic review and meta-analysis of randomised controlled trials of psychological interventions to improve glycaemic control in patients with type 2 diabetes. *The Lancet* 2004; **363**(9421): 1589–1597.

Jayasinghe S. Yoga in cardiac health; a review. *European Journal of Cardiovascular Prevention and Rehabilitation* 2004; **11**(5): 369–375.

Kainz K. Avoiding patient self-blame. *Complementary Therapies in Medicine* 2003; *11*: 46–48.

Kerr D, Gillam E, Ryder J, Trowbridge S, Cavan D, Thomas P. An Eastern art form for a Western disease: randomised controlled trial of yoga in patients with poorly controlled insulin-treated diabetes. *Practical Diabetes International* 2002; **19**: 164–166.

Khalsa S. Yoga as a therapeutic intervention: a bibliometric analysis of published research studies. *Indian Journal of Physiology and Pharmacology* 2004; **48**(3): 269–285.

Kostic

Lorig K, Ritter P, Laurent D, Fries J. Long-term randomized controlled trials of tailored-print and small-group arthritis self-management interventions, *Medical Care* 2004; **42**: 346–254.

Lustman P, Anderson R, Freedland K, de Groot M, Carney R, Clouse R. Depression and poor glycemic control: a meta-analytic review of the literature. *Diabetes Care* 2000; **23**: 934–942.

Malhotra V, Singh S, Singh K, Gupta P, Sharma S, Madhu S. *et al.* Study of yoga asanas in assessment of pulmonary function in NIDDM patients. *Indian Journal of Physiology and Pharmacology* 2002a; **46**(3): 313–320.

Malhotra V, Singh S, Tandon O, Madhu S, Prasad A, Sharma S. Effect of yoga asanas on nerve conduction in type 2 diabetes. *Indian Journal of Physiology and Pharmacology* 2002b; **46**(3): 298–306.

McGrady A, Horner J. Role of mood in outcome of biofeedback assisted relaxation therapy in insulin dependent diabetes mellitus. *Applied Psychophysiology and Biofeedback* 1999; **24**: 79–88.

Mollema E, Snoek F, Ader H, Heine R, van der Ploeg H. Insulin-treated diabetes patients with fear of self-injecting or fear of self-testing: psychological comorbidity and general well-being. *Journal of Psychosomatic Research* 2001; **51**: 665–672.

Nash J, Skinner T. Eating disorders in type 1 diabetes mellitus. *Practical Diabetes International* 2006; **22**: 139–145.

Polonsky W. Alexandra: American Diabetes Association, 1999.

Pouwer F, Beekman A, Nijpels G, Dekker J, Snoek F, Kostense P. *et al*. Rates and risks for co-morbid depression in patients with Type 2 diabetes mellitus: results from a community-based study. *Diabetologia* 2003; **46**: 892–898.

Ratner

Rosengren A, Hawken S, Ounpuu S, Sliwa K, Zubaid M, Almahmeed W. *et al*. Association of psychosocial risk factors with risk of acute myocardial infarction in 11119 cases and 13648 controls from 52 countries (the INTERHEART study): case-control study. *Lancet* 2004; **364**: 953–962.

Rubin R. Hypoglycaemia and quality of life. *Canadian Journal of Diabetes Care* 2002; **26**: 60–63.

Rubin RR, Peyrot M Psychological issues and treatments for people with diabetes. *Journal of Clinical Psychology* 2001; **57**: 457–478.

Skinner T, Murphy H, Huws-Thomas M. Diabetes in adolescents. In: Snoek FJ, Skinner TC (eds), *Psychology in Diabetes Care*, pp 27–51.

Snoek F. The mind matters. *Diabetes Spectrum* 2001; **14**: 116–117.

Snoek F, van der Ven N, Lubach C, Chatrou M, Ader H, Heine R. *et al*. Effects of cognitive behavioural group training (CBGT) in adult patients with poorly controlled insulin-dependent (type 1) diabetes: a pilot study. *Patient Education and Counselling* 2001; **45**: 143–148.

Stenstrom U, Goth A, Carlsson C, Andersson P. Stress management training as related to glycemic control and mood in adults with Type 1 diabetes mellitus. *Diabetes Research and Clinical Practice* 2003; 147–152.

Surwit R, van Tilburg M, Zucker N, McCaskill C, Parekh P, Feinglos M *et al*. Stress management improves long-term glycemic control in type 2 diabetes. *Diabetes Care* 2002; **25**: 30–34.

Taylor EP, Crawford J, Gold A. Design and development of a scale measuring fear of complications in type 1 diabetes. *Diabetes/Metabolism Research and Reviews* 2005; **21**: 264–270.

van der Ven N, Hogenelst M, Tromp-Wever A, Twisk J, van der Ploeg H, Heine R. *et al*. Short-term effects of cognitive behavioural group training (CBGT) in adult Type 1 diabetes patients in prolonged poor glycaemic control: a randomized controlled trial. *Diabetic Medicine* 2005; **22**: 1619–1623.

Viner R, Christie D, Taylor V, Hey S. Motivational/solution-focused intervention improves HbA1c in adolescents with Type 1 diabetes: a pilot study. *Diabetic Medicine* 2003; **20**: 739–742.

Weinger K, Schwarts E, Davis A, Rodriguez M, Simonson D, Jacobson A. Cognitive behavioural treatment in type 1 diabetes: a randomised controlled trial (abstract). *Diabetes* 2002; **51**: A439.

Yasar S, Mulassay T, Madacsy L, Korner A, Szucs L, Nagy I *et al*. Sympathetic-adrenergic activity and acid-base regulation under acute physical stress in type I (insulin-dependent) diabetic children. *Hormone Research* 1994; **42**: 110–115.

Yeh G EDDRPRS. Use of complementary and alternative medicine among persons with diabetes mellitus: results of a national survey. *American Journal Public Health* 2002; **92**: 1648–1652.

8 Energy Therapies

Geraldine Milton

8.1 Introduction

This chapter focuses on the possible benefits and potential harms of bioenergetic therapies in the management of diabetes and vascular disease particularly 'natural healing', Therapeutic Touch (Krieger–Kunz method), Healing Touch, Reiki, Qi gong and magnetic therapy. Commonly used energy therapies are:

- acupuncture and acupressure, see Chapter 10;
- colour and light therapy such as Aurasoma;
- Feng shui;
- flower remedies (Bach and Australian bush flower essences);
- Healing Touch;
- kinesiology or muscle testing, which is used to assess the state of the energy system;
- pranic healing;
- Qui gong;
- reflexology, see Chapter 13;
- Reiki;
- Shiatsu;
- Therapeutic Touch.

Each modality acts via a different mechanism but they all aim to re-establish or maintain a balanced energy flow. There is very little research to specifically support or challenge the use of bioenergetic therapies in the management of people with diabetes or vascular disease. However, there is a growing body of credible evidence to support the following:

- The existence of electromagnetic and subtle energy fields in living organisms. Factors that alter the subtle energy fields and electromagnetic fields can affect the structure and function of bodily systems (Tiller, 1987; Oschman 2000; Oschman 2003).
- Manipulating, changing, channelling or running energy, which is said to occur during bioenergetic treatments, have the potential to restore significant cellular

function (Oschman 2000). Restoration of cells throughout the body includes vascular, retinal, kidney, heart, pancreas, or skin cells, which is relevant to diabetes and vascular disease.

- Significant areas of the brain appear to be activated in people who are 'sent' healing energy from a distance (Achterberg *et al.* 2005).
- All healers produce similar brain patterns when they are in an altered state and performing healing treatments (Beck 1969, in Oschman 2000).
- More experienced healers generally have better results in experimental studies (Wilkinson *et al.* 2002).
- Healers tend to emit extremely low frequency energy waves from their hands (ELF of 0.3–30Hz). Artificially induced ELF frequencies have been used to stimulate capillary and fibroblast proliferation, bone growth, nerve regeneration, neurite outgrowth from cultured ganglia, ligament healing, to reduce skin necrosis, and to create synergic effects with nerve growth factor (Zimmerman 1990; Seto *et al.* 1992; Oschman 2000).
- Many people have a natural innate ability to heal by placing their hands on another person, which has been recognised by numerous cultures throughout the ages, and may be separate from faith healing within a religious context. Many 'healers' are often unaware of their ability, which is very relevant when selecting subjects to give treatments or mimic treatments in research on bioenergetic therapies (Grad 2004). Krieger and Kunz claim that everybody has an innate ability to 'heal' and can be taught how to 'send' healing energy to another person.

There is a growing perception that all medicine is energy medicine and that energy medicine 'holds the key to the future of the entire medical enterprise' (Oschman 2003). Oschman claims there are three reasons for this trend. First, the increasing awareness in medical science that 'the electrical and magnetic fields as well as light and sound affect cellular processes and can be used to stimulate healing in various tissues'. Second, there is a rapidly growing acceptance of complementary, alternative and integrative medicine. Third, sports medicine has contributed to the growth of energy medicine, particularly in the area of human performance. Athletes and their trainers are highly motivated to explore all available practical and acceptable approaches to enhance athletic potential in the competitive global sporting environment. However, health professionals and members of the community are still sceptical about the existence and efficacy of therapies that claim to work through energy, energy fields and synergism via a unique structural organisation of molecular components.

Gerber (2001) believes doctors do not accept the existence of subtle life force energy because there are no 'currently acceptable scientific models, which explain their existence and function'. However, Gerber maintains there is a scientific model that supports the existence of a subtle life force in the body, which is generally overlooked by conventional health professionals. For example, Gerber cites the well-known equation attributed to Einstein that energy and matter are dual expressions of the same thing ($E = MC^2$) and that objects or living things only appear solid because the molecular structure that creates synergy is denser than ethereal matter. From Gerber's perspective, human beings are beings of energy, and exposure to subtle energies influences their cellular growth patterns. Thus, repatterning and reorganising disordered energy fields is the key to treating recurring conditions, rather than predominantly using medicines, 'magic bullets', or quick fix plumbing such as unclogging clogged arteries, all of which is the mainstay of modern medicine. He also claims that science's inability to deal with the concept of vital forces 'animating the human frame' is partly due to the historical conflict between Eastern and Western belief systems.

8.2   Brief History of Energy Field Medicine within a Western Context

Energy field theory is not new within early models of medicine in Western cultures. For example, Paracelsus (1493–1541), the famous Swiss doctor said to have reformed medical thought, believed that man had two bodies; one of flesh and blood, and the other an energy body, known as the astral body (Brennan 1987). Paracelsus stated the vital force 'was not enclosed within an individual but radiated within and around him or her like a luminous sphere which could be made to act at a distance' (The Academy of Parapsychology and Medicine 1992). Franz Anton Mesmer (1733–1815), the founder of mesmerism, a precursor of clinical hypnotism, is also a well known but more controversial scientist who published his memoirs on his discovery of 'animal magnetism'. In 1773, Mesmer began using magnets in healing and his patients frequently noticed unusual currents coursing through their bodies prior to the onset of a 'healing crisis' that led to a cure. Even more significantly, he claimed he could produce the same phenomena without magnets simply by passing his hands above the patient's body (Brennan 1987; Oschman 2000). The energy movement appears similar to techniques currently used in Therapeutic Touch, Healing Touch and Qi gong, which will be discussed later in the chapter.

Mesmer was ridiculed and faced 'animosity, malicious rumours, slander and fear' when he invited other scientists to witness his work with 'incurable cases'. Three scientific commissions, one of whom included Benjamin Franklin, investigated Mesmer's work and concluded the reported effects were the imagination of his patients, 'not from any real magnetic effects' (Oschman 2000). The Faculty of Medicine in Vienna accused Mesmer of practising magic and expelled him (Brennan 1987). Given the growing scientific evidence now emerging that supports the phenomenon of bioenergetic healing therapies, Mesmer's work may need to be re-evaluated and he may be considered a courageous pioneer in the field of bioenergetics in the future.

Kaptchuk (1996) claimed that Mesmer's followers rapidly split into two denominations: lower and higher mesmeric interpretation. The lower 'made the force analogous to a physical electromagnetic vibration that resembled more recognised scientific energies' and the higher interpretation was less conventional because it regarded the force as ethereal and linked to mystical and occult traditions. It could be argued that the division still exists. Both positions attract different critics and supporters. Harold Burr from Yale School of Medicine studied electromagnetic fields in nature, which he called electrobiology. Burr believed 'fields of life' are the basic blueprints for all living things and that they reflect physical and mental conditions and therefore can be used for diagnostic purposes (Oschman 2000). In 1932, Burr began a series of 'controversial studies into the role of electricity in development and disease'. An early experiment, which continued for years, connected various trees at his home to voltmeters believing that 'all living things . . . are formed and controlled by fields that can be measured by standard detectors' (bioenergetics) (Oschman 2000). Burr found the electric field of trees changes in advance of weather patterns and other atmospheric phenomena.

In a subsequent study in 1935, Burr described the detection of ovulation by monitoring the substantial voltage changes during the ovulation cycle and in 1936 he began a series of studies on the relation between electrical fields and cancer in mice. Large voltage changes were detected with electrodes 10 days to two weeks before the tumours appeared. Burr's work is now highly recommended for the 'serious student . . . of biomedical research . . . exploring the role of energy fields in health and disease'. His work shows electromagnetic changes take place within all living things in response to stress, normal physiological processes and during illness (Oschman 2000).

Martha Rogers, a renowned nursing theorist and a physicist, had a strong influence on contemporary nursing in the 1970s and 1980s through her conceptual framework of nursing as the 'Science of Unitary Human Beings'. She asserted that human beings must be perceived in terms of their wholeness and as more than and different from the 'sum of their parts'. Rogers described an energy field as the fundamental unit of living. The field is a unifying concept and is dynamic and infinite. She maintained that human beings and the environment do not *have* energy fields, they *are* energy fields (Rogers 1989). Furthermore, she argued that human beings are not biological, physical, or psychosocial fields, they are irreducible. The fields are continuously open and each individual has their own unique pattern and their field is 'integral with its own unique environmental field'. From Rogers' perspective, therefore: 'a person is not an isolated energy field, but lives in an environmental energy field with which there is constant interaction . . . a change in one of the fields produces a change in the other' (Lewis 2000).

8.3   Effects of Geomagnetic Earth Rhythms on Health and Wellness

Living organisms are part of the energy environment of the planet in which they live, however, not all regions on earth are energetically beneficial and some local energy fields could be detrimental. Many cultures try to counteract harmful energies. For example, Western cultures are becoming more aware of a form of Chinese geomancy, Feng shui, which aims to create positive energy in individuals' work and living environments (Gerber 2001). Some of the earth's geomagnetic rhythms are slow and others are fast (in the extremely low frequency ELF) range called geomagnetic micropulsations caused by the Schumann resonance. The Schumann resonance is created by the sum of the lightning activity around the world and ranges in frequency from 1–40Hz (ELF) (Oschman 2000).

Eccles (2005) refered to the phenomenon noted by many scientists from space flight research, that depriving astronauts of the electromagnetic wave between the earth's surface and ionosphere, leads to abnormal body functioning. Others living on the planet may also react in the same way in certain environments. For example, in 1968, Wever *et al.* observed hundreds of subjects living in two underground rooms shielded from external rhythms of light, temperature, sound and pressure (Oschman 2000). Sleep–waking rhythms, body temperature, urination, and other physiological activities were monitored. One of the rooms had an electromagnetic shield that reduced geomagnetic rhythms by 99 per cent. All subjects developed longer and irregular or desynchronised or chaotic physiological rhythms. Those in the magnetically shielded rooms developed significantly longer and irregular rhythms. The only field pulsed into the shield around the rooms that normalised the physiological rhythms was a very weak 10Hz electrical field. As noted at the beginning of the chapter, Therapeutic Touch and other energy therapists tend to emit very low frequency energy (ELF) of 0.3–30Hz when they are in a healing state, with most of the activity in the range of 7–8 Hz (Zimmerman 1990, in Oschman 2000).

8.4 Electromagnetic and Subtle Energy Within Living Organisms

How does manipulating, changing, channelling or running subtle energy, the basis of bioenergetic therapies, potentially improve health and well-being? Oschman (2000) maintains vibrational or subtle energy, such as that emitted by healers, can restore significant cellular function throughout the living matrix that is designed to absorb information at a vibratory level. The living matrix can convert the information into signals that can be readily transmitted to lymph, blood, muscle, bone, organs, skin and connective tissue and throughout the nervous and immune system.

Living matrix

The invention of the electron microscope was a significant development in health care. It led to a very different picture of cells from that previously taught in health science courses. The cell is not a bag of fluid that just contains a nucleus and organelles. Scientists now know that cells are filled with a cytoplasmic matrix or cytoskeleton composed of filaments, tubes, fibres and trabeculae, with very little water, all of which link to the nuclear envelope, nuclear matrix and genes (Oschman 2000). Oschman described the crystalline system, which pervades all living organisms and the way electrical energy moves through the body so rapidly. Enzymes are delicately attached to structures within cells and are detached by biochemical homogenisation techniques. The surface of the cell is connected to the extracellular matrix by connective tissue and the cytoplasmic matrix is also linked to the nuclear envelope, nuclear matrix and genes. A whole series of transmembrane linking molecules or integrins have been discovered and the entire interconnective tissue has been called the 'living matrix'.

Scientists previously thought information was processed by neurohormones reacting with cell surfaces while others cross the cell membrane to affect cell functioning. However, many hormones deliver messages to cell surfaces and activate production of a second messenger within the cells that activate cellular activities (Oschman 2000). Therefore, there are two languages of communication in living systems. One is chemical and the other is energetic (electrical and electronic).

Resonance

> At the level of the atom we know that electrons whirl about the nucleus in certain energetically defined orbits. In order to move an electron from a lower to a higher orbit, a quantum of energy with very special frequency characteristics is required. An electron will only accept energy of the appropriate frequency to move from one energy level to another. If the electron falls from the higher to the lower orbit, it will radiate energy of that very same frequency.
>
> (Gerber 2001)

The resonance principle is fundamental to MRI and EMR imaging systems used in diagnostic procedures. Gerber gave a simple easily verified example of resonance. If two violins are placed at opposite ends of a small room and the E string is plucked on one of them, the violin on the other side of the room will also begin to vibrate 'and sing'. In a clinical context Gerber (2001) maintained that the energy essence of homeopathic remedies carries a 'subtle-energy signature of a particular frequency' and a skilled homeopath matches treatment with the energetic frequency of the ill patient. The resonance effect applies to all bioenergetic therapies that are applied to facilitate healing. Oschman (2000) claimed:

> we now know that all parts of the [human living] matrix set up vibrations that move about within the organism, and that are radiated into the environment. These vibrations or oscillations occur at many different frequencies, including visible and near visible light frequencies.

These are apparently not subtle phenomena but large vibrations. Furthermore, 'their effects are not trivial, because living matter is highly organised and exceedingly sensitive to the information conveyed by coherent signals' (Oschman 2000). Like Gerber, Oschman (2000) claimed that each molecule, cell tissue and organ has an ideal resonant frequency that coordinates its activities and complementary therapists are able to directly influence the body's systemic defence and repair mechanisms by manipulating and balancing the vibratory circuits.

8.5   Effects of Subtle and Electromagnetic Energy on Body Structure and Function

In relation to the effect of the subtle energy on the body's structure and function, Tiller presented three equations to explain how living organisms operate (Gerber 2001). The first is a traditional model where structural defects were thought to arise out of chemical imbalances, that is, function affects structure, which affects the chemistry of cells, and vice versa, see Figure 8.1 a. The second equation incorporates knowledge from more recent studies on the interactions between structure and electromagnetic fields. For example, studies have shown that small direct electric currents (DC) applied to leukocytes in vivo produce cell regeneration. On the other hand, larger current densities cause cell degeneration. This phenomenon demonstrates the 'less is more' principle, which is discussed later in the chapter. Tiller gave another example: bone receiving non-uniform stress over an extended period of time will grow new trabeculae in the precise location to support the new stress distribution. Therefore, Tiller believed that equation 1 must be replaced by equation 2. See Figure 8.1 b.

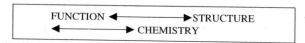

(a) Function affects structure, which affects the chemistry of cells, and vice versa

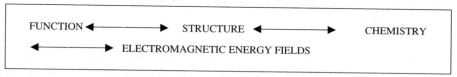

(b) Function affects structure which affects chemistry, which in turn affects the electromagnetic energy fields

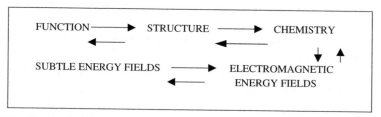

(c) Explanatory framework of how energy therapies can bring about change to affect an individual's well-being

Figure 8.1   Three equations to explain how living organisms operate through the effect of subtle energy on the body structure and function developed by Professor William Tiller from Stanford University in 1987.

However, Tiller offered a third equation (Figure 8.1 c) as a more reasonable explanation for a living organism cell. He argued that equation 2 was obviously defective because it overlooked mental effects. For example, individuals are capable of enormous strength and remarkable feats under hypnosis and acute stress. Practitioners of Aikido and Zen Yoga disciplines show a conscious link between the mind and structure and function and biofeedback studies show that the mind can control bodily functions and body repair. Tiller labelled these and other fields not clearly discriminated 'subtle energy fields'. Each item in the reaction chain maintains its conditions of homeostasis with the support from the item on its right. The development of a serious imbalance in any particular part of the chain leads to obvious disruption of homeostasis for the item to the left over time (Tiller 1987, in Gerber 2001).

Tiller's third equation provided another explanatory framework of how energy therapies can bring about change and affect an individual's well-being. Tiller's equations also leave open the possibility that fluctuations in subtle energies can sometimes be detected by healing therapists. Oschmann (2000) stated:

Suppose accumulated physical and/or emotional injury or trauma impairs continuity. The application of healing energy, whether from a medical device or from the hands of an energy therapist, would then open the network to the flow of energy and information. Once the whole network is functioning, natural biological communications could flow freely through the entire system, from the extracellular matrix, across the cell membrane, through the cytoskeleton, to the nucleus and on to the gene level, and in the opposite direction as well.

8.6   Brief Overview of Eastern Perspectives of Energy Healing

Western cultures have only recently begun to accept bioenergetic therapies and most conventional practitioners are still sceptical about their health benefits. Working with energy flows such as Chi, Ki or prana is generally integrated within the mainstream health care of most Eastern cultures, see Chapters 10 and 11. It is also possible that fluctuations in these subtle energies can sometimes be detected by healing therapists.

Another key concept of Chinese philosophy is the belief that energy polarity is expressed by Yin and Yang.

A scientific explanation consistent with the duality of Yin and Yang was provided by Tiller (1987) who differentiated between the duality of the physical and etheric human body. Tiller maintained that one part of the duality, which 'is electrical in nature and travels at velocities less than that of electromagnetic light, is of positive energy and positive mass' and forms the physical part of the body. This seems to correspond with Yin energy. The second part is magnetic in nature and 'travels at velocities greater than that of electromagnetic light' is of negative mass and energy and forms the etheric part of the vehicle for example the body.

This is similar to the Chinese perception of Yang energy. The total sum of these dual energies is zero.

Barbara Brennan, a former researcher at NASA, maintained that when Yin and Yang are balanced, the body exhibits physical health, but when they are unbalanced, disease results (Brennan 1987). This point is relevant to the practice of Therapeutic and Healing Touch where the practitioner aims to clear and rebalance the energy field through and around the client's body to enhance their wellness and facilitate healing.

8.7 Energy Medicine in Health Care and Relevance to Diabetes and Vascular Disease

The description of energy medicine given by the National Center for Complementary Medicine (NCCAM) is used in this part of the chapter. NCCAM is the US Federal Government's lead agency for CAM research and has posted five background reports on CAM categories on their website, one of which focuses on energy medicine. NCCAM acknowledged their overview is a summary of the scientific perceptions of energy medicine at the time it was posted rather than a comprehensive description. NCCAM divided energy medicine into two distinct areas: The first 'veritable' refers to bioelectromagnetic-based therapies that can be measured and the second 'putative' energy fields (biofields), which they claim have not yet to been measured.

Veritable therapies

Veritable therapies involve the unconventional use of electromagnetic fields such as pulsed fields, magnetic fields, or alternating current or direct current fields. Practitioners using this approach may use visible light, magnetism, monochromatic radiation such as laser beams, and rays from different parts of the electromagnetic spectrum. They may also utilise sound to create mechanical vibrations as treatment. The belief is that manipulating specific wavelengths and frequencies may promote health and treat disease. NCCAM identified four commonly used therapies in this category: magnetic therapy, millimetre wave therapy, sound energy therapy and light therapy.

- *Magnet therapy*: Chen (2002) focused the effects of magnets on blood glucose and eye function in diabetic subjects by attaching magnets to the auricular acupuncture points and showed blood glucose levels reduced and eye conditions improved. However, it is difficult to interpret how improvements were measured or ascertained. NCCAM noted that until recently very little well-structured research has been conducted into the effects of magnetic therapy. NCCAM does refer to a study that showed dilated microvessels constrict when exposed to a magnetic field (Morris and Skalak 2003). These results suggest magnetic therapy might benefit patients with oedema or ischaemic conditions, although further studies are needed to verify these benefits. If there are benefits, magnetic therapy may have a place in the management of diabetic retinopathy, renal impairment, cardiovascular disease, and other long-term complications.

- *Millimetre wave therapy*: Millimetre wave therapy uses low power millimetre waves (MW) irradiation and has been used by medical practitioners in Russia and Eastern Europe since 1977. Oschman (2003) differentiates between the traditional extremely high millimetre wave frequency range of 30–300 GHz and the therapeutic very low frequency range of $\leqslant 10\text{mW}/\text{cm}^2$ used in MW therapy. According to Pakhomov *et al.* (1998), MW is beneficial for over 50 diseases and conditions alone or in combination with other therapies. In both animals and humans, local exposure to these low power waves appear to stimulate tissue repair and regeneration, alleviate stress and pain, and accelerate recovery from a wide range of diseases and conditions. Pakhomov *et al.* conducted a comprehensive review of the uses of MW and discovered >1000 MW centres operating in the former Soviet Union and over three million people had received MW by 1995. MW has been used extensively to treat skin conditions, in wound healing, various types of cancer, gastrointestinal and cardiovascular diseases and psychiatric conditions (Rojavin and Ziskin 1998, cited by NCCAM). MW has also been shown to augment T cell immunity in vitro, but there is little understanding of the mechanism of action in these conditions (Logani *et al.* 2004, cited in NCCAM 2005). If all of these benefits are supported by quality research, MW treatment should be readily available to all health professionals to improve quality of life and long-term prognosis of people with diabetes and vascular disease. NCCAM recently established a centre to study the effects of MW therapy.
- *Sound energy therapy*: Sound energy therapy is also known as vibrational or frequency therapy (NCCAM 2005). The best known of these therapies is music therapy, which has been shown to reduce pain, relieve anxiety and affect blood pressure. There are numerous meditation tapes on the market that use music alone or music in combination with imagery. Gerber (2001) cited a well-known study by a Swiss researcher, Hans Jenny, who experimented on liquids with a sound transducer, which is relevant because most of the human body is made up of liquid. Jenny found sonic generators induced beautiful symmetrical shapes on a water droplet as long as the sound emitted by the transducer was moving through the drop and different sounds created different patterns. If Jenny is correct, the key to using sound in healing would be to know which sonic frequency should be applied to the body to facilitate healing particular health problems, and how the sounds should be applied.
- *Light therapy*: Natural or artificial light has long been used to treat a variety of health problems, the best known of which is seasonal affective disorder (SAD). There is little current evidence to show that light therapy improves depression or sleep disorders, although it is generally believed to be beneficial in these conditions (Culliton *et al.* 1997).

Energy medicine involving putative energy fields

NCCAM claims that putative energy fields or 'biofields' cannot currently be reproducibly measured, although this could be debated in light of the wealth of research referred to by authors such as Oschman and Gerber, discussed previously. Nevertheless, NACCM (2005) acknowledges that biofield therapy approaches are among the most controversial of CAM practices because of the lack of convincing biophysical evidence, despite their growing popularity.

8.8   Bioenergetic Therapies

Healers provide one of the oldest and most widespread forms of health care in many cultures, including faith healing, laying-on-of-hands, and ritual Shamanism (Rankin-Box 2001). Lay healers claim that religious faith does not influence the healing process (Rankin-Box 2001). Many healers believe that they are born with a natural ability to transmit healing energy, others believe the gift was sent to them, for example, Australian Aboriginal medicine men the author worked with in remote areas of Australia, see Chapter 12. Aboriginal healers claim their healing ability came to them in their sleep when they were young and they may lose it again when they are very old. Others who use therapies such as Therapeutic Touch (Krieger–Kunz method), Healing Touch, Reiki and Qigong have learned or enhanced their healing skills by attending courses, by mentorship or initiation, see Table 8.1. Warber *et al.* (2004) undertook extensive interviews with energy therapists from a variety of disciplines and concluded that biofield therapists share a common energetic world view, wherein they must surrender to a universal energy while simultaneously creating a therapeutic alliance with the client who is also an active agent in healing process. Table 8.1 outlines some of the main research in bioenergetic therapies.

Extremely low frequency waves and healing

Smith's findings that healers do not seem to emit a strong electromagnetic field, can be explained by Zimmermans research at the University of Colorado in Denver, USA. Zimmerman (1990) used a magnetometer that detected Extremely Low Frequency (ELF) electromagnetic fields. In the 1980s, Zimmerman conducted a series of experiments using a SQUID detector, which is highly sensitive and detects the weakest of the human biomagnetic fields (Oschman 2000). In Zimmerman's study, a TT practitioner entered a magnetically sealed chamber containing a SQUID detector and a baseline recording of his hand was made. The practitioner then relaxed into the meditative or 'centre' state, which is the focus of the TT method, see Table 8.1. Immediately the SQUID detected a large biomagnetic field emanating from the practitioner's hand. The field was so strong that the amplifiers and recorder had to be readjusted in order to record the energy field. This was the strongest ELF biomagnetic field Zimmerman had encountered in his years of medical research using SQUID detectors. It is important to note that

Table 8.1 Some of the main research into bioenergetic therapies: (a) Therapeutic Touch (TT) (Krieger–Kunz method); (b) Reiki; (c) Healing Touch; and (d) Qi gong.

Therapy and practice	Research	Treatment
(a) TT. Taught TT by recognised TT teacher over a 14–21 hour workshp for levels one, intermediate and advanced levels. There is an expectation these levels be repeated with different teachers, TT practitioners attend regular TT (peer reviewed) treatment sessions and show evidence of ongoing professional development. In Australia, TT is developing a national body (State bodies exist in South Australia, Tasmania and Victoria). While accredited competencies have been written, the Australian TT community are considering Cert. IV and diploma levels for professional practice. The intention of the practitioner is crucial to this practice, and usually begins with the intention of the TT practitioner to help or to heal the client. The premise being that 'energy' follows thought. The aim is to help to facilitate flow and balance in the client's energy field to promote wellness and wellbeing, and to reduce pain and anxiety. The overall aim is to facilitate an environment for the client to 'heal' themselves. (Heal in this sense is to make whole).	Has an impressive bibliography – from evidence-based research to a series of anecdotal case studies. Developed by Dolores Krieger and Dora Kunz. TT originated from nursing studies when Krieger was undertaking her PhD – is one of the most researched of all the bioergetic therapies. Early studies showed improvement in haemoglobin, immune function, wound healing, pain reduction, and reduced anxiety following a TT treatment. Subsequent studies have suggested that the nervous and circulatory systems are particularly receptive to TT with reduction in hypertension and tachycardia, and improvement in circulation for conditions like Raynard's disease. Improved arterial circulation with peripheral vascular disease also seen by author Some case studies show improved bone growth, resolution of phantom limb pain after amputation, and benefits to clients with chronic fatigue. Many of the early studies had problems with research design. A meta-analysis of TT research shows mixed findings in terms of efficacy. Some show significant benefits and some do not. In many studies the TT practitioner only gives 5–10 minutes of treatment rather than completing the treatment when a balanced field is achieved. This may skew some studies to show that TT treatment is not significantly effective when potentially it may be.	Usually 20 minutes in length, although less but more frequently if the client is acutely ill. Most of treatment actually non-touch. Practitioners prepare for giving treatments by 'centring' themselves or attaining a meditative-like state. (Step 1) Assessing the energy field follows (approx 2 minutes) although assessment is done frequently during TT. When assessing, the TT practitioner's intention is one of paying attention to subtle differences in perceptions of temperature, texture and flow of energy as they gently sweep their hands approximately 10–30 cms above the skin surface of the client. (Assessment is not essential, and inexperienced practitioners tend to vary in their ability to sense the field). The third step is unruffling the field, and the intention of the practitioner is to smooth and clear the energy field of irritation and congestion. The forth step is to modulate the energy, with the specific intention of rebalancing the energy flow when findings such as congestion, irritation or deficit have been detected, or are likely to occur. e.g. over adrenal glands if clients are stressed.

The final step is reassessing the energy field. Throughout and after the treatment the comfort and response of the client is paramount.

Treatment given in chair, bed or on treatment table. Explained to client what Reiki is and what the treatment procedure entails:

- Reiki practitioners do not diagnose;
- Use universal energy, not practitioner's personal energy with treatments.
- Reiki is the 'healer' not the practitioner.
- Practitioner will place their hands on client's body in a basic sequence – or in some cases, hands held briefly just above the body first in each position;
- Client usually fully clothed during treatment.
- Reiki practitioners are also taught to treat themselves – and encouraged to give a Reiki treatment to themselves daily.

Practitioners prepare themselves for treatment usually by attaining a meditative like state. Treatment usually lasts about a hour, but may be 20–30 mins, especially if client in seated position. Clients may be invited for frequent treatments daily/weekly depending on client's needs. Recipients with chronic conditions tend to benefit from a more prolonged series of treatments.

See table 2 for examples of some Reiki research. Reiki appears to induce a profound and prolonged relaxation response, pain relief, deepened awareness of spiritual connection with reduction in anxiety, tension and aggression. (Chapman and Milton 2002. Galeb, 2003. Kajsa Krishni Borang, 1997).

It also tends to elicit self awareness in clients who receive a treatment. This was seen to be a significant factor in assisting with counselling for clients in a drug and alcohol program in Melbourne. (Chapman and Milton 2002).

Some of the current research being undertaken in Australia includes Reiki support for cancer patients at Browne's Cancer Support Centre at Sir Charles Gardiner Hospital in Perth, Western Australia. Research is also being conducted at 'Bloomhill Cancer Help' in Buderim in Queensland. (Frew 2006).

No meta-analysis of Reiki research found at time of publication. It is expected that far more research on Reiki healing will soon take place as Reiki treatment is being given more frequently in health care settings. With the development of competencies for Reiki treatment practitioners, and with greater cohesion of Reiki groups and organizations, it will be easier to undertake Reiki research by minimizing variables inherent in the discipline.

(b) Reiki

Reiki. The System of Reiki. Since founded by Mikao Usui in Japan in the early 1920s, various lineages and forms of Reiki have emerged. Representatives of Reiki organizations and practices in Australia are co-operatively developing National competencies for Reiki treatment practitioners, with support from the Community Services Health Industry Skills Council.

If these draft Cert IV and Diploma qualifications are endorsed, they will become the nationally recognised standard for Reiki practitioners who wish to work in community services or health care settings in Australia. Participation in the validation of the Draft qualifications by stakeholders such as Reiki practitioners, and potential employers and associations, is vital to ensure broad industry acceptance of qualifications. (National Reiki Reference Group: www.nrrg.org.au)

Reiki courses are usually conducted over a 14–21 hour workshop – practitioners are 'initiated' by a Reiki 'Master', for levels one, and a similar length of time

Table 8.1 (Continued)

Therapy and practice	Research	Treatment
for level two. Level three or Master's level is usually through extensive mentorship of the student by one or more recognised Reiki Masters.		Reiki fundamentally differs from many other complementary therapies in that it is both a spiritual practice and healing art. The essential philosophical basis of Reiki incorporates both these dimensions in the practice of Reiki (*Report by Reiki Australia: Reiki Treatment Practice Draft 1 qualifications* 2005)
(c) Healing Touch Healing touch (HT) is taught in the American Holistic Nurses Association's Certificate Program, or in courses throughout the world endorsed by the AHNA. It is a holistic therapy that purports to work within the human energy system to clear blockages and restore balance in the body. From the viewpoint of a HT practitioner, healing is the process of altering mental, physical, emotional, and spiritual health positively Blends the energetic techniques of a number of practices, including some aspects of Therapeutic Touch. in addition to a number of other techniques (i.e. Brennan;	Sample from Healing Touch International website: • Arom, M.D & MacIntyre, B. 2002. Shorter hospital stay by patients undergoing coronary artery bypass surgery after HT (25 ICU patients) • Gilbert *et al.*, 2002. Use of healing touch in improving the quality of life among the dying. Reported that physical symptoms decreased compared to the control group who received standard care. The HT group also experienced increased relaxation, pain relief, spiritual benefit, increased calmness and improved breathing. 55 subjects in a Hospice and Palliative care centre were involved in the study. • Merritt, P. A combination of HT, massage and reflexology were tested in DIABETIC patients. Reported 70 per cent decrease in blood sugar when	Like TT and Reiki, treatment is given with clients fully clothed, either sitting or lying. Practitioners center themselves before treatment, and a key part of HT is that energy follows intent. Like TT, clients are assessed by the practitioner's hands 'sweeping' gently through the energy field of the client, while paying attention to subtle differences in energy flow, temperature, irritation and blankness in the field. The quality of healing is effected by the intent of the healer, the information obtained during assessment, the ability of the healer to influence the energy system of another person, and the openness of the client

Hover-Kramer et al.; Joy; Mentegen and Bulbrook).

The aim is to assess and if necessary rebalance the energy field of clients to promote wellness and restoration of health, and reduce pain and anxiety, Healing Touch International provides international standards of practice. Mentgen founded the systematic practitioner certification training program consisting of five clinical levels of practitioner training. Levels 1, 11A, 11B, 111A and 111B, and one instructor level (1V).

using combined therapies by 38 points, and 77 per cent of the subjects receiving HT had warming of hands suggesting improved circulation.

A meta-analysis of HT research conducted by Wardell & Weymouth (2004) showed HT used in diverse clinical settings including treatment of patients with various types of pain, cancer, cardiovascular disease, HIV, mental health problems and postoperatively. The analysis showed none of the findings were conclusive, especially those submitted to the HTI research program – they lacked vital information.

(d) Qi gong

Chinese Qi gong (trans; 'vital energy') is an ancient healing discipline, that McGee et al. (1996) claim has emerged from centuries of secrecy in the early 1980s. Written records go back 4000 years. Qi gong had been banned during the cultural revolution in China.

Has been some spectacular cures or remissions of cancers and skull/vertebral fractures published by the media in China. Most of the research has been conducted in China, and often abstracts have only been available in the West for review.

Diseases and medical conditions studied in which beneficial effects of Qigong have been reported include.

Qigong practitioners believe that energy is emitted from the body, and but not necessarily from the hand.

There are several forms of qi gong.

Internal Qi gong refers to Qigong practice or to cultivate by oneself optimal health of both mind and body (Jang and Lee, 2004). e.g. Guo Lin Gong is a walking form for self healing. Usually practiced for about 30 minutes a day, plus another 30 minutes of meditation. (McGee et al. 1996).

Table 8.1 (Continued)

Therapy and practice	Research	Treatment
The discipline consists of breathing techniques and mental exercises, usually accompanied by physical exercises. Qi gong balances subtle energy systems in the body. Tai Chi and marshal arts are based on the pronciples of Qi gong. It is Qi gong that approximately eighty million people in China practice every morning in groups and parks. (McGee et al. 1996). Theory based on the theories of Traditional Chinese Medicine. Qi or life force flow through the meridian pathways. According to TCM, when energy is flowing through the body at notmal levels and in balance, the body stays healthy. When imbalances or blockages occur, physiology is affected and illness and disease occur.	Aging; allergy; asthma; bone fractures; cancer; cardiovascular disorders; cervical spondylosis; circulation; diabetes; digestion disorders; gallstones; gastrointestinal disorders; headaches; hepatitis; hormone balance; hypertension; immunodeficiencies; impotency; inflammation; injuries; joint diseases; kidney disorders; liver disorders; lung disorders; lung disorders; mental health; myopia; paralysis; personality; stroke; tumours. (McGee et al. 1996). The inappropriate application of Qi gong or the inability to terminate the exercise has been reported to cause minor, mostly short-lived symptoms. In rare cases Qigong induced mental disorder is a recognised complication in China, with rare occurrence of abnormal violent behaviour. (Ernst, 2002a)	External Qi gong, where patients are treated by a Qi gong practitioners or master on a regular basis. A Qi gong Master is defined as a person who has learned to emit healing energy from the body and they have proven success in healing with qi energy. (McGee et al. 1996) During treatment, the qigong practitioner emits or directs their qi energy with the specific intention of helping patients clear blockages in the flow of energy in the body, and move bad qi out of the body to get rid of disease. (Jang & Lee, 2004).

these are very low frequency waves (ELF) not the high frequency (HF) waves emitted from mobile phones and electrical overhead lines, which have attracted controversy because of perceived risks to the health of individuals exposed to them over time. Zimmerman was unable to produce biomagnetic pulses when he tested practitioners not skilled in energy therapies under the same research conditions.

Interestingly, signals from the TT practitioner pulsed at a variable frequency ranging from 0.3Hz to 30Hz, with most of the activity in the range of 7–8 HZ, which is consistent with the earth's geomagnetic field. In other words, the signal the TT practitioner emitted was not steady or constant, it moved through a range of frequencies (Oschman 2000). This is the same range as the ELF that biomedical researchers are finding effective to commence healing in a variety of soft and hard tissues. Oschman (2000) claimed that, in general, organisms are able to respond to extremely small changes in the electromagnetic environment. This reflects clinical and behavioural research that validates the less is more principle that underpins energetic interactions (Oschman 2005). For example, artificially induced ELF frequencies have been used to stimulate capillary and fibroblast proliferation and reduce skin necrosis at a low 15, 20 and 72 Hz. ELF has been shown to stimulate bone growth (7Hz), nerve regeneration (2Hz), neurite outgrowth from cultured ganglia (2Hz), ligament healing (10Hz), and create synergic effects with nerve growth factor (25 and 50 Hz) (Sisken and Walker 1995), all of which may be relevant to diabetes and vascular disease.

Seto et al. (1992) conducted a similar study to Zimmerman in Japan but used a simple magnetometer rather than a SQUID detector and confirmed that an extraordinarily large biomagnetic field (10^{-3} gauss, which is 1000 times stronger than the normal biomagnetic fields) emanated from the three of 37 subjects studied. However, they recognised that the magnetometer was set to pick up electromagnetic signals in the 2Hz–30 Hz band and was not sensitive enough to detect the usual low human frequencies (10^{-6}). Therefore, the fields of the other 34 subjects were negative. The three subjects who emitted large ELF frequencies were described as:

- Male high school teacher who had not had any practice for external Qi emissions until the study. However, he said he had a great interest in Qi emissions and was able to feel the flow of Qi. The researchers postulated that his interest in Qi might have activated his latent ability to emit an extraordinary large biomagnetic field.
- Female Buddhist who had been practising as a healer. The researchers were unaware of her occupation until the end of the study.
- Female who worked as an 'aesthetic salon consultant' who had studied Qi gong for six months prior to the study (Seto et al. 1992).

The researcher concluded these people's ability to emit extraordinary large amounts of Qi is sometimes innate and sometimes obtained through education and practice such as Qi gong exercises. However, they emphasised that not all people practising external Qi emission are able to radiate the extraordinary large bio-magnetic field strength shown by the subjects in the study and indicated the will to emit energy was crucial to the ability to do so, although they admit the physical mechanism remains unknown. For example, in the study they sent a signal to subjects to interrupt Qi emissions after 90 seconds of emitting Qi. At this point researchers became aware of a reduced amplitude on the oscilliscope for the three subjects able to emit large ELF waves that reduced the wave length to almost control level. Seto *et al.*'s finding supports the claims of many biofield therapist such as TT practitioners that energy follows thought. Seto *et al.* were unable to find the internal body current that corresponded to the extremely large current emitted from these subjects. They concluded that individuals able to emit extraordinary large biomagnetic field strength use Qi or energy currents, which are never derived from the internal sources alone.

Therapeutic Touch, Krieger–Kunz method

TT (Krieger–Kunz method) is a contemporary interpretation of the ancient art of laying on of hands based on the learned skill of consciously directing or sensitively modulating human energies. It was derived from several ancient healing practices and is based on the fundamental assumption that there is a universal life energy that sustains all living organisms. Krieger developed the Krieger/Kunz TT method as part of her doctoral thesis in 1979 in conjunction with Dora Kunz (theosophist and healer) and introduced the method to the health sciences field through a Master's degree programme entitled *Frontiers of Nursing* at New York University. A basic assumption of TT is that healthy individuals have a free flowing energy field and the energy flow changes when physical distress such as pain or emotional disturbance is present. The aim of a TT treatment is to facilitate client well-being by assessing, modulating and ultimately rebalancing the energy field, if necessary. Two major premises underpin TT. First, compassion with and intention to help and to heal are necessary requirements for healing. Second, intention follows thought.

TT has been widely researched at Master's, doctoral and post-doctoral levels. Early studies were criticised on methodological grounds. Many studies show a positive outcome, some show no significant benefits, and a few indicate minor discomfort following treatments. Methodological flaws include:

- The short time for which treatment was delivered, possibly for logistic reasons, which may not achieve optimum outcomes because the treatment was incomplete.
- The studies undertaken with well individuals such as university students tended to have little or no significant benefits compared to studies when TT was given to ill individuals.
- The health and well-being of the TT practitioner on the day of the study.
- TT practitioner membership of a recognised professional organisation that could assess their TT training and experience.
- The potential healing ability of those giving placebo TT.

Krieger (1993) stated TT is taught in more than 80 hospitals and universities throughout North America and practised in 78 countries throughout the world.

In Australia, TT is practised at Monash and Victoria Universities in Melbourne, Victoria, and at Flinders University in Adelaide, South Australia. Courses have also been offered in most states within Australia, see Table 8.1 for more information on TT research, practice, and treatment.

Early TT studies

Krieger decided to expand Grad's work by studying the effects of the laying on of hands on human haemaglobin values. She reasoned that haemoglobin is the oxygen-carrying pigment of the red blood cells, which transfers oxygen to the tissues in the body and that both chlorophyll and haemoglobin are tetrapyrroles with a similar stereochemical structure. She wondered whether human haemoglobin level would increase in people treated by the same healer used to demonstrate chlorophyll increased when barley seeds were irrigated with water treated by a healer (Grad 1965). The major difference between the two substances is that the haemaglobin molecule centres on iron and the chlorophyll molecule has magnesium atoms at its centre. There are also some differences in the side chains (Krieger 1975).

Krieger conducted her first pilot study in 1971 using 19 ill people in the experimental group and nine in the control group. The ages and sexes of the groups were comparable. Her substantive hypotheses was that the mean haemoglobin values of the experimental group would exceed their before-treatment haemoglobin values after receiving laying on of hands and that the mean haemoglobin values of the control group at comparable times would not be significantly different. Estabany provided the healing. The hypotheses were confirmed; there was a significant increase in the haemoglobin levels of the treated group compared to controls $p = 0.01$ (Krieger 1975). Krieger undertook a larger study in 1972 with 43 ill people in the experimental group and 33 controls. The groups were comparable in age and sex distribution. The hypotheses were again confirmed $p > 0.01$ (Krieger 1975). The research was again replicated in 1973 but this time possible confounding variables that could affect haemoglobin values such as the practice of medication, yoga, breathing exercises, biorhythm change, smoking, diet and medications, were controlled for. The hypotheses were confirmed $p > 0.001$.

Kramer compared the effects of casual touch and TT on stress levels in 30 children aged two years and under admitted for acute illness or surgery without regard to deviations in cognitive or psychosocial development. Stressful experiences included painful and non-painful procedures; being forcibly held; departure of parents; and being awakened from sleep. Stress reduction was measured using pulse rate, galvanic skin response, and peripheral skin temperature. Data were collected when the child became stressed, TT was administered and measurements recorded three minutes after the intervention and again after six minutes. Interventions were administered when the parents were not present and only the researcher was in the room. Children settled faster after stressful events when they received TT. Kramer suggested it would only take a few minutes to give TT and reduce childhood stress, provide comfort, and reduce length of stay in hospital. It could be extrapolated that TT might be beneficial for children with diabetes who become stressed having insulin injections or blood glucose tests.

More recently TT has been reported to lower blood pressure; reduce oedema; ease abdominal cramps, nausea, post-operative pain, tension and migraine headaches, phantom limb pain, and lower back pain, resolve fevers; improve the immune system; stimulate growth in premature infants, and accelerate fracture and wound healing, as well as with the common cold and other infections (Boguslawski 1980; Wright 1987; Krieger, 1993; Ching, 1993). Despite this body of research, further research is needed.

Healing Touch (HT)

Healing Touch (HT) is an energy-based hands-on therapeutic approach to healing (Mentegen and Bullbrook 1994). The aim of HT is to restore harmony and balance in the energy system to encourage self-healing. HT was developed by Janet Mentegen to prepare nurses and other health workers to work with bioenergetic healing techniques. HT blends the energetic techniques of a number of practices, including some aspects of TT and a number of other techniques from the work of Brennan, Hover-Kramer *et al.*, Joy, and Mentegen and Bullbrook. Like TT, HT practitioners centre themselves before beginning a treatment. They undertake a physical assessment including the energy field, then provide HT followed by a grounding phase. The following study illustrates the benefits and possible risks of HT and raises issues about HT future research.

Slater (1996) conducted a study into the safety, elements and effects of HT on chronic non-malignant abdominal pain. Twenty-three people who had undergone abdominal surgery at least four weeks prior to taking part in the study who continued to experience pain associated with the surgery participated in the study. More than 50 per cent had been in pain for more than a year after surgery, one for > nine years. Subjects received three different treatments on separate days: HT provided by an experienced HT practitioner; mimic HT, which appeared to be the same as HT was given by 'naïve providers', and interviews were also conducted. The order in which the interventions were provided was randomly selected. Quantitative changes were measured using the Melzack Pain Questionnaire (MPQ) and qualitative data about both the providers and recipient's experiences were documented. All three treatments were safe for the recipients and providers. The naïve providers experienced more discomfort than the HT providers. Subjects experienced more nausea, headaches, dizziness, and drowsiness after HT than after the naïve treatment. Slater concluded that HT was uncomfortable for some people but not unsafe and HT given by experienced and naïve providers achieved similar effects on pain relief.

The findings are contradictory in that subjects reported more relaxation and pain relief after HT than naïve treatment, and the researcher suggested that people in pain might evaluate their pain using criteria other than the sensation of pain. Another conclusion relevant for future research was a recommendation that naïve providers should not be used in this type of research because unlike HT, TT and Reiki practitioners may not have been trained to protect themselves from uncomfortable experiences during treatments. It is the author's view that consideration should also be given to the possibility that some naïve providers may also be latent healers. Furthermore, the wellness of the HT (or any other biofield therapist) providing treatment should also be considered. Research outcomes are likely to be less favourable if the energy therapist is not feeling well, such as from a cold or other viral infections (Grad 2004).

Healing or improvement response

HT practitioners and other biofield therapists such as TT and Reiki practitioners may well interpret the increased discomfort noted in Slater's study such as nausea, dizziness and drowsiness as a 'healing or improvement response', which is generally considered to be a temporary physical response to treatment. People are generally encouraged to drink additional fluids for the first 12–24 hours after TT, HT, and Reiki treatments because increasing the vibrational energy assisted by the emission and resonance of ELF signals from the therapist's hands during treatment could release toxins from diseased cells. Releasing toxins is a natural healing process and is necessary for cells to regain optimum function, and is consistent with Oschman's review of cellular function and healing described earlier.

Hiroshi Doi, a revered Japanese Reiki Master and founder of the Usui Reiki form of Gendai Reiki-ho, emphasised the importance of explaining the post-healing changes to patients before a Reiki treatment:

> Sometimes the condition or the symptoms of a receiver get worse after healing. Some receivers have fever, have more excretion, get eczema or feel pain. You should not worry about this as it is the process of restoration to health called improvement reaction
>
> (Hiroshi Doi 2000, English translation version)

Thus, it is common for people to experience mild usually physical responses after energy treatments. Practitioners of energy therapies such as HT, TT or Reiki need to discuss possible responses with their clients. This is particularly relevant for people with diabetes who require insulin or other medication because the blood glucose levels may change and medicines may need to be adjusted more frequently, especially in the first week after treatment. However, this phenomena could also occur after many other complementary therapies.

Reiki

Reiki is an ancient healing art whose origins can be traced to Nepal and the Himalayas. Mikao Usui, a Japanese Buddhist scholar, who gave it the name by which it is now known throughout the world, rediscovered it at the end of the nineteenth century. The term is used to describe the energy of this healing art as well as its forms of practice within the traditional systems (Chapman and Milton 2002), see Table 8.1 for information about Reiki education and practice. Dr Ranga Premaratna, Head of the Reiki Jin Kei Do Lineage, and former post-doctoral research scientist in food microbiology, defined Reiki energy as:

> Reiki is a Japanese word composed of two characters or 'Kanji'. . . . REI most simply defined as spirit and KI as energy (in Chinese, chi or qi). The combined meaning of the two characters, REIKI, is Spiritual Energy or a higher form of energy. But in practice Reiki is translated as Universal Energy, Universal Life Force or Universal Energy Field.

Research into Reiki healing is limited but may increase as Reiki treatments are increasingly being given in hospitals and other health care settings. Two contrasting Reiki research studies are presented to illustrate outcomes of treatment and raise some of the issues regarding research design that may need to be addressed in future studies. Shiflett *et al.* (2002) undertook a pilot study with patients in a post-stroke rehabilitation unit. The aims of the study were to evaluate the effectiveness of Reiki as an adjunct treatment for patients with subacute stroke, receiving standard rehabilitation as inpatients and evaluate a double-blind procedure for training Reiki practitioners. A third aim was to determine whether Reiki and sham practitioners could determine which category in the double blind study they were allocated to. Four conditions: Reiki Master, Reiki practitioner, sham Reiki, and no treatment (historic control) were studied. Subjects received up to 10 treatments over a two and a half-week period. Reiki did not have any clinically useful effect on stroke recovery in subacute hospitalised patients receiving standard rehabilitation therapy. However, selective positive effects on mood and energy were noted that were not the result of attentional or placebo effects.

The interesting and unique approach to Reiki research in this study merits a brief exploration, particularly in relation to training and blinding of practitioners. The Reiki Master trained a total of 14 health professionals in the techniques of Reiki treatment. The requirement for Reiki 1 training is that practitioners are initiated into Reiki by a Reiki Master who uses specific symbols, breath, and touch in a ritualistic manner. However, only half of the trainees in the study were initiated by the Reiki Master who sat across the room from them while they sat together 'in a quiet meditative state'. The initiation method was conducted by a technique used in distance healing. None of the 14 trainees were told who had been initiated to 'blind' the Reiki and sham Reiki practitioners. On completion of the study, but before being told what category they were in, the touch practitioners were given a questionnaire to determine whether they believed they had been initiated. They were also asked whether they noticed any sensations in their hands during treatment and to indicate their beliefs about whether their patients had benefited from treatment. Surprisingly, in several cases sham Reiki practitioners reported greater frequency of feeling heat in the hands compared to Reiki practitioners ($t = 2.44$, $p < 0.03$). Reiki practitioners were more likely to feel cold hands

$(t = -1.84, \ p < 0.10)$. Reiki practitioners were less confident about whether they were initiated than non-Reiki practitioners $(t = -2.12, \ p < 0.06)$.

In such a small study, these findings are not unusual in the author's experience. Many people have an innate healing ability, particularly those working as health professionals who generally are highly motivated from compassion. From the perspective of TT, anybody can learn how to send healing energy. The method of initiation may also have compromised the internal validity of the study because distance initiations are unusual but not unknown, and many Reiki Masters believe that all initiates need to be touched by the Reiki Master to seal the initiation for it to be sustained. Shiflett *et al.* (2002) do not indicate how long after the initiation the touch therapists began treating the patients. Furthermore, if the touch therapists were sitting so close together, it seems feasible from a shared environmental energy point of view, that those not being initiated would also experience some change in the energy flow from the distant initiation that could also affect them. In the author's experience, in a Reiki clinic at a drug rehabilitation centre in Melbourne, the energy changed substantially when four or five residents were receiving Reiki treatment at the same time in a moderate sized room. The quality of energy in the room was calming, peaceful and pleasant to experience according to both the centre staff and those receiving treatment. It would be important to have more comment from the Reiki community about the appropriateness of initiating practitioners in this way for future research.

Kumar and Karup conducted the second study in India in 2003. Changes in the isoprenoid pathway folllowing transcendental meditation and Reiki healing in seizure disorder were monitored. Fifteen patients with refractory seizure disorder defined as ILAE classification – 1E-generalized seizures – tonic clonic. Patients with persistent seizures, or on three or more anti-epilectic drugs in full dosage, and total compliance over a period of three years were included in the study. Subjects were selected randomly from the epilepsy clinic at the Medical College Hospital in Travindrum. Age range was 20–30 years, with eight males and seven females. Patients with diabetes, hypertension, cardiac, renal and hepatic diseases were excluded. They received a Reiki-like treatment three times a week and underwent one hour of transcendental meditation each day. At the end of three months they were clinically assessed to estimate seizure frequency.

An equal number of age- and sex-matched healthy subjects served as controls and were randomly selected from the town population. They were free from any systemic diseases. All patients and controls were on the same types of diets. Biochemical parameters assessed at the start and end of the three months were plasma HMG CoA reductase, serum digoxin, serum magnesium and RBC membrane Na + -K + ATPase activity. The serum levels of tyrosine, dopamine, noradrenaline, tryptophan, serotonin and quinolinic acid were also assessed. Fasting blood was taken from each patient. RBCs were separated within an hour of collection of the blood to estimate membrane Na + -K + ATPase. Serum was used to estimate HMG CoA reductase activity. Plasma serum was used for the other parameters.

Results showed a significant reduction in seizure frequency. Blood chemistry results showed that the activity of HMG CoA reductase and the concentration of serum digoxin that were increased prior to the interventions, reduced post-therapy and the RBC membrane Na + -K + ATPase activity and serum magnesium that were reduced pre-therapy, actually increased post-therapy. Likewise, concentrations of serum tryptophan, quinolinic acid and serotonin that were elevated prior to the study fell and thyrosine, dopamine and noradrenaline that were initially low increased post-study. The researchers concluded that results provide evidence regarding quantal perception and brain function because the ELF waves emitted from the healer are too weak to be transferred by normal sensory perceptive mechanisms. They also believe the study provides evidence about the regulation of metabolic processes by quantally perceived, low levels of EMF-(ELF) induced changes in neuronal transmission. It would be interesting to conduct a similar study for patients with diabetes to determine whether Reiki, with or without meditation, could have a positive effect on blood glucose regulation over a prolonged period of time.

Qi gong

Chinese Qi gong is an ancient healing discipline that has emerged from centuries of secrecy in the early 1980s. For approximately 900 years people in China have gathered every morning to practise a form of Qi gong called taiji (tai chi chuan), see Table 8.1. Most of the research into Qi gong has been undertaken in China and is difficult to obtain. Information about research studies often comes from abstracts from papers presented at conferences. For example Jing *et al.* (1996) on the effect of Qi gong on 31 subjects with type 2 diabetes. A group of middle-aged older subjects who practised regular Qi gong were observed over a year. Body weight did not change, fasting blood glucose reduced from an average of 10.19 ± 3.29 mmol/L, to 6.93 ± 1.32 mmol.L (p,0.001). Cholesterol levels fell from 6.75, ± 1.32 mmol/L to 5.51 ± 1.16 mmol?L (p,0.001). Triglyceride levels levels fell from 2.80 ± 1.01 mmol/L to 1.34 ± 0.71 mmol/L (p, 0.001). Serum insulin levels (by IRI) fell from 16.604 ± 6.005 MCU/L to 12.62 ± 14.85 MCU/L (p, 0.05). Severe obstruction of nail-microcirculation was greatly improved. This research raises the possibility that people with type 2 diabetes may be able to manage their disease with Qi gong exercises and without medicines.

Safety of magnet and energy therapies

These therapies are generally low risk, however, some precautions are necessary:

- Magnets may affect other equipment such as MRI machines, pacemakers and defibrillators, watches, hearing aids and metallic prostheses. People using magnets and other people in close proximity must be informed about the possible effects on the functioning of these instruments. Magnets should be

stored away from computers and other materials, for example, magnetic strips on credit cards.
- Magnets should not be dropped or heated because their strength can be reduced.
- Store different strength magnets separately.
- Magnets should not be placed on the abdomen for 60–90 minutes after a meal or during pregnancy (Springhouse Corporation 1999).

8.9 Homeopathy

Homeopathy is essentially an energy therapy (Ellison and MacGregor 2001). Samuel Hahnemann (1755–1843) was responsible for the systematic investigation of the effects of homeopathy but the roots can be traced back to the writings of Hippocrates. The term 'homeopathy' is derived from the Greek *homeo*, which means similar and *pathos*, which means suffering. Homeopathic practitioners treat illnesses using substances that produce a similar state in a healthy person, based on the theoretical principles of the 'law of similars'. The law of similars states that 'a substances which can produce a totality of symptoms in a health person is capable of removing that totality of symptoms in an unwell patient' (Ellison and MacGregor 2001). Hahnemann undertook a series of 'provings' in substances in healthy volunteers primarily students, family and friends who became known as provers to determine the medical value, effects, and dose. Hahnemann's provings were essentially phase 1 trials (Shalts 2006). The term proving is derived from the German 'Prufung' meaning to test and experiment.

Homeopathic practitioners consider illness to be an imbalance of vital forces that manifest as unique physical and psychological responses. Therefore, not all patients with the same diagnosis will present exactly the same way and management will need to be individualized. Practitioners use homeopathic principles in different ways such as classical and use the traditional spelling 'homoeopathy' or modern and use the more familiar spelling 'homeopathy'. In some countries homeopathy practice is restricted to medical doctors, for example, France, Germany and Russia. Homeopathic medicines are used in very low dilutions based on the assessment of the individual to assist their natural healing potential, which Hahnemann referred to as their 'vital force'. The basic principles of homeopathy are shown in Table 8.2.

Unlike many other complementary therapists, homeopathic practitioners do not undertake extensive diagnostic testing. They observe the patient very carefully and take a detailed history and description of their symptoms to identify any underlying pattern of symptoms. The components of homeopathic prescribing, treatment and healing processes are described in the *Organan of Medicine: The Rational Art of Healing* (Haehl 1922). Once the relevant symptoms are identified, the homeopath consults a 'medical repertory' of symptoms. The repertory is divided into sections that correspond to each body system, which are referred to as 'rubrics'. Each rubric lists medicines known to evoke the symptoms described by the patient through Hahnemann's systematic provings. Once a short list of potential medicines

Table 8.2 The basic principles of homeopathy.

- Like cures like. *Similia similibus curentur* or 'The Law of Similars'.
- One remedy at a time.
- Minimum dose and potency – small doses stimulate, moderate doses inhibit, large doses kill. The more dilute the preparation, the greater the potency – the 'Law of the Infinitesimal Dose'.
- The law of the direction of the cure (Hering's Law) – return to health follows a predictable pattern which occurs layer by layer treating the most recent symptom to the oldest.
- The Doctrine of Miasms.
- The Principle of Vital force.
- Holistic, individual approach.

is obtained, the practitioner consults a *Homeopathic Materia Medica* to determine the closest symptom match in a process known as Simillimum. The medicines are selected for their constitutional effect, their effects specific to the disorder, and according to individual needs. That is, they are prescribed according to the 'psychometric totality of symptoms', which reflects the physical and psychological aspects of illness. The medicine is then administered usually in a single dose. However, other symptoms or imbalances may emerge and require assessment and treatment.

Homeopathic medicines

Homeopathic medicines are derived from plants, mineral, and animal sources, diseased tissues, conventional medicines and non-physical sources such as magnetic fields and electric currents. The medicines are prepared in water or alcohol according to a method known as 'succussing', which involves diluting and shaking the preparation according to a specific protocol, see Table 8.3. The effectiveness of homeopathic medicines beyond placebo is frequently debated. However, homeopathy has been shown to be effective over placebo in several systematic reviews and meta-analysis especially for treating influenza, allergic conditions, childhood diarrhoea and post-operative ileus (Reilly *et al.* 1994; Linda *et al.* 1997; Ernst 2002; Jonas *et al.* 2003). Some of these trials have methodological problems and often only demonstrate small effect.

However, Shang *et al.* (2005) compared 110 homeopathic trials matched with 110 conventional medicine trials randomly selected from the Cochrane Controlled Trials Register that included respiratory tract infections, asthma, gastrointestinal disease and neurological disorders. Trials of 'a lower quality' demonstrated more beneficial treatment effects in both groups. When 'higher quality' trials were compared, there was a non-significant benefit for homeopathy (odds ratio 0.88) but a significant benefit for conventional medicines (odds ration 0.58) where an odds ration of < 1 indicated a beneficial effect. The clinical application of Shang *et al.*'s review is difficult to estimate.

Table 8.3 Steps in preparing a homeopathic medicine (succussion). The dilution process reduces the amount of the original material in the preparation to the point where even a trace may not remain (i.e. none of the original material remains).

Step	Process
1.	One part of the chosen material is pulverised and ground (solids) or dissolved (liquid). The preparation is then diluted in a solvent, such as alcohol, water or sugar, either $9^{(1x)}$ or 99 parts$^{(1c)}$.
2.	The preparation 1x or 1c is further diluted a second time by taking one part of the first dilution and adding another 9 or 99 more parts of the same solvent to produce 2x or 2x dilution.
3.+	The process is repeated until the desired potency is obtained 3x or 3c, 4x or c, etc. After the dilutional process a specified number of shakes or succession is carried out at each level.

Notes: The dilutional process is known as potentisation.
* x = 10 ** x = 100

Homeopathy and diabetes and vascular disease

Very few randomised control trials address homeopathy use in the management of diabetes and cardiovascular disease. A review of its use in stroke and hypertension provided insufficient evidence to conclude either a positive or negative effect (Whitmont and Mamtani 2005). Anecdotal evidence exists for a beneficial effect in a range of cardiovascular conditions such as angina, arrhythmias, congestive cardiac failure, coronary artery disease, hypertension, hypotension and tachycardia. Jayasuriya (no date) provides very detailed information about homeopathic remedies used to treat a large range of conditions but only briefly mentions diabetes. Preparations Jayasuriya listed for cardiac or heart diseases are shown in Table 8.4. He suggests a range of preparations depending on the accompanying symptoms.

Safety of homeopathic medicines

Homeopathic medicines are manufactured according to strict guidelines in countries such as Australia, the USA, the UK and New Zealand. There are few side effects and these are usually mild and resolve quickly. They include headaches, skin rashes, and gastrointestinal symptoms. There are no reports of toxicity in the literature when qualified practitioners use homeopathy but there are at least two reports of serious adverse events due to self-treatment or treatment delivered by inadequately qualified practitioners (Shalts 2006).

The alcohol base of some medicine may be contraindicated in some individuals when water-based preparations should be selected. Some homeopathic tablets contain lactose that could affect blood glucose levels, conventional medicines may interfere with the actions of homeopathic medicines and some practitioners recommending not using them in children younger than 5 or in the long term (Springhouse Corporation 1999). Regular blood glucose monitoring should be undertaken.

Table 8.4 Homeopathic preparations used to treat cardiac and vascular disease The preparations are chosen according to Homeopathic principles.

Cardiac	Vascular
Arsenicum album	*Crataegus*
Ammonium carbonicum	*Gelsemium sempervirens*
Arnica montana	*Glonoin*
Belladonna atropa	*Natrum muriaticum*
Bryonia alba	*Sulphur*
Cactus grandifloras	
Cimicifuga racemosa	
Digitalis	
Glonoine	
Kalium bichromium	
Latrodectus mactans	
Magnesia phosphorica	
Tubacum	

Source: Based on Jayasuriya

8.10 Summary

A broad range of energy medicine practices have been discussed in this chapter. Energy medicine is probably safe for most people with diabetes provided the safety issues outlined are considered. However, research to support any benefit or risk is limited. There is evidence that all body systems are receptive to biofield therapies, particularly the circulatory, lymphatic, endocrine, nervous and immune systems and these therapies are safe when they are given by qualified, experienced therapists, However, temporary healing response reactions have been recorded following treatment by untrained people. TT, Reiki and HT can all be given as self-treatments or by family members. In addition, distance healing methods can be arranged by a therapist, although these methods are more controversial.

Research and anecdotal evidence suggests that biofield therapies could offer numerous benefits to individuals with diabetes and vascular disease. For example, in the author's own experience, fortnightly treatments of a patient lying awake for long periods with severe leg pain at night from peripheral vascular disease was relieved using TT and the patient was able to regain mobility and walk to the day room again after two treatments. In a drug and alcohol rehabilitation centre in Melbourne, one client returned for a second Reiki treatment a week later. Three other residents saying, 'Whatever you gave him last week, can we have some too?' followed him. He had apparently been aggressive and withdrawn before the Reiki, but after the treatment was relaxed and approachable and more willing to talk with the centre counsellors. These two case scenarios are offered as an invitation to researchers to investigate these outcomes on a larger scale.

Finally, Guthrie and Gamble support using energy-based therapies in diabetes based on few known side effects and the potential for multiple benefits. However, they emphasise the importance of blood glucose monitoring to determine whether medications need to be adjusted. They note: 'Catecholamines such as epinephrine and norepinephrine, when released by the body in response to the use of an energy therapy, increase lipolysis and thermogenesis, resulting in increasing energy expenditure and potential for weight change' (Guthrie and Gamble 2001).

References

Achterberg J., Cooke KBS, Richards T, Standish LJ, Kozak L, Lake J. Evidence for correlations between distant intentionality and brain function in recipients: a functional magnetic resonance imaging analysis. *The Journal of Alternative and Complementary Medicine* 2005; **11**(6): 965–971.

Beck R. Mood modification with ELF magnetic fields: a preliminary exploration. Archaeus 4:48. In: Oschman JL. *Energy Medicine: The Scientific Basis*. Edinburgh: Churchill Livingstone, 2000.

Boguslawski M. Therapeutic Touch. A facililitator of pain relief. *Topics in Clinical Nursing*. 1980; 27–37.

Borang KK. Principles of Reiki. London: Thorsons, 1997.

Bouligand Y. Liquid crystals and their analogs in biochemical systems. In: Liebert L (ed.) Liquid crystals. *Solid State Physics* 1978; **14** (supplement): 259–294.

Brennan B. *Hands of Light: A Guide to Healing through the Human Energy Field*. Toronto: Bantam Books, 1987.

Chapman E, Milton G. Reiki as an intervention in drug and alcohol withdrawal and rehabilitation: almost a decade of experience. Paper presented at Brave new world, WFTC 21st World Conference. Melbourne, 17–22 February 2002.

Chen Y. Magnets on ears helped diabetics. *Am J Chin Med*. 2002; **30**(1): 183.5. (Abstract).

Ching M. The use of touch in nursing practice. *The Australian Journal of Advanced Nursing* 1993; **10**(4): 4–9.

Culliton PD, Boucher TA, Carlson GA. Substance misuse. In: Watkins, A (ed.) *Mind-Body Medicine: A Clinician's Guide to Psychoneuroimmunology*. New York: Churchill Livingstone, 1997.

Eccles NK. A critical review of randomized controlled trials of static magnets for pain relief. *The Journal of Alternative and Complementary Medicine* 2005; **11**(3): 495–509.

Ellison E, MacGregor P. Homoeopathy: How does it work? *Diversity*. 2001; **2**(5): 18–25.

Ernst E. Investigating the safety of complementary medicine. In: Lewith G, Jonas W, Walach, H (eds) *Clinical Research in Complementary Therapies*.

Gallob R. Reiki: a supportive therapy in nursing practice and self-care for nurses. *Journal of New York State Nurses Assoc* 2003; **Spring – Summer**: 34.

Gerber R. *Vibration Medicine: The Handbook of Subtle-Energy Therapies*, 3rd edn. Rochester: Bear & Co., 2001.

Grad B. A telekinetic effect on plant growth II. Experiments involving treatment of saline in stoppered bottles. *International Journal of Parapsychology* 1964; **6**: 473–498.

Grad B. Some biological effects of the laying on of hands: a review of experiments with animals and plants. *The Journal of the American Society for Psychical Research* 1965; **59**(2): 95–129.

Grad B. Discussion of Grad's research on healers and healing. Vision and Reality Conference. The Therapeutic Touch Network of Ontario 5–7 Nov. Markham.

Guthrie DW., Gamble M. Energy therapies and diabetes mellitus. *Diabetes Spectrum: American Diabetes Association Inc* 2001; **14**: 149–153.

Haehl R. Samuel Hahnemann: his life and work. In: Jonas W, Jacobs H (eds), *Healing with Homeopathy: A Doctor's Guide*. New York, Warner Books, 1922.

Horrigan B. Interview: Dolores Krieger, RN, PhD. Healing with therapeutic touch. *Alternative Therapies* 1998; **4**(1).

Hover-Kramer, P *Healing Touch: A Guidebook for Practitioners*, 2nd edn. Albany, NY: Thompson Learning, 2002.

Jang H, Lee M. Effects of Qi therapy (External Qigong) on premenstrual syndrome: a randomized placebo-controlled study. *The Journal of Alternative and Complementary Medicine* 2004; **10**(3): 456–462.

Jayasuriya A. *Clinical Homeopathy*, 4th edn. Sri Lanka: Medicina Alternative International, (no date).

Jing Y, Li X, Wang Z *et al*. Observations on effects of 31 cases of diabetes treated by huichunggong, Shandong Institute of TCM, Shandong Province, Jinan 250014, China. Presented at the Second World Conference for Academic Exchange of Medical Qigong, Beijing (Abstract). In: McGee, C. Sancier, K, and Yew Chow, E. (eds), *Fundamentals of Complementary and Alternative Medicine*, New York: Churchill Livingstone, 1996.

Jonas B, Kapchuk T, Linde K. A critical overview of homeopathy. *Annals of Internal Medicine* 2003; **138**: 393–399.

Joy B. *Joy's Way*. New York: GP Putnam, 1979.

Kaptchuk TJ. Historical context of the concept of vitalism in complementary and alternative medicine. In: Micozzi M (ed.), *Fundamentals of Complementary and Alternative Medicine*. New York: Churchill Livingstone, 1996.

Kramer NA. Comparison of Therapeutic Touch and casual touch in stress reduction of hospitalized children. *Pediatric Nursing*. 1990; **16**(5).

Krieger D. Therapeutic Touch: the imprimatur of nursing. *American Journal of Nursing*. 1975; **75**(5): 784–787.

Krieger. D. *Accepting Your Power to Heal*. Rochester: Bear and Co., 1993.

Krieger D. Dolores Krieger, RN, PHD. Healing with Therapeutic Touch. Interview by Bonnie Horrigan. *Alternative Therapies*. 1998; **4**(1).

Kumar RA, Karup PA. Changes in the isoprenoid pathway with transendental meditaion and Reiki healing practices in seizure disorder. *Neurology India*. 2003; **51**(2): 211–214.

Lewis D. Spiritual dimensions of Therapeutic Touch: Sacred space. *The International Journal of Spirituality and Health*. 2000; **1**(5).

Linda K, Clausis N, Ramirez G. Are the clinical effects of homeopathy placebo effects? A meta-analysis of placebo controlled trials. *Lancet* 1997; **350**: 834–843.

Mentegen J, Bullbrook M. *HT Healing Touch Level 1 Notebook*. Carrboro, NC: North Carolina Center for Healing Touch, 1994.

Merritt P, Randall D. The effect of healing touch and other complementary therapies on diabetes. (Abstract) *Healing Touch International Research Survey*. Lakewood CO; Healing Touch International Inc., 2002.

McGee CT, Sancier K, Yew Chow E. Qigong in traditional Chinese medicine. In: Micozzi MS (ed.), *Fundamentals of Complementary and Alternative Medicine*, New York: Churchill Livingstone, 1996, pp. 225–242.

Morris CE, Skalak TC. Effects of static magnetic fields on microvascular tone in vivo. Abstract presented at Experimental Biology Meeting; April; San Diego, CA. In National Centre for Complementary and Alternative Medicine (NCCAM). http://www.nccam.nih.gov/health/backrounds/energymed.htm. Accessed 19/12/05.

National Centre for Complementary and Alternative Medicine (NCCAM) http://www.nccam.nih.gov/health/backrounds/energymed.htm. Accessed 19/12/05.

National Reiki Reference Group. www.nrrg.org.au

Oschman JL. *Energy Medicine: The Scientific Basis*. Edinburgh: Churchill Livingstone, 2000.

Oschman JL. *Energy Medicine in Therapeutics and Human Performance*. Sydney: Butterworth Heinemann, 2003.

Oschman JL. Energy and the healing response. *Journal of Bodywork and Movement Therapies*, 2005; **9**(1): 3–15.

Pakhomov AG, Akyel Y, Pakhomova ON, Stuck BE, Murphy MR. Current state and implications of research on biological effects of millimeter waves: a review of literature, *Bioelectromagnetics* 1998; **19**(7): 393–413.

Premaratna RJ. *Reiki Jin Kei Do Stage 1 Manual*. Sydney, Australia, 1999.

Rankin-Box D. Healing. In: Rankin-Box D. (ed.) *The Nurse's Handbook of Complementary Therapies*. 2nd edn. Edinburgh: Bailliere Tindall, 2001.

Rassmussen H. *The Calcium and CAMP as Synarchic Messengers*. New York: John Wiley & Sons, 1981.

Reilly D, Taylor M, Beatte N. Is evidence for homeopathy reproducible? *Lancet* 1994; **II**: 1–86: 1601–1606.

Report by Reiki Australia. *Reiki Treatment Practice Draft 1 qualifications* 2005; p10.

Rogers ME. Nursing: a science of unitary human beings. In: Riehl-Sisca J (ed.), *Conceptual Models for Nursing Practice*. Norwalk: Appleton & Lange, 1989; pp. 181–188.

Rojavin MA, Ziskin MC. Medical application of millimetre waves. *QJM: Monthly Journal of the Association of Physicians* 1998; **91**(1): 57–66.

Samarel N. The experience of receiving therapeutic touch. *Journal of Advanced Nursing* 1992; **17**: 651–657.

Seto A, Kusaka C, Nakazato S, Huang W, Sato T, Hisamitsu T, Takenshinge C. Detection of extraordinary large bio-magnetic field strength from human hand. *Acupuncture and Electro-Therapeutics Research International Journal* 1992; **17**: 75–94.

Shalts E. Homeopathy: a brief overview with examples. *Alternative Medicine Alert* 2006; **9**(2): 17–23.

Shiflett SC, Nayak S, Bid C, Miles P, Agostinelli S. Effect of Reiki treatments on functional recovery in patients in post stroke rehabilitation: a pilot study. *The Journal of Alternative and Complementary Medicine* 2002; **8**(6): 755–763.

Sisken BF, Walker J. Therapeutic aspects of electromagnetic fields for soft-tissue healing. In: Blank, M. (ed.), *Electromagnetic Fields: Biological Interactions and Mechanisms*. Washington, DC: American Chemical Society, 1995; pp 277–285.

Slater VE. Safety, elements, and effects of healing touch on chronic non-malignant abdominal pain. University of Tennessee. PhD, 1996. Abstract.

Smith J. The influence on enzyme growth by the 'laying on of hands'. In: *The Dimensions of Healing: A Symposium*. Los Altos, CA: The Academy of Parapsychology and Medicine, 1972.

Springhouse Corporation. *A Nurse's Handbook of Alternative and Complementary Therapies*. Springhouse Corporation, Pennsylvania, 1999.

Tiller W. Foreword. In: Gerber R *Vibrational Medicine: The Handbook of Subtle Energy Therapies*, 3rd edn. Rochester: Bear & Co. 2001; pp. 12–16.

The Academy of Parapsychology and Medicine. *The Dimensions of Healing: A Symposium*. Los Altos, CA: The Academy of Parapsychology, 1992.

Warber S, Cornelio D, Straughn J, Kile G. Biofield energy healing from the inside. *Journal of Alternative and Complementary Medicine* 2004; **10**(6): 1107–13.

Wardell DW, Engebretson J. Biological correlates of Reiki Touch healing. *Journal of Advanced Nursing* 2001; **33**(4): 439.

Wardell D, Weymouth K, Review of studies of healing touch. *Journal of Nursing Scholarship* 2004; **36**(2): 147–154.

Wever R ELF-effects on human circadian rhythms. In: Persinger MA (ed.), *ELF and VLF Electromagnetic Field Effects*. New York: Plenum Press, 1974; pp. 101–144.

Whitmont R, Mamtani R. Homeopathy with a special focus on treatment of cardiovascular disease. In: *Complementary Therapies for Cardiovascular Disease*. Mosby, St Louis: Elsevier 2005; pp. 232–247.

Wilkinson DS, Knox PL, Chatman JE, Johnson TL, Barbour N, Mykes Y, Reel A. The clinical effectiveness of healing touch. *The Journal of Alternative and Complementary Medicine.* 2002; **8**(1): 33–47.

Wright S. The use of Therapeutic Touch in the management of pain. *Nursing Clinics of North America* 1987; **22**(3): 705–713.

Zimmerman J. Laying-on-of-hands healing and therapeutic touch: a testable theory: BEMI currents. *Journal of the Bio-Electro-Magnetics Institute* 1990; **24**: 8–17.

Acknowledgments

Eileen Chapman, Reiki Master, Melbourne, Victoria, Australia.

Jim Frew, Reiki Master at Mornington Peninsula, Victoria. Australia

The Therapeutic Touch Network of Victoria, Australia.

Useful websites

Bastyr University in Seattle. 25 years of CAM studies. http://www.bastyr.edu/research/projects/default.asp?view=CompletedResearchStudies

Complementary and Alternative Medicine (NCCAM). http://www.nccam.nih.gov/health/backrounds/energymed.htm

Healing Touch International website. Accessed December 2005.

National Training Information Services, Australia. http://www.ntis.gov.au/

Nurse Healer Professional Associates for information on Therapeutic Touch. http://www.therapeutic-touch.org/

Quackwatch website http://www.quackwatch.com

Reiki Australia http://www.reikiaustralia.com.au/

Subtle Energies and Energy Medicine Journal. http://www.issseem.org/journal.html www.therapeutic-touch.org

Therapeutic Touch. Crystal Hawk in Canada has good linkages on this site. http://www.therapeutictouch.com/

9 Herbal Medicines and Interactions with Conventional Medicines Used to Manage Diabetes

Lesley Braun

9.1 Introduction

Herbal medicine, sometimes known as phytotherapy, can be broadly defined as the science and art of using botanical medicines to prevent and treat illness, and the study and investigation of these medicines. Herbal medicine is one of the oldest forms of medicine and has been used to alter the course of disease and promote better health since antiquity. Over the centuries, empirical knowledge about herbal medicines slowly accumulated to form a body of evidence commonly referred to as 'traditional evidence'. Traditional evidence accumulates on the basic tenets of good clinical practice, that is, the careful observation of people, their environment and the diseases they acquire, see Chapter 2. Cumulative experiences and informed trial and error lead to the accumulation of a large and diverse information base, which continues to grow in many countries.

More recently, scientific evidence has supported and extended the traditional evidence base. Today, evidence is also derived from scientifically designed laboratory, animal and human studies. Increasingly, randomised controlled trials, meta-analyses and systematic reviews are being undertaken and provide additional information about the pharmacological actions, clinical effects, and safety of herbal medicines. In the past, most herbal medicines research was conducted in Europe and Asia where there is a rich tradition of use. With the advent of specialist complementary medicine research centres such as the National Center for Complementary and Alternative Medicine in the United States, more research is being initiated in other countries. However, a general lack of resources, infrastructure, government funding and financial incentives to invest in the research and development of herbal medicines has slowed the research effort and many herbal medicines still require investigation. Importantly, herbal medicines occur naturally in the environment, making it difficult, if not impossible to patent them, which is a major disincentive to financial investment into herbal research because there is no guarantees that costs can be recuperated because of the way patents protect investments.

Interestingly, a significant number of modern conventional medicines were originally derived from plants. For example, morphine from *Papaver somniferum* is widely regarded as the first medicine to be produced from a plant. It was developed in the early 1800s and eventually led to the development of the opiate class of medicines. Investigation into the herb meadowsweet (*Filipendula ulmaria*) ultimately yielded salicylate medicines, modern digoxin preparations were derived from the foxglove (*Digitalis officinalis*) and Metformin from goat's rue (*Galega officinalis*). Some pharmaceutical companies continue to scour nature for potential medicine sources.

Recently, the drug Taxol was produced from the Yew tree (*Taxus brevifolia*) and currently trials are being conducted on star anise (*Illicium verum)* to determine its potential to cure avian influenza (*Bangkok Post*, October 2005). Star anise is a source of shikimic acid from which the medicine tamiflu is made. Although these discoveries are significant, they are more applicable to the way conventional medicines are used. Conventional medicines are distinctly different from herbal medicines even when they are derived from the same plants. Herbal medicines are prepared in a range of formulations shown in Table 9.1.

Table 9.1 Formulations of herbal medicines. Herbal medicines are available in various dose forms depending on the indications for use and the body system being treated. Herbal medicines can be individually compounded or purchased as preformulated blends.

Formulation type	
Tincture or extract	Usually formulated in alcohol or liquid glycerin. The therapeutic properties disperse into the alcohol or glycerine.
	Alcohol-based tinctures often have an unpleasant taste.
	Alternatively, liquid glycerin is used. These formulations are known as glycerites and are sweet and feel warm in the mouth but do not affect blood glucose levels. Excess doses can have a laxative effect.
	Tinctures and extracts can be administered in tea or water or externally on a compress.
	They have along shelf life.
	Tinctures have a higher alcohol content than extracts. The label should state whether the base is alcohol or glycerin.

Capsules or tablets	These may be freshly prepared for use within twenty four hours. They are made from the dried and powered form of the herb and are not as potent as tinctures. It is important that the tablets are formulated soon after the herbs are harvested because their therapeutic content degrades soon after harvesting.
	Tablets and capsules also contain fillers often soy or millet flour, binders for example magnesium stearate or dicalcium phosphate, which absorb water and enable the tablet to be broken down and absorbed more readily after administration.
	Tablets can be ingested whole or mixed with fruit juice of food.
Lozenges	Lozenges are rich in nutrients and dissolve easily in the mouth. They usually have a sweet taste and usually contain vitamin c. Various formulations such as cough suppressants and decongestants are available.
Teas	These can be made form most herbs and formulated as:
	• Infusion where the herb is steeped in hot water forr 3–5 minutes, usually the leaf and stems are used.
	• Decoction where the herbs are placed in gently boiling water for 15–20 minutes usually used for roots and barks.
	The herbal material can be placed in muslin bags, tea balls, or herbal teacups. Metal containers are not usually used.
	The taste depends on the chemical content of the herbs. Usually 1–2 teasponns of prepared herb are used for a single cup of tea and should be strained before use.
Juices	Obtained by squeezing the juice form the herbs in a juicer after washing in cold running water.
	They are best used immediately but can be stored in the refrigerator for 1–2 days. Thyeyare ideal for compresses or administered in drinks where a few drops are used.
Essential oil vapours	Commonly used to deliver essential oils see chapter 6. Some cultures burn herbs and inhale the smoke or 'smoke' the body.
Baths	Bags of herbs or essential oils are used in carrying agents such as *Aloe vera* ain the bath as a cleanser, to induce relaxation and reduce tension, alleviate pain and skin irritation, and warm cold muscles.
	Herbal infusions or tinctures or extracts can also be used.
Compresses and poultices	A compress consists of fresh herbs, which are usually wrapped in moist linen or gauze before applying to the affected area. They are used to reduce bleeding, pain, swelling, bruising either hot or cold depending on the indication. Care needs to be taken if people have insensate feet due to peripheral

Table 9.1   (Continued)

Formulation type	
	neuropathy to prevent burns. Alternatively the cloth can be soaked in an herbal infusion and wringing out excess moisture before applying. Poultices are moist pastes made by crushing herbs and applying to the affected area directly or wrapped in a cloth. Essential oils can be applied as either compresses or poultices. In the latter they can be mixed in clay. In both cases they are left in place for short periods and repeated applications may be needed.
Ointments and salves	These preparations are used topically for a range of conditions such as wound care and skin irritation. Beeswax and lanolin are commonly used bases into which the herbs, tinctures or essential oils are blended.

9.2   Differences between Herbal and Conventional Medicines

Herbal medicines are chemically complex entities and can be described as naturally occurring chemical cocktails, much like food or wine. Herbs contain hundreds of different 'phytochemicals' such as various macronutrients (fats, carbohydrates, proteins and enzymes) and micronutrients (vitamins and minerals). In addition, secondary metabolites are present in plants and are believed to function in the plant as a natural defence against herbivores, pathogens, insect attack and microbial degradation. Some of these metabolites are produced in response to injury, infection or are required for signalling, fertilisation and regulating growth. The secondary metabolites are compounds such as tannins, isoflavones, bitters and flavonoids and largely dictate the pharmacological activities of a herb.

The growing conditions, methods of harvesting, processing and storing herbs can influence the final chemical profile of the resultant herbal product. For example, a herbal extract prepared in the traditional way as a water-ethanolic extract can result in a very different medicine from a modern herbal extract prepared with chemical solvents, even though both are derived from the same plant. In some instances, the chemical variations that result can be significant and can alter the pharmacological activity and/or safety of the final product. The herb kava kava illustrates this point: generally kava kava prepared in the traditional manner is considered to be safe and well tolerated, however, kava kava preparations that have been manufactured with acetone solvents have been associated with serious adverse effects and toxic reactions. As a result, it is important to take note of the type of herb used, the part of the plant used, and the method of preparing the final medicine when evaluating the scientific literature about specific herbal medicines and assessing adverse medicine reactions.

Considering that most herbs contain several active constituents, which have different modes of action, work at different sites, and have different pharmacokinetic profiles, it is easy to understand how a herbal medicine can have a variety of unrelated actions and indications for use. In addition, intraherbal interactions among constituents, such as synergy or quenching, sometimes produce important clinical effects and may contribute to a herb's therapeutic index and tolerability. As such, predicting the clinical effects of a herbal medicine by only considering the actions of one key constituent is unlikely to be entirely accurate.

A number of different complementary medicine systems employ herbal medicines as a component of the overall treatment. These systems have developed over generations in different parts of the world, guided by different cultures and tend to vary in their philosophies and application of treatment. Two notable systems are Chinese Medicine (CM), which developed in China, and Ayurvedic medicine from India, see Chapters 10 and 11. These complex health-care systems involve formal diagnostic methods and treatment and often use herbal medicines as an important part of a more comprehensive management approach. As a result, a single herb may be prescribed in different ways, depending on the indication for use and the medicine system in which it is prescribed.

Although herbs can be prescribed as single entities, herbal polypharmacy is often considered essential to good practice. The rationale for prescribing multiple herbal medicines together is to individualise treatment and utilise beneficial interactions among herbs and their constitutents. For instance, two herbs with mild sedative effects might be prescribed together to take advantage of a pharmacodynamic interaction that achieves a greater sedative effect than if either herb was used alone. The herbal literature variously describes these herbs as relaxants or tonics. Herbal polypharmacy (possibly first practised by Paracelsus who included ~ 60 ingredients in his *Galenicals*) has reached a high level of sophistication in CM where some formulas contain up to 20 different herbs.

In contrast, most conventional medicines contain a single, highly purified, often artificially produced chemical with a known structure, function and pharmacokinetic profile. They are developed, understood and used within the framework of a single medical system; therefore, opinions about mechanisms of action, safety and efficacy do not vary appreciably. Polypharmacy is a potential safety issue and thus the number of medicines used at the same time should be kept to a minimum in order to reduce the risk of adverse interactions/reactions. There are instances where polypharmacy is necessary such as chemotherapy, or when one drug is used to offset the side effects of another. Another exception is the management of diabetes and its complications and comorbidities where polypharmacy is frequently necessary and may well be best practice.

Importantly, newly developed chemical entities have no history of use and therefore no empirical evidence is available to help determine safety or efficacy, the appropriate dose, dose range, or dose interval. As a result, all new medicines must go through extensive testing to determine these aspects. Undoubtedly, the research process is very costly, requires the application of highly specialised knowledge and infrastructure, as well as many years of concentrated effort. However, it is also extremely lucrative because the company that finances the development, research and marketing of a new entity can patent the product. In some countries, the commercial manufacture, availability and commercial advertising of herbal medicines are regulated differently from pharmaceutical medicines, see Chapter 3.

9.3   Similarities between Herbal Medicines and Conventional Medicines

Like conventional medicines, evidence of efficacy and safety comes from in vitro, in vivo and clinical testing and significant therapeutic and adverse effects are possible. Informed prescribing and accurate dispensing of herbal medicines improve patient safety and promote beneficial outcomes. Careful patient observation, supervision and follow-up are essential to good practice. The World Health Organization (WHO) continues to develop publications and documents relating to the quality, safety, efficacy and use of medicinal plants including:

- *Basic Tests for Drugs: Pharmaceutical Substances, Medicinal Plant Materials and Dosage Forms* (1998);
- *Good Manufacturing Practices: Supplementary Guidelines for the Manufacture of Herbal Medicinal Products* (1996);
- *Guidelines for the Appropriate Use of Herbal Medicines* (1998);
- *Quality Control Methods for Medicinal Plant Materials* (1998);
- *WHO Monographs on Selected Medicinal Plants Volume 1* (1999) and *Volume 2* (2001);
- *Research Guidelines for Evaluating the Safety and Efficacy of Herbal Medicines* (1993).

The WHO monographs include a section about the levels of medicinal use to differentiate between herbal medicines supported by quality research and those based on traditional use. A number of herbal monographs are available on the Internet and contain important information somewhat similar to conventional medicine prescribing information in books such as the Australian Medicines Handbook and the British National Formulary.

In Australia, the manufacture of herbal medicinal products is conducted under the same code of Good Manufacturing Practice (GMP) required of pharmaceutical medicine manufacture. This means herbal medicine products produced under the GMP are manufactured to the same standard as conventional medicines, which is indicated by an AUST L or AUST R number, which must be displayed on the packaging of all herbal or conventional medicines. Listed products (Aust L) are considered lower risk than registered products (Aust R) and include most herbal medicines.

In the United Kingdom, the British Herbal Pharmacopeia provides quality control standards together with guidance about appropriate and safe use. Not every country has a code of GMP and those that do may have quite different standards from those expected for conventional medicines. It is recommended that practitioners become familiar with the quality control standards required of the herbal medicines available in their country and determine which products are manufactured to acceptable standards.

In Australia, all potentially toxic therapeutic substances, those likely to cause severe adverse reactions or are open to abuse, are scheduled. Herbal and pharmaceutical medicines are assessed and scheduled according to the same criteria. Products deemed sufficiently safe are available over the counter (OTC) without a medical prescription. This system enables the public to have greater access to medicines and an opportunity to prevent illness, treat and manage their health without the need to consult a doctor or complementary medicine practitioner in the first instance. This is empowering for patients and promotes greater self-awareness, self-care and personal responsibility but can also lead to delays in appropriate diagnosis and management. Like all medicines, if used incorrectly, herbal medicines can result in adverse events, therefore, professional advice is recommended especially for high risk people or people who are not sure how to select and use medicines.

9.4 Herbal Medicines and Diabetes

It is sobering to find that diabetes has been recognised since ancient times. For instance, as early as 700–200 BC two types of diabetes were recorded in India (Chapter 10), one of which was diet related and the other was described as genetic. Diabetes has also been recognised in China for thousands of years, where it is attributed to yin deficiency and treated using an integrated approach, which is more complex than just lowering blood glucose. At least 30 different herbal medicines are frequently used in CM to manage associated diabetes in Chinese medicine syndromes and complications and several of these medicines have outstanding potential as effective medicines, see Chapter 11.

Due to the chronic nature of diabetes, people with diabetes and their health-care practitioners are given ample time to implement important therapeutic strategies to improve, manage and eliminate the effect of modifiable risk factors for future diseases and complications. As indicated in Chapter 2, an increasing number of people are considering complementary and herbal medicines as part of this approach (Dunning 2003; Yeh *et al.* 2003). A national study of 2,055 people with diabetes conducted in the US between 1997 and 1998 reported that about one-third of respondents used complementary medicine to treat diabetes (Yeh *et al.* 2002). The main therapies used were nutritional and spiritual therapies, herbal medicines, massage and meditation. Interestingly, 43 per cent were referred to complementary therapists by their doctor, which indicates a degree of acceptance and willingness to collaborate for the benefit of the patient.

People with diabetes use numerous herbal medicines to improve their diabetes management, prevent or treat complications or address other health concerns such as intercurrent illnesses. Some of the medicines are plant-based foods whereas others are traditional herbal medicines with a history of traditional use in diabetes. Increasingly, the herbal therapies used are being subjected to scientific investigation. A systematic review published in 2003 identified 108 human trials of herbs and nutritional supplements that lower blood glucose. Most trials investigated the effects of the herb/s or supplement as adjuncts to conventional treatment.

Herbs shown to reduce blood glucose in over 50 per cent of controlled trials are:

- *Trigonella foenum* (fenugreek)
- *Coccinia indica* (ivy gourd)
- *Panax quinquefolius* (American ginseng)
- *Streptocantha opuntia* (nopal or prickly pear cactus)
- *Gymnema sylvestre*
- cinnamon
- aloe vera
- *Momordica charantia* (bitter melon, fuzzy melon or bitter gourd).

Based on expert opinion, anecdote, case report and/or clinical trial evidence, many other herbal medicines show potential or obvious benefit in the management of diabetes and its comorbidities and complications such as:

- *Vaccinium myrtillus* (bilberry)
- *Arctium lappa* (burdock)
- *Taraxacum officinalis* (dandelion)
- *Harpagophytum procumbens* (Devil's claw)
- *Hydrastis canadensis* (goldenseal)
- *Ginkgo biloba*
- *Allium sativum* (garlic)
- *Aesculus hippocastanum* (horse chestnut)
- *Althea officinalis* (marshmallow)
- *Silybum marianum* (St Mary's thistle)
- *Rosmarinus officinalis* (rosemary)
- *Urtica dioica* (nettle)
- *Marrubium vulgare L.* (white horehound)
- *Pinus pinaster ssp. atlantica* (Pycnogenol)
- *Plantago ovata* (psyllium).

The herbal medicines discussed in the remainder of this chapter were selected because they are commonly used in Western countries as well as their countries of origin, or there is some evidence to support their use. However, the list is not exhaustive and others medicines with actual or potential application to diabetes management are used. It would be prudent for clinicians to become familiar with the herbal medicines popular among the people in their country/practice area and consider the risks and benefits associated with each one.

Trigonella foenum (fenugreek) was described in early Greek and Latin pharmacopoeias for hyperglycemic states and has been used as a popular condiment in India for generations. The hypoglycaemic activity of fenugreek has been demonstrated in numerous studies involving experimentally induced diabetes (both type 1 and type 2) in rats, dogs, mice, rabbits and humans (Ribes *et al.* 1984; Madar *et al.*, 1988; Riyad 1988; Alarcon-Aguilara *et al.* 1998; Sharma *et al.* 1990; Raju 2001; Vats *et al.* 2002) and can be described as slow but sustained (Puri *et al.* 2002). These studies demonstrate that fenugreek significantly reduces fasting blood glucose, serum insulin, HbA_{1c} and urinary glucose levels. However, several different fenugreek preparations, various doses and different treatment time frames were used in the studies, which makes it difficult to interpret the results. Besides lowering blood glucose levels, *Trigonella* significantly reduced serum triglycerides and increased HDL cholesterol in type 2 diabetes in at least one randomised double-blind placebo-controlled study (Gupta *et al.* 2001).

Fenugreek exerts its glucose-lowering effect by delaying gastric emptying, reducing carbohydrate absorption and modulating glucose utilisation (al Habori *et al.* 2001). Results from in vivo experiments suggest it also increases tissue sensitivity to available insulin (Puri *et al.* 2002). Thus, it has similar actions to the alpha-glucosidase inhibitors and insulin sensitisers. The active component responsible for these activities is associated with the defatted part of the seed, which is rich in fibre-containing steroidal saponins and proteins (Valette *et al.* 1984; Ribes *et al.* 1986).

With regard to interactions, studies in which patients were concomitantly using fenugreek and conventional glucose-lowering medicines report positive effects in terms of glucose control and no adverse events, which suggests the combination is safe and may be beneficial. However, there is a potential for hypoglycaemia to occur when two or more glucose-lowering agents are used together and patients need to be educated about monitoring their blood glucose levels and how to recognise, treat and prevent hypoglycaemia.

Coccinia indica (ivy gourd) grows wild in Bangladesh and many parts of the Indian subcontinent. It is traditionally used to treat 'sugar urine' in Ayurvedic medicine. *Coccinia indica* appears to have an insulin-mimetic activity and produces no adverse effects (Kamble *et al.* 1998). Numerous in vivo studies demonstrate significant hypoglycemic activity, which has been confirmed in at least one double blind and one open clinical study involving people with type 2 diabetes (Azad *et al.* 1997; Grover *et al.* 2002). Beneficial effects have been reported within six weeks of treatment and it is well tolerated.

Panax quinquefolius (American ginseng) has been investigated in healthy subjects and those with type 2 diabetes after a standard glucose tolerance test (Vucksan *et al.* 2000; Vucksan *et al.* 2001). Doses between 1 and 3 g effectively reduced post-prandial glycaemia in both groups on a short-term basis. Additionally, reductions in fasting blood glucose and HbA_{1c} have been observed in eight-week trials. The glucose-lowering activity of American ginseng is partly due to a sulphonylurea-like activity (stimulates insulin production) (Rottshteyn and Zito 2004).

Panax ginseng (Korean or Asian ginseng) has a similar but different chemical make-up to American ginseng and according to one double-blind study in type 2 diabetes, also reduces fasting blood glucose levels (Sotaniemi *et al.* 1995), most likely by increasing tissue sensitivity to insulin.

Momordica charantia (bitter melon) is a gourd-like vegetable indigenous to subtropical and tropical regions of South America and Asia. It has been a popular folk remedy for diabetes in South-East Asian countries for centuries. Extract of fruit pulp, seed, leaves and the whole plant of *Momordica charantia* have demonstrated glucose-lowering effects in various animal models (Grover *et al.* 2002). One in vivo study using an aqueous extract of fresh unripe whole fruits at a dose of 20mg/kg body weight reduced fasting blood glucose by 48 per cent, an effect comparable to that of glibenclamide (Virdi *et al.* 2003). Four clinical trials have shown that bitter melon juice, fruit, and dried powder exert a moderate glucose-lowering effect, however, these studies were not randomised or double-blinded, Basch *et al.* 2003). It is postulated that the pharmacological effects are mediated through several mechanisms such as delaying gastric emptying and slowing gastrointestinal transport of glucose, increasing the efficiency of glucose uptake and storage in skeletal muscle and liver, down regulation of enzymes required for gluconeogenesis, and renewal of beta cells (Ahmed *et al.* 1998; McCarty 2004).

Gymnema sylvestre is a traditional Ayurvedic herb also known as gudmar, merasingi or periploca of the woods. The glucose-lowering activity was first confirmed in animal models in 1930 and has since been reconfirmed in several experiments (Srivastava *et al.* 1985; Shanmugasundaram *et al.* 1990). Two non-randomised studies have been conducted in diabetes (Baskaran *et al.* 1990; Shanmugasundaram *et al.* 1990). One study using an oral extract of *G. sylvestre* leaves (400 mg) for 18–20 months in addition to conventional oral diabetic treatment (glibenclamide or tolbutamide) showed significant effects in people with type 2 diabetes. Treatment resulted in a significant reduction in fasting blood glucose (174 ± 7 *vs.* 124 ± 5 mg/dL), HbA_{1c} (11.91 ± 0.3 *vs.* 8.48 ± 0.13 per cent) and glycosylated plasma protein levels (3.74 ± 0.07 *vs.* 2.46 ± 0.05 μg hexose/mg protein) whereas no changes were observed in the control group. A study involving 27 people with type 1 diabetes found that the same extract of *Gymnema sylvestre* reduced insulin requirements and fasting blood glucose for all participants. $HbA1_c$ and glycosylated plasma protein levels were significantly lower after treatment with the herb.

Cinnamon: in the past decade, in vitro studies have revealed that cinnamon extract mimics the effect of insulin and improves insulin receptor function (Qin *et al.* 2003). A recent randomised trial investigating the effects of cinnamon in type 2 diabetes demonstrated clinically significant glucose-lowering effects. The study involved 60 people divided into six groups. Groups one, two and three consumed 1, 3 or 6 g of cinnamon daily whereas groups four, five and six were given the equivalent number of placebo capsules and acted as controls (Khan *et al.* 2003). After 40 days of treatment, all three cinnamon doses reduced mean fasting serum glucose by 18 per cent to 29 per cent, triglycerides by 23 per cent to 30 per cent, LDL cholesterol by 7 per cent to 27 per cent, and total cholesterol by 12 per cent to 26 per cent. No significant changes were observed in the placebo groups.

These studies suggest many herbal substances are known or suspected to exert significant pharmacological effects that are beneficial in diabetes management, however, large controlled studies are still required to define their place in practice. Although the discussion so far has focused on individual herbs, in practice, herbs are often prescribed in combination and several specific herbal combinations are now being tested in clinical trials. For example, a study involving 40 people with diabetes showed that the CM herbal combination Jin Pi Jang Tang Pain significantly reduced fasting and post-prandial blood glucose levels after two months of treatment. The CM herbal combination, Jiang Tang Sang reduced glucose and lipid levels and blood pressure in 30 people with type 2 diabetes.

Many fixed commercial herbal formulations are available and are becoming more common; some also contain vitamin and/or mineral supplements. Not all of them have rigorous research to support their glucose-lowering or other effects, see Chapter 2, for some examples of Ayurvedic fixed herbal medicine combinations. Labelling on these products is often inadequate and it can be difficult to determine the composition of some preparations, especially when they are not subject to GMP codes.

The Modernised Chinese Medicine International Association (MCMIA) was convened to establish standard Chinese medicine preparations using modern biomedical techniques, which will make it easier to establish safety, efficacy and toxicity data as well as identify possible and actual adverse events associated with Chinese herbal medicines. The Australian government is preparing a catalogue of prescription, non-prescription and complementary medicines that will be available on-line to the general public as well as health professionals, which is in the final phases of testing at the time of writing. Recently, Fratkin's (1997) book describing Chinese patent herbal formulas was published in English.

9.5 Herbal Medicines and Vascular Disease

A number of herbal medicines such as grapeseed extract (*Vitus vinifera*), horse chestnut seed (*Aesculus hippocastanum*), French maritime pine bark (*Pinus pinaster ssp. atlantica*), bilberry (*Vaccinium myrtillus*), garlic (*Allium sativum*) and *Ginkgo biloba* have been used successfully to treat various aspects of vascular disease. The following information discuss several selected herbal medicines, however, many others worthy of consideration are also available.

Horse chestnut seed extract (*Aesculus hippocastanum*) is a popular European herbal treatment for chronic venous insufficiency, which is characterized by oedema of the lower extremities, pruritis, pain, atrophic skin changes, varicosity and ulceration. Its use in this condition is well supported by research and the treatment is well tolerated. A systematic review of 13 randomised, double-blind, controlled clinical studies found that horse-chestnut seed extract alleviates signs and symptoms of chronic venous insufficiency, however, more rigorous clinical studies are still required (Pittler and Ernst 2004). The most important constituents responsible for the pharmacological activity of the extract are collectively known as asaescin.

The herb is well tolerated with the incidence of adverse effects ranging from 0.9–3.0 per cent, mainly gastrointestinal disturbances (ESCOP 2003). Patients should be advised to monitor their blood glucose levels when horse chestnut seed extract is commenced to avoid hypoglycemia because glucose-lowering activity has been reported in a rat study, however, the clinical significance of the finding is unknown (Yoshikawa *et al.* 1996).

Pycnogenol is the patented name of a water extract of the French maritime pine bark (*Pinus pinaster ssp. atlantica*) whose main constituents are procyanidins and phenolic acids. It has been subjected to numerous clinical studies involving various conditions such as hypercholesterolaemia, gingival bleeding and male infertility, and has been most effective in treating chronic venous insufficiency (Rohdewald 2002). Pycnogenol is reported to reduce pain and oedema associated with the condition and is best tolerated when taken with food. Pycnogenol has antioxidant, anti-inflammatory and immunomodulation effects and possibly vasodilatory effects on small vessels.

Pycnogenol has also been investigated in the treatment of retinopathy in five clinical studies (Schonlau *et al.* 2001). One multicentre study involving, 1169 people with diabetic retinopathy showed Pycnogenol slowed progression of the disease and improved visual acuity to a degree (Schonlau *et al.* 2001). A smaller randomised, double-blind study also demonstrated that treatment with Pycnogenol delayed progression of retinopathy, retained retinal function and significantly improved visual acuity. Improvements in retinal vascularisation and reduced endothelial permeability and leakage were also observed (Spadea *et al.* 2001).

Garlic (*allium sativum*) is used to treat various vascular diseases and reduce cardiovascular risk factors such as hyperlipidemia, hypertension and increased plasma viscosity. A meta-analysis of 13 clinical trials concluded that garlic shows significant but modest cholesterol-lowering effects (Stevinson *et al.* 2000). According to a review of 37 randomised trials, the effects may be short-lived and disappear within six months (Mansoor 2001). In vitro studies suggest the mechanism of action involves deactivating HMG-CoA reductase by enhancing phosphorylation (Liu *et al.* 2002).

There has been some investigation into the effects of garlic on dyslipidemia in people with diabetes. A 12-week randomised, single-blind, placebo-controlled study involving 70 type 2 diabetic patients with newly diagnosed dyslipidemia found that oral supplementation with 300 mg garlic containing 1.3 per cent allicin twice per day in combination with a diet and exercise plan resulted in a significant reduction in total cholesterol compared to placebo (Ashraf *et al.* 2005). Several clinical studies suggest garlic has mild antihypertensive effects (Silagy and Neil 1994; Andrianova *et al.* 2002), however, this effect is not consistently reported in the literature.

Overall, the evidence regarding garlic is difficult to assess because many studies have methodological flaws, use different garlic formulations/preparations and different time frames, therefore, long-term studies that investigate doses and preparation variations are still required to clarify the best way to use this herb in practice.

Ginkgo biloba is a popular herbal medicine and is taken to prevent and/or treat poor peripheral circulation, chilblains, cognitive decline and claudication.

It has been the subject of dozens of randomised controlled trials, for example, Pittler and Ernst (2000) and Mouren *et al.* (1994). *Gingko* contains several different active constituents and exerts its effects through multiple mechanisms. A number of these mechanisms provide a basis for its role in vascular disease. More specifically, *Ginkgo* promotes peripheral blood flow through arteries, veins and capillaries. Under randomised, cross-over study conditions, it has been shown to increase microcirculatory blood flow one hour after administration (Jung *et al.* 1990). Several mechanisms of action have been proposed: nitric oxide (NO) release, activation of Ca^{2+}-activated K^+ (K_{Ca}) channels, and prostacyclin release (Nishida 2003).

A meta-analysis of eight clinical trials found a significant difference in the increase in pain-free walking distance in favour of *Ginkgo biloba* over placebo in intermittent claudication (Pittler and Ernst 2000). An earlier randomised study measured transcutaneous partial pressure of oxygen during exercise and demonstrated that a dose of 320mg/day of EGb 761 taken for four weeks significantly reduced the degree of ischaemia by 38 per cent compared to placebo (Mouren *et al.* 1994).

Several old studies suggest that *Ginkgo biloba* may prevent retinopathy and peripheral necrosis in people with 'severe diabetes' (Doly *et al.* 1986; Lanthony and Cosson 1988). In addition, neuroprotective effects have been demonstrated in a variety of studies ranging from molecular and cellular, to animal and human, however, the mechanisms responsible for these effects and the application to clinical diabetes care are not well elucidated (Smith *et al.* 2002).

Ginkgo biloba is well tolerated with a side effect profile similar to placebo. Gastrointestinal upset, headaches, and dizziness have been reported in less than 0.001 per cent of cases. The small possibility of causing gastrointestinal upsets needs to be considered if *Gingko* is combined with other herbal or conventional medicines that also produce such symptoms, for example, metformin and when gastroparesis is present. Although *Ginkgo* has a vasodilatory effect, it does not appear to alter heart rate or blood pressure, affect cholesterol and triglyceride levels or increase intraocular pressure (Chung *et al.* 1999).

Recent case reports suggest *Ginkgo* should be used with caution in people with known risk factors for cerebral haemorrhage and epilepsy until further investigation can clarify its safety in these conditions (Benjamin *et al.* 2001; Granger 2001). *Ginkgo* exerts PAF antagonist activity in some test models, therefore, it should be discontinued at least one week prior to major surgery to reduce the increased risk of bleeding. Whether the herb interacts with Warfarin is controversial and randomised trials have found no evidence to support such an interaction ((Engelsen *et al.* 2003; Jiang *et al.* 2005).

While many of these studies suggest at least some herbal medicines could have a role in managing the metabolic abnormalities associated with diabetes and its complications, more research is needed to determine the exact role and the most appropriate method to use them, especially given the effectiveness and safety of conventional medicines.

Other formulations that might be used by people with diabetes

As well as the range of fixed formulations of glucose-lowering herbs and supplements already mentioned, people with diabetes might use fixed formulations to control weight, which often contain *Hoodia gordonii* cactus extracts, and to treat erectile dysfunction, which often contain horny goat weed. Preparations that contain iodine, for example, some kelp preparations can affect their thyroid function and consequently blood glucose levels. There is little quality evidence to support the benefit of these formulations.

9.6   Herbal interactions

The pharmacological effect of an herbal medicine results from the interplay between various factors:

- intraherbal interactions among the constituents within a herb.
- interactions between the herb and the vehicles it is formulated in during processing and manufacture;
- interaction between the product and person receiving it;
- interactions between the foods, drugs and other conventional and herbal medicines an individual takes concomitantly.

In practice, interactions can be harnessed to produce beneficial outcomes and managed or avoided to reduce harm, see Chapter 3.

A pharmacological interaction refers to an alteration of the usual predicted effect of one substance when it is used concomitantly with another. Put another way, when a pharmacological or clinical response to a combination of medicines is different from that anticipated when one considers the activity of either agent given alone. Usually the term 'interaction' has a negative connotation when referring to medicines because they can lead to toxicity or reduce or enhance the effects making clinical outcomes difficult to predict (Braun and Cohen 2005).

An understanding of the mechanisms involved is essential to provide a rational basis for interpreting, preventing, treating or beneficially manipulating specific interactions and is essential when classifying or grading interactions. Currently, much information about conventional medicine – herb interactions derives from case reports, theoretical reasoning based on known or suspected pharmacology of the substance, and in a few cases, formal studies. As such, it is important to remember that a great deal of the information available is still speculative and the clinical significance of predicted interactions is often unknown.

In clinical practice, not every person who takes potentially interacting substances experiences an adverse effect. It is difficult, however, to predict which people are at greatest risk. Some of the characteristics of both people consuming medicines and the medicine that appear to increase the risk of harmful interactions are:

- medicines with a narrow therapeutic index (NTI), for example, digoxin, warfarin, lithium, barbiturates, phenytoin;
- old and frail people;
- children;
- people with renal or hepatic disease;
- people already taking multiple medicines;
- people prone to allergies;
- people who consult multiple practitioners;
- inadequate communication between patients and practitioners;
- inadequate communication between complementary and conventional practitioners;
- those using products not manufactured under strict manufacturing standards and codes;
- self-selection of OTC products without professional assistance, especially when an accurate diagnosis has not been made.

9.7 Pharmacokinetic Interactions

Pharmacokinetic, pharmacodynamic and physicochemical interactions are possible between herbal and conventional medicines. Pharmacokinetics refers to the quantitative analysis of the medicine's absorption, distribution, metabolism, and excretion.

Pharmacokinetic interactions occur when there is an alteration to any of these four processes causing a change in the amount and persistence of available medicine at receptor sites or target tissues. As a result, the type of effect seen remains unchanged, however, the strength or duration of effect may alter. Multiple mechanisms can be involved in this type of interaction making clinical predictions difficult.

Altered drug absorption can occur through a number of mechanisms and result in a changed rate of absorption and/or extent of absorption. A reduced rate of absorption can lead to a 'sustained release' effect, whereas reduced extent of absorption is particularly problematic for drugs with a NTI. Gums and mucilages such as guar gum and psyllium are examples of substances known or suspected to have an effect on drug absorption and are used in diabetes management by both conventional and complementary practitioners to modify the absorption of carbohydrates from the gut and sometimes, promote satiety and weight loss.

One double-blind study found that guar gum slowed the absorption rate of digoxin but did not alter the extent of absorption, whereas penicillin absorption was both slowed and reduced (Huupponen et al. 1984). The mucilage content is weakly lipid soluble and forms an additional physical barrier that needs to be traversed before the medicine can enter the systemic circulation. Whether other mucilages also have a clinically significant effect on the rate and/or extent of absorption of other medicines is currently unknown. In practice, this interaction can be minimised by separating the time of administration of each medicine by three to four hours.

Most medicine metabolism occurs in the liver in two apparent phases known as phase 1 and phase 2. Although many enzymes are responsible for phase 1 reactions, the most important enzyme group is the cytochrome P-450 system (CYP). Many factors can interfere with CYP activity such as the ingestion of environmental contaminants, certain food constituents, beverages, herbs and conventional medicines. If CYP substrates are taken at the same time as a substance that induces or inhibits that CYP, a pharmacokinetic interaction can occur.

Many medicines used in diabetes management are metabolised by CYP enzymes, mainly CYP3A4 and CYP2C9. CYP inhibitors and CYP inducers have significantly changed plasma levels of sulphonylureas, meglitinide derivatives and thiazolidinediones respectively, in studies of healthy volunteers (Scheen 2005). The resultant effect is either enhanced or reduced glucose-lowering activity and hypoglycemia or poor metabolic control respectively. Alternately, metformin is not significantly metabolised in humans and there are no clinically relevant metabolic interactions with other medicines.

The herb St John's wort provides a good example of a herbal substance capable of interacting with a variety of medicines through a pharmacokinetic mechanism. Clinical studies have confirmed that long-term administration of St John's wort significantly induces CYP, particularly CYP3A4 (Roby et al. 2000; Wang et al. 2001). It appears that the hyperforin component of the herb is a potent ligand for the pregnane X receptor, which regulates expression of CYP3A4 mono-oxygenase. In this way, hyperforin increases the availability of CYP3A4, resulting in enzyme induction (Moore et al. 2000). Examples of CYP 3A4 substrates are alprazolam, codeine, erythromycin and simvastatin.

More recently, research involving volunteers with type 2 diabetes suggests CYP induction effects associated with *Ginkgo biloba* that could lead to increased hepatic clearance of insulin (Kudolo 2001). In this case, the interaction would result in reduced insulin-mediated glucose metabolism and elevated blood glucose levels. Although this interaction needs to be tested further in clinical studies, caution is advised. Medicine excretion occurs via several routes kidneys, colon, saliva, sweat, breast milk and lungs. If a medicine is chiefly eliminated by one pathway, alterations to that particular pathway can theoretically have a significant influence on its excretion.

9.8 Pharmacodynamic Interactions

When one substance alters the sensitivity of tissues to another substance, a pharmacodynamic interaction is said to occur. This type of interaction results in additive, synergistic or antagonistic drug effects and is widely harnessed in practice to improve clinical outcomes. Pharmacodynamic interactions do not always produce wanted results. For instance, the combined use of a glucose-lowering medicine with a glucose-lowering herb may result in additional hypoglycemic effects. If unsupervised, the interaction can increase the risk of a hypoglycemic episode, however, under supervision the interaction may be avoided, managed or manipulated to improve therapeutic outcomes and reduce conventional medicine doses or dose intervals. In addition, pharmacodynamic interactions can produce other unwanted effects such as when two medicines with overlapping toxicities or side effects are used together, thereby increasing the risk of harm.

9.9 Using Herbal Medicines in Practice and Avoiding Adverse Herb–Medicine Interactions

Herb–medicine interactions involving medicines used in diabetes management are an important issue; particularly since lack of glycaemic control is associated with numerous diabetic complications. Several surveys have found that people with diabetes also use herbal medicines in addition to their conventional medicines thereby presenting the possibility of interactions. A Canadian survey of 502 people with diabetes found that 78 per cent were taking prescribed medication for their diabetes, 44 per cent were taking OTC supplements such as multivitamins, and 31 per cent were taking complementary medicines, mainly garlic (allium sativum), Echinacea (Echinacea spp.), *Ginkgo biloba*, and St John's wort (*Hypericum perforatum*) (Ryan *et al.* 2001).

It is important for clinicians to be aware of the risks and benefits associated with herbal medicines and become an information source people with diabetes or at least know to whom and how to refer them to obtain appropriate information. Promoting open communication about complementary medicine use is essential in order to effectively consider benefits, risks and safety and avoid misdiagnosis or inappropriate prescribing due to unknown complementary medicine use. Open communication furthers the patient–practitioner relationship and enables clinicians to learn from their patient's experiences with herbal medicines.

Besides having access to herbal medicine resources, it is worthwhile becoming familiar with a herbal medicine practitioner in the practice area because they may have valuable experience, information and insight, which can help guide patients and practitioners appropriately. Lastly, keep in mind the factors that increase a person's risk of experiencing a harmful herb–medicine interaction such as older people, children, people taking multiple medicines, those with poor renal or liver function, those seeking advice from multiple health-care professionals and not disclosing their use of complementary medicines and when NTI drugs are involved. People with diabetes who choose to add herbal medicines to their conventional management plan should be encouraged to use products manufactured under strict manufacturing standards and codes and inform all their healthcare providers about use.

Identifying a potential herb–medicine interaction

Although some herb–drug interactions can be manipulated to produce beneficial outcomes for patients such as improved quality of life or reduced drug requirements, interactions can also produce unwanted effects, see Table 9.2. An herb–medicine interaction should be considered when:

Table 9.2 Factors that could indicate an herb-medicine interaction with special reference to diabetes and cardiovascular disease.

Clinical situation	Comments
When a patient with previously stable blood glucose readings suddenly becomes unstable (either reduced or raised levels)	Are they taking a herb with hypoglycemic activity? Has their diet significantly changed? Have they stopped taking a herbal medicine with hypoglycemic effects?
When a patients lipid levels suddenly change (for better or worse)	Are they taking a herb which affects lipid levels? Has their diet significantly changed?
When a previously effective medicine becomes ineffective or the drug dose must be increased to maintain a therapeutic effect	Are they taking a herb which can reduce the bioavailability of the drug, increase its metabolism or excretion?
When a previously well tolerated medicine is now poorly tolerated i.e. side effects start to develop	Are they experiencing adverse effects due to a herbal medicine or the interaction of both medicines?

- a previously stable patient suddenly experiences a significant change in their condition for better or worse;
- a previously effective treatment that was well tolerated becomes poorly tolerated or is no longer as effective;
- when the dose of a previously effective treatment must be increased to maintain therapeutic effect.

If one or more of these clinical scenarios occurs, and an interaction is suspected, it is important to confirm the suspicion by asking the patient in an open and non-judgemental way about their use of any complementary, 'natural' or herbal medicine. If they are unsure, ask them to bring in all the medicines they are taking so you can check the product labels for TGA or equivalent listed ingredients.

If an interaction produces a beneficial effect, it may be preferable for the patient to continue taking the combination. In the case of herbal glucose-lowering medicines, blood glucose levels can start to fall within several days to weeks, depending on the herbal medicine being used. Patients should continue to carefully monitor blood glucose levels and clinicians should consider lowering doses of conventional glucose-lowering agents if appropriate. Considering that some herbal treatments also produce favourable effects on lipid levels, lipids should also be monitored and medicines adjusted if necessary. Clinicians need to monitor the patient closely and measure HbA_{1c} after three months in order to ensure that metabolic targets are attained and maintained. Likewise, the metabolic targets should be the same as those required of conventional medicines.

If an interaction produces an unwanted effect such as an adverse reaction, the herbal medicine should be discontinued. A sample of the herbal medicine should be collected from the patient and, ideally, submitted for chemical analysis.

A detailed report should be submitted to the national adverse event reporting programme.

References

Ahmed I, Adeghate E, Sharma A, Pallot D, Singh J. Effects of *Momordica charantia* fruit juice on islet morphology in the pancreas of the streptozotocin-diabetic rat. *Diabetes Research and Clinical Practice* 1998; **40**: 145–151.

Alarcon-Aguilara F, Roman-Ramos R, Perez-Gutierrez S, Aguilar-Contreras A, Contreras-Weber C, Flores-Saenz J. Study of the anti-hyperglycemic effect of plants used as antidiabetics. *Journal Ethnopharmacology* 1998; **61**: 101–110.

Al Habori M, Raman A, Lawrence M, Skett P. In vitro effect of fenugreek extracts on intestinal sodium-dependent glucose uptake and hepatic glycogen phosphorylase A. *International Journal of Experimental Diabetes Research* 2001; **2**: 91–91.

Andrianova I, Fomchenkov I, Orekhov A. Hypotensive effect of long-acting garlic tablets allicor (a double-blind placebo-controlled trial). *Ter. Arkh.* 2002; **74**: 76–78.

Ashraf R, Aamir K, Shaikh A, Ahmed T. Effects of garlic on dyslipidemia in patients with type 2 diabetes mellitus. *Journal Ayub Medical College Abbottabad* 2005; **17**: 60–64.

Azad Khan A, Akhtar S, Mahtab H. *Coccinia indica* in the treatment of patients with diabetes mellitus. *Bangladesh Medical Research Council Bulletin* 1979; **5**: 60–56.

Basch E, Gabardi S, Ulbricht C. Bitter melon (*Momordica charantia*): a review of efficacy and safety. *American Journal Health System Pharmacology* 2003; **60**: 356–359.

Baskaran K, Kizar A, Radha S, Shanmugasundaram E. Antidiabetic effect of a leaf extract from *Gymnema sylvestre* in non-insulin-dependent diabetes mellitus patients. *Journal Ethnopharmacology* 1990; **30**: 295–300.

Benjamin J, Muir T, Briggs K, Pentland B. A case of cerebral haemorrhage: can *Ginkgo biloba* be implicated? *Postgraduate Medical Journal* 2001; **77**: 112–113.

Chung H, Harris A, Kristinsson J, Ciulla T, Kagemann C, Ritch R. *Ginkgo biloba* extract increases ocular blood flow velocity. *Journal Ocular Pharmacological Therapy* 1999; **15**: 233–240.

Doly M, Droy-Lefaix M, Bonhomme B, Braquet P. Effect of *Ginkgo biloba* extract on the electrophysiology of the isolated retina from a diabetic rat. *Presse Medicine* 1986; **15**: 1480–1483.

Dunning T. Complementary therapies and diabetes. *Complementary Therapies in Nursing and Midwifery* 2003; **9**: 74–80.

Engelsen J, Nielsen J, Hansen K. Effect of Coenzyme Q10 and *Ginkgo biloba* on warfarin dosage in patients on long-term warfarin treatment: a randomized, double-blind, placebo-controlled cross-over trial. *Ugeskr Laeger* 2003; **165**: 1868–1871.

ESCOP. *Hippocastani semen*, ESCOP monographs. Thieme: ESCOP, 2003; pp. 248–256.

Fratkin J. 1997 *Chinese Herbal Patent Formulas*. Pelanduk Publications, Jalan, Malaysia.

Granger A. Ginkgo biloba precipitating epileptic seizures. *Age and Ageing* 2001; **30**: 523–525.

Grover J, Yadav S, Vats V. Medicinal plants of India with anti-diabetic potential. *Journal of Ethnopharmacology* 2002; **81**: 81–100.

Gupta A, Gupta R, Lal B. Effect of *Trigonella foenum-graecum* (fenugreek) seeds on glycaemic control and insulin resistance in type 2 diabetes mellitus: a double blind placebo controlled study. *Journal of the Association of Physicians India* 2001; **49**: 1057–1061.

Huupponen R, Seppala P, Iisalo E. Effect of guar gum, a fibre preparation, on digoxin and penicillin absorption in man. *European Journal Clinical Pharmacology* 1984; **26**: 279–281.

Jiang X, Williams K, Liauw W, Ammit A, Roufogalis B, Duke C, Day R, McLachlan A. Effect of ginkgo and ginger on the pharmacokinetics and pharmacodynamics of warfarin in healthy subjects. *British Journal of Clinical Pharmacology* 2005; **59**: 425–432.

Kamble S, Kamlakar P, Vaidya S, Bambole V. Influence of *Coccinia indica* on certain enzymes in glycolytic and lipolytic pathway in human diabetes. *Indian Journal of Medical Science* 1998; **52**: 143–146.

Khan A, Safdar M, Ali Khan M, Khattak K, Anderson R. Cinnamon improves glucose and lipids of people with type 2 diabetes. *Diabetes Care* 2003; 3215–3218.

Kudolo G. The effect of 3-month ingestion of Ginkgo biloba extract (EGb 761) on pancreatic beta-cell function in response to glucose loading in individuals with non-insulin-dependent diabetes mellitus. *Journal of Clinical Pharmacology* 2001; **41**: 600–611.

Lanthony P, Cosson J. The course of color vision in early diabetic retinopathy treated with *Ginkgo biloba* extract: a preliminary double-blind versus placebo study. *Journal French Ophtalmology* 1998; **11**: 671–674.

Liu L, Yeh Y. S-alk(en)yl cysteines of garlic inhibit cholesterol synthesis by deactivating HMG-CoA reductase in cultured rat hepatocytes. *Journal Nutrition* 2002; 1129–1134.

Madar Z, Abel R, Samish S, Arad J. Glucose-lowering effect of fenugreek in non-insulin dependent diabetics. *European Journal Clinical Nutrition* 1988; **42**: 51–54.

Mansoor G. Herbs and alternative therapies in the hypertension clinic. *American Journal of Hypertension* 2001; **14**: 971–975.

McCarty M. Does bitter melon contain an activator of AMP-activated kinase? *Medical Hypotheses* 2004; **63**: 340–343.

Moore L, Goodwin B, Jones S, Wisely G, Serabjit-Singh C, Willson T, Collins J, Kliewer S. St. John's wort induces hepatic drug metabolism through activation of the pregnane X receptor. *Proceedings Natural Academy Science U.S.A* 2000; **97**: 7500–7502.

Mouren X, Caillard P, Schwartz F. Study of the anti-ischemic action of EGb 761 in the treatment of peripheral arterial occlusive disease by TcPo2 determination. *Angiology* 1994; **145**: 413–417.

Nishida S, Satoh H Mechanisms for the vasodilation induced by *Ginkgo biloba* extract and its main constituent, bilobalide, in rat aorta. *Life Science* 2003; **72**: 2659–2667.

Persaud S, Al Majed H, Raman A, Jones P. *Gymnema sylvestre* stimulates insulin release in vitro by increased membrane permeability. *Journal Endocrinology* 1999; **163**: 207–212.

Pittler M, Ernst E. *Ginkgo biloba* extract for the treatment of intermittent claudication: a meta-analysis of randomized trials. *American Journal of Medicine* 2000; **108**: 276–281.

Pittler M, Ernst E. Horse chestnut seed extract for chronic venous insufficiency. *Cochrane Database Systematic Reviews* 2004; CD003230.

Puri D, Prabhu K, Murthy P. Mechanism of action of a hypoglycemic principle isolated from fenugreek seeds. *Indian Journal Physiology Pharmacology* 2002; **46**: 457–462.

Raju J, Gupta D, Rao A, Yadava P, Baquer N. *Trigonella foenum graecum* (fenugreek) seed powder improves glucose homeostasis in alloxan diabetic rat tissues by reversing the altered glycolytic, gluconeogenic and lipogenic enzymes. *MolecularCell Biochemistery* 2001; **224**: 45–51.

Ribes G, Sauvaire Y, Baccou J, Valette G, Chenon D, Trimble E, Loubatieres-Mariani M. Effects of fenugreek seeds on endocrine pancreatic secretions in dogs. *Annals of Nutrition Metabolism* 1984; **28**: 37–43.

Ribes G, Sauvaire Y, Da Costa C, Baccou J, Loubatieres-Mariani M. Antidiabetic effects of subfractions from fenugreek seeds in diabetic dogs. *Proceedings of the Society Exp. Biology and Medicine* 1986; **182**: 159–166.

Riyad M, Abdul-Salam S, Mohammad S. Effect of fenugreek and lupine seeds on the development of experimental diabetes in rats. *Planta Medica* 1988; **54**: 286–290.

Roby C, Anderson G, Kantor E, Dryer D, Burstein A. St John's Wort: effect on CYP3A4 activity. *Clinical Pharmacology Therapy* 2000; **67**: 451–457.

Rohdewald P. A review of the French maritime pine bark extract (Pycnogenol), a herbal medication with a diverse clinical pharmacology. *International Journal Clinical Pharmacology Therapeutics* 2002; **40**: 158–168.

Rotshteyn Y, Zito S. Application of modified in vitro screening procedure for identifying herbals possessing sulfonylurea-like activity. *Journal Ethnopharmacology* 2004; **93**: 337–344.

Ryan E, Pick M, Marceau C. Use of alternative medicines in diabetes mellitus. *Diabetic Medicine* 2001; **18**: 242–245.

Scheen A. Drug interactions of clinical importance with antihyperglycaemic agents: an update. *Drug Safety* 2005; **28**: 601–631.

Schonlau F, Rohdewald P. Pycnogenol for diabetic retinopathy: a review. *International Ophthalmoogy* 2001; **24**: 161–171.

Shanmugasundaram E, Gopinath K, Radha S, Rajendran V. Possible regeneration of the islets of Langerhans in streptozotocin-diabetic rats given *Gymnema sylvestre* leaf extracts. *Journal Ethnopharmacology* 1990a; 265–279.

Shanmugasundaram E, Rajeswari G, Baskaran K, Rajesh Kumar B, Radha S, Kizar A. Use of *Gymnema sylvestre* leaf extract in the control of blood glucose in insulin-dependent diabetes mellitus. *Journal Ethnopharmacology* 1990b; **30**: 281–294.

Sharma R, Raghuram T, Rao N. Effect of fenugreek seeds on blood glucose and serum lipids in type I diabetes. *European Journal of Clinical Nutrition* 1990; **44**: 301–306.

Silagy C, Neil H. A meta-analysis of the effect of garlic on blood pressure. *Journal Hypertension* 1994; **12**: 463–468.

Smith J, Burdick A, Golik P, Khan I, Wallace D, Luo Y. Anti-apoptotic properties of *Ginkgo biloba* extract EGb 761 in differentiated PC12 cells. *Cell Molecular Biology* 2002; **48**: 699–707.

Sotaniemi E, Haapakoski E, Rautio A. Ginseng therapy in non-insulin-dependent diabetic patients. *Diabetes Care* 1995; **18**: 1373–1375.

Spadea L, Balestrazzi E. Treatment of vascular retinopathies with Pycnogenol. *Phytotherapy Research* 2001; **15**: 219–223.

Srivastava Y, Nigam S, Bhatt H, Verma Y, Prem A. Hypoglycemic and life-prolonging properties of *Gymnema sylvestre* leaf extract in diabetic rats. *Israeli Journal Medical Science* 1985; **21**: 540–542.

Stevinson C, Pittler M, Ernst E. Garlic for treating hypercholesterolemia: a meta-analysis of randomized clinical trials. *Annals Internal Medicine* 2000; **133**: 420–429.

Valette G, Sauvaire Y, Baccou JC, Ribes G. Hypocholesterolaemic effect of fenugreek seeds in dogs. *Atherosclerosis* 1984; **50**: 105–111.

Vats V, Grover J, Rathi S. Evaluation of anti-hyperglycemic and hypoglycemic effect of *Trigonella foenum-graecum* Linn, *Ocimum sanctum* Linn and *Pterocarpus marsupium* Linn in normal and alloxanized diabetic rats. *Journal Ethnopharmacology* 2002; **79**: 95–100.

Virdi J, Sivakami S, Shahani S, Suthar A, Banavalikar M, Biyani M. Antihyperglycemic effects of three extracts from *Momordica charantia*. *Journal Ethnopharmacology* 2003; **88**: 107–111.

Vuksan V, Sievenpiper J, Koo V, Francis T, Beljan-Zdravkovic U, Xu Z, Vidgen E. American ginseng (*Panax quinquefolius L*) reduces postprandial glycemia in nondiabetic subjects and subjects with type 2 diabetes mellitus. *Archives of Internal Medicine* 2000; **160**: 1009–1013.

Vuksan V, Sievenpiper J, Wong J, Xu Z, Beljan-Zdravkovic U, Arnason J, Assinewe V, Stavro M, Jenkins A, Leiter L, Francis T. American ginseng (*Panax quinquefolius L.*) attenuates postprandial glycemia in a time-dependent but not dose-dependent manner in healthy individuals. *American Journal of Clinical Nutrition* 2001; **73**: 753–758.

Wang Z, Gorski J, Hamman M, Huang S, Lesko L, Hall S. The effects of St John's wort (*Hypericum perforatum*) on human cytochrome P450 activity. *Clinical Pharmacology Therapy* 2001; **70**: 317–326.

Yeh G, Eisenberg D, Davis R, Phillips R. Use of complementary and alternative medicine among persons with diabetes mellitus: results of a national survey. *American Journal of Public Health* 2002; **92**: 1648–1652.

Yeh G, Eisenberg D, Kaptchuk T, Phillips R. Systematic review of herbs and dietary supplements for glycemic control in diabetes. *Diabetes Care* 2003; **26**: 1277–94.

Yoshikawa M, Murakami T, Matsuda H, Yamahara J, Murakami N, Kitagawa I. Bioactive saponins and glycosides. III. Horse chestnut. (1): The structures, inhibitory effects on ethanol absorption, and hypoglycemic activity of escins Ia, Ib, IIa, IIb, and IIIa from the seeds of *Aesculus hippocastanum* L. *Chemistry Pharmacology Bulletin* (Tokyo) 1996; **44**: 1454–1464.

10 Ayurvedic Management of Diabetes

Devaka Fernando

10.1 Introduction

Ayurveda as described in the classical treatises is one part of an evolving system of medicine. Over the last millennium, Ayurveda probably evolved and interacted with other systems of medicine brought into India by invaders. These medical systems include Greek medicine when Alexander the Great invaded India and Unani medicine following the Mogul invaders. British physicians in India and Sri Lanka and missionaries were particularly interested in learning local systems of medicine (Muller 1985).

Although the British actively denounced Indian medicine and promoted Western medicine following the educational reforms in 1835 (Porter 1997), the expense of shipping pharmaceuticals from England encouraged British physicians in India to experiment with local remedies. However, with the development of a formal pharmacopoeia in 1858, the concept of a legally enforceable standard of medicines was established. In the broader setting of suppressing indigenous arts, skills and technology state support for Ayurveda ceased. However, when India (1947) and Sri Lanka (1948) gained independence from British rule, Ayurveda was recognised as an official form of medicine along with allopathy, homeopathy, naturopathy, Unani Tibb and Siddha, a variant of Ayurveda practised in the Tamil-speaking region of India. Ministries of Indigenous Medicine have been established for many decades but until recently there been little investment in research.

Ayurvedic medicines have been in use for millennia. In recent years there conventional practitioners have become increasingly interested in herbal medicines because they have increased in popularity in the developed world. In the USA self-prescribed herbal medicine use increased from 2.55 per cent to 12.1 per cent between 1990 and 1997 (Fisher and Ward 1994; Eisenberg *et al.* 1998) and frequency of consultations with herbal medicine practitioners rose from 10.2 per cent to 15.1 per cent, see Chapter 2. A similar increase has been reported in Europe (Astin 1999).

Complementary Therapies and the Management of Diabetes and Vascular Disease   Editor Trish Dunning
© 2006 John Wiley & Sons, Ltd.

A variety of herbal medicines, including Ayurvedic herbs, are used to manage diabetes, see Chapters 9, 11 and 14. Few people with diabetes use over the counter (OTC) or CAM alone but many use them concurrently with conventional medicines such as sulphonylureas and metformin but do not tell their doctors (Leese et al. 1997; Mills 2001). In Edmonton, Canada, 44 per cent of patients take OTC medicines and 31 per cent take alternative medicines (Ryan et al. 2001). It is evident that many people with diabetes are attracted to CAM medicines despite the considerable extra cost of such treatment (Egede et al. 2002).

The complex nature of managing diabetes and the emphasis on empowered self-care and an increasing dissatisfaction with multi-medicine management, may contribute to the attraction of CAM, which is seen as more holistic than conventional medicine. Diabetes health professionals need to discuss CAM use with their patients and have some knowledge of other systems of medicine in order to provide effective patient-centred care according to modern diabetes management philosophies. The aim of this chapter is to provide an overview of Ayurveda and the available scientific evidence for its application to diabetes management.

10.2 Ayurveda

Ayurveda is derived from Sanskrit words meaning knowledge (*veda*) of life (*ayus*). The *vedas* contain details of substances, qualities and actions that enhance longevity. Ayurvedic medicine is practised in India and Sri Lanka and is believed to have originated in the Vedic period around 1500 BC. The descriptions of its principles and practice are recorded in the Vedas or the great books of knowledge. Ayurveda probably evolved as an *upaveda* or subsidiary body of knowledge of the *Atharvaveda*, one of four Vedic books, the others being *Rigveda, Yajurveda and Samaveda* (Porter 1997; Hardy et al. 2001).

The most important sources of information about Ayurvedic practices are the major treatises, the *Charaka Samhita* and the *Susrutha Ayurveda* (Lad 1999; Wujastyk 1995). The first chapter of the third treatise of the *Sutrasthana* (place of aphorisms) written by *Vagbhata*, is regarded widely as a succinct and clear summary of the principles of Ayurveda in the form of a rhythmic verse. Written records were in Pali and Sanskrit, the ancient languages of India, which occupied a place in India similar to that of Greek and Latin in Western Europe. However, most of the information about Ayurveda was conveyed orally where the art and science of Ayurvedic practice were passed on from master to pupil. The oral tradition was taught and learned by memorising verses. Lolimbaraja compiled the Vaidyajivana (*Life of Medicine*) in the sixteenth century. The Vaidyajivana consists of one hundred verses and is the best known summary. The popularity of the Vaidyajivana over the longer treatise with students resulted in inexperienced practitioners being referred to as 'doctors by a hundred stanzas' (Wujastyk 1995).

The *Charaka Samhita* consists of eight position papers or *sthanas*:

1. *Sutra* (aphorism), which deals with the origin of Ayurveda and the general principles, and philosophy.

2. *Nidana*, which discusses the diagnosis, causes and symptoms of disease.
3. *Vimana*, which is concerned with measurement of an environment of the body such as physiology.
4. *Sharira*, which focuses on the body especially anatomy, embryology, metaphysics, and ethics.
5. *Indriya*, the sense organs.
6. *Cikitsa* or treatment.
7. *Kalpa*, which describes methods of preparing medicines.
8. *Siddhi* or purification therapy.

Diseases are described using a structured format that addresses:

- *Nidhana* (aetiology);
- *Samprapti* (pathogenesis);
- *Purvarupa* (prodromal phenomena, i.e. indicators of high risk);
- *Rupa* (clinical picture, signs and symptoms);
- *Upasaya* (sensitivity to treatment);
- *Aushada* (therapeutics) (Lad 1985, 1995, 1999; Hardy 2001).

Principles of Ayurveda

Ayurveda is based on the assumption held in its spiritual base that there is a close relationship between the individual and the universe. This relationship is reflected in Ayurveda being widely regarded as having an holistic approach to a person with a health problem rather than a problem in a person. The study of Ayurveda and its practice involves maintaining the harmony of a number (*sankhya*) of factors.

The inter-relationship of the nine categories of matter or *dravayas* and the five great elements or *mahabhutas* determines health. The *dravayas* are: *dik* direction or space, *kala* time, *athma* soul/spirit and *manasa* mind.

This forms the cornerstone of the *Panchabhuta* or five elements philosophy, which teaches that the basic energy of life occurs as five great elements (*mahabhutas*): ether or space, air, fire, water, and earth.

All five elements present in the world are also present in each individual but vary in proportion and composition depending on age, presence of illness, and physiological changes such as pregnancy. The five elements are perfectly balanced in health and any disturbance of the balance produces ill health, the degree of which is proportional to the disturbance. In the human body the five elements combine with each other and produce defects, known as *doshas*.

The *doshas* govern the status of the body and are collectively referred to as the *tridosha*. Ether and air combine to form *vata*; fire and water combine to form *pitta*; and water and earth combine to form *kapha* (Lad 1985, 1995, 1999). *Vata* governs physical processes such as respiration, circulation, and voluntary action and is of particular relevance during exertion and exercise. In addition, *vata* may have a role in mental activity such as motivation, enthusiasm and concentration. *Pitta* plays a role in physical phenomena such as digestion and metabolism. *Kapha* maintains body cohesiveness by providing it with a fluid matrix and maintaining 'oiliness' and stability. *Kapha* plays a role in physical phenomena such as the promoting physical strength, integrating the structural elements of the body to achieve stability, and maintaining smooth joint mobility.

Although the *doshas* are said to be associated with organ systems, they exist in each organ system with one predominant *dosha* in each organ. Thus *vata* predominates in respiration, *pitta* in digestive juices and *kapha* in mucous. However, the *doshas* are not identical to the Hippocratic humours of wind, bile and phlegm.

Individual constitution – *Prakriti*

Prakriti is a Sanskrit word denoting the constitution or nature of each individual. *Prakirti* in turn determines *ahankara* or self-identity. *Ahankara* is said to produce expressions of individuality in those with similar *prakirti*. An individual *ahankara* is influenced by three attributes (*guna*), which are activity (*rajas*), equilibrium (*sattva*), and inertia (*tamas*). *Tamas* represents input from the senses: sound, touch, form, taste and odour, which are, in turn, influenced by the components of the environment the *panchamahabhutas*. *Sattva* develops into the mind, the five senses (hearing, touch, sight, taste and smell). The five actions are speech, action of hands, action of feet, action of reproductive organs and action of excretory organs.

Health is defined as the functioning as one unit in one place and one time of the five great elements, five senses and five activities and the thinking mind. It is a composite of physical, emotional and spiritual state of an individual rather than an absence of disease. The approach to maintaining health is considered to be a primary objective of the individual.

> An intelligent person should therefore specially devote himself to those endeavors which assure the body's well being. The whole body is truly the support of one's well-being, since humans are established in the body. Leaving everything else one should take care of the body, for in the absence of the body there is the total extinction of all that characterizes embodied beings.
>
> (*Charaka Nidhanasthana* 6/6–7, cited in Svoboda 1995)

An individual's *prakriti* makes a contribution at conception in that the individual is born with a dominant *vatha*, which determines their personality and body type. The basic constitution is influenced by extrinsic factors such as diet, lifestyle, behaviour, emotions, and the seasons. Changes in constitution are termed *vikurti*. *Doshas* changes occur throughout life depending on age and physiological states such as adolescence, puberty, pregnancy, in different phases of the menstrual cycle and in response to food, exercise, lifestyle and environmental factors.

Combinations of the *doshas* determine individual susceptibility to such influences. There is a relationship between different spaces (*desha*), which could be either terrestrial environment (*bhumi*) or within the body (*deha*). Hence environmental factors (from *bhumi*) such as food, water, sunlight, touch, odours, tastes, sights, sounds, emotions and thoughts may affect an individual's body (*deha*) and evoke a response determined by his *prakirti*. The ability to adapt is determined by an internal 'fire' (*agni*), which is determined by the harmony of the *doshas*.

This fire can cope with change and is balanced if the *doshas* are in harmony (*samaagni*). If *doshas* are unbalanced, the fire may be insufficient (*mandaagni*), intense (*tiksha agni*) or toxic (*visamagni*) leading to a change or mutation (*vikurti*) in the constitution (*prakirti*) and cause illness. Depending on their ability to withstand external stress without disrupting the harmony of *doshas*, constitutions (*prakirti*) are classified as *uttama* (superior), *madhya* (average) or *hina* (weak or small).

Dominance of any one *dosha* with a weak constitution (*hina prakirti*) and diminished ability to deal with environmental stress (*mandaagni*) leading to *vikurti* in the inherited constitution may predispose the individual to certain illnesses. According to Ayurveda, it is possible to anticipate any potential risks of *vikurti* by identifying the nature of the disturbed *dosha* by observing and assessing the manifestations of the predisposing *hina prakirti*. Thus, prescribing appropriate remedies can prevent illness.

Tissues and excretions – *dhatu and mala*

The *doshas* are only one of three principal body divisions in Ayurveda. The other two are seven *dhatus* or tissues and three *malas* or excretions. The dhatus are responsible for the entire structure of the body and maintain the functions of different organs. The seven *dhatus* are:

1. *rasa* (plasma)
2. *rakta* (blood)
3. *mansa* (muscle)
4. *medas* (fat)
5. *asthi* (bone)
6. *majja* (marrow and nerves)
7. *shukra* and *artava* (reproductive tissues).

The three *malas* are *sveda* (sweat), *purisha* (faeces), and *mutra* (urine). Ayurveda practitioners consider that the origin of most diseases is due to either an exogenous or endogenous *dosha* imbalance or an inherent or acquired weakness of the tissues. Vabhata explains the relationship among the *doshas, dhatu* and *mala*. The word *dosha* means defect. Thus *dosha* is not regarded as a structural component but a flaw in the organism that has the potential to harm the organism if it is present in abnormal amounts. In health, the person's metabolic ability/fire (*agni*) ensures the *doshas* are in balance. Thus, the *doshas* continuously flow out of the body through *malas*. The key concept is that the *doshas* must flow out of the body. When healthy amounts of *mala* are produced, *doshas* do not accumulate within the body and cause ill health. Thus, the *doshas* differ from the classical Hippocratic humours of air, bile and phlegm. The *doshas* are described as invisible forces whose presence in the body can be inferred.

Pathogenesis of illness

Ancient societies believed that that health was determined by fate. Ayurveda asserted that everything has an effect and that fate was a result of previously performed actions or inactivity that in turn led to the conclusion that such events could be avoided or prevented. In Ayurveda, illness is said to develop in six stages. An individual's *prakirti* determines their susceptibility. A person with a *hina prakirti* (weak constitution) has limited ability to counter external threats (*agnimandhya*), which in turn obstructs the pathways (*margavarodha*) and *doshas* become unbalanced. *Dosha* imbalance may be due to inappropriate thought (*pagnaaparadha*) leading to inappropriate actions.

These factors set in motion a six-stage process of developing an illness. In the phase of accumulation, one or more *doshas* accumulate in the diseased organ and create an imbalance of doshas. In case of digestive illness, *kapha* accumulates in the stomach, *pitta* in the small intestine or *vata* in the colon. If untreated, *doshas* continue to accumulate and exert pressure on the diseased organ and intensify the symptoms produced. If the *dosha* imbalance caused by accumulation of one or the other *dosha* is not corrected, the *doshas* escape from the diseased organ, change their properties (*gathi*) and create disease throughout the body. The escaped *doshas* tend to settle in a part of the body where the *dhatus* have been weakened by previous illness or heredity.

Before *doshas* spread out to other parts of the body the disease is considered to be silent in terms of symptoms and signs, but various *purvarupa* or premonitory non-clinical factors may be present and can lead to a high index of suspicion. However, once the *doshas* change location, the illness becomes clinically evident, manifesting in the *rupa* or clinical picture. The specific illness results from the status of the dominant *dosha* and *dhatu* involved (Lad 1995; Lad 1999).

According to the Astagahrdaya Sutrasthana, the three *doshas* pervade the body and work in every part of it but they are particularly concentrated in the tissues where they are produced. They produce ill health by the six-point mechanism described previously (Svoboda 1995).

It is tempting to draw parallels with current concepts of pathophysiology. Metabolites produced by normal physiological activities such as carbon dioxide, bilirubin and creatinine are produced in different tissues and excreted by different organs. Accumulation of these metabolites can occur due to specific organ dysfunction and lead to disease if they accumulate and spread into the systemic circulation. Failure of each organ produces distinct clinical features in the late stages but experts may recognise more subtle early features. According to Ayurveda, *dosha* excess cannot be demonstrated by clinical examination and observation. It can only be inferred. Modern medical practice requires particular metabolites to be demonstrable in excessive amounts (outside normal limits). However, the presence of excess carbon dioxide, urea or bilirubin can be inferred from a physical examination and history but demonstration requires biochemical tests that were not available to early Ayurvedic physicians.

10.3 Ayurvedic Diagnosis

Ayurvedic diagnosis is based on the assumption that the basic elements of life are continuous. Disease processes occur due to a reaction between an imbalance of *doshas* and weakened tissues (*dhatus*) and may be influenced by the environment. These interactions can produce a spectrum from order (health) to disorder (disease). Ayurvedic practitioners have very precise methods for understanding the disease process at a preclinical stage (*purvarupa*) before any overt signs of the disease are obvious. By recognizing *purvarupa* it is thought possible to determine the nature of future health or predisposition to ill health. Regularly monitoring the interactions helps the practitioner detect *purvarupa* before *rupa* develops and enables timely remedial or preventive measures to be implemented, which is an important aspect of Ayurveda (pers. comm. with traditional healers working with Ritigala Economic Advancement Foundation Allagollewa Sri Lanka (REAFASL)).

Physical examination is preceded by *Prashna* (questioning). Ayurvedic texts recommend that the practitioner ask about the patient's family, occupation, social status, lifestyle and symptoms, seek information from family members to establish/clarify the facts. Details about the tone of voice and body language also need to be considered when assessing an individual. The practitioner then proceeds to examine the patient and their environment, consider suitable management options, prepare the medicines, and commence treatment. Classical clinical examination in Ayurveda is called *Ashta Sthana Pariksha* or eight-position examination and includes assessing the state of the *doshas* as well as various physical signs (*rupa*), the tissues (*dhatu*), and excretions (*mala*). It is recommended that the nine doors (eyes, ears, nostrils, mouth, anus and penis or vulva) and their secretions be examined. The components of the examination include:

- *Nadi pariksha* (examining the pulse).
- *Mutra pariksha* (examining the urine).
- *Sparsha* (touch).
- *Pitta* (assessing digestive secretions).
- *Kapha* (assessing mucous and mucoid secretions).
- *Mala pariksha* (examining the stools).
- *Jihva pariksha* (examining the vital signs of life).
- *Sabda pariksh* (listening to body sounds).

The texts refer to using smell (*gandha*), colour (*varna*), and taste (*rasa*) as important aspects of Ayurvedic diagnosis. Using these methods, the Ayurvedic practitioner is expected to determine the symptoms and signs of imbalance and disease and prescribe appropriate management strategies to correct imbalances (Lad 1985, 1995, 1999; pers. comm. REALFASL).

Ayurvedic management practices

Ayurvedic practitioners identify an individual's constitutional type before initiating management. Medicines are prescribed on the basis of a patient's constitution as well as on the disease or *doshas* imbalance they are suffering from. An Ayurvedic physician is expected to consider everything that might affect the patient's health including their activities, the time of the day, and the season. In other words, patients are viewed as individuals in relation to their environment.

Ayurvedic therapy often begins with *shodhana* (cleansing) in which emotional or physical toxins are eliminated or neutralised. If *shodhana* is neglected, the toxins will penetrate deeper into the tissues. Cleansing can occur on either an emotional or physical level or both. To promote the emotional release of toxins Ayurvedic practitioners recommend dealing with negativity by observing it and then releasing it. For example, when anger appears, the person should be counselled to be completely aware of their anger, watch the feeling as it unfolds, and then let the anger go. Conventional anger management specialists use similar anger management techniques.

The physical release of toxins requires different techniques. For ailments such as excess mucus in the chest and gas in the intestines, the physical release of toxins is achieved through *panchakarma* or five actions: vomiting, purgation, fluid restriction or diuresis, laxatives, medicated enemas, intranasal medicines, and blood-letting. Treatment may be preceded by a massage with medicated oils and with steam treatments to initiate the detoxification process. Cleansing processes eliminate *ama* or undigested food and help maintain the health and proper functioning of the individual.

Once *shodhana* is accomplished, *shamana* or palliative treatment is used to reduce the intensity of a disease. *Shamana* is usually carried out using herbs such as ginger, cinnamon, and black pepper in conjunction with fasting (*ksud nigraha*), fluid restriction (*trut nigraha*), exercise (*vyayama*), breathing exercise (*prananyama*), sunbathing/phototherapy (*atap seva*) and rejuvenation therapy (*rasayana*) to maintain health. In addition, dietary and lifestyle interventions are initiated according to which *doshas* are disturbed and the *prakriti* (physical and mental constitution) of the individual. Spiritual nurturing (*sattyavajaya*) and physical exercise (*vyayama*) are necessary aspects of holistic management.

10.4　Principles of Preparing Ayurvedic Herbal Medicines

Ayurvedic herbs are classified according to five major properties: *rasa* (taste), *guna* (physical properties), *veerya* (potency), *vipaka* (effectiveness), and *prabhava* (efficacy). *Rasa* is divided into six major tastes: *madhu* (sweet), *amla* (sour/acid), *lavana* (salty), *katuka* (pungent), *tiththa* (bitter), and *kashaya* (astringent):

- *Guna* represents the more physical aspects of a medicinal substance.
- *Veerya* represents the active principle or potency of a medicine. Factors such as growth conditions, harvesting technique, and storage affect a herb's *veerya*.

- *Vipaka* is the quality a substance takes on after it has been acted on by the body.
- *Prabhava* refers to the unique effect of a medicine on the body. Ayurvedic practitioners have observed that medicines may have the same *rasa, guna, veerya,* and *vipaka* and yet act differently in the body. The medicine's *prabhava* accounts for the differences.

Single medicines are rarely used in Ayurveda where the balance or action of a formula is valued. Ayurvedic pharmacy assumes that substances are combined in such a way that their natural attributes synergistically enhance the action of the whole formulation. Harnessing these attributes is based on understanding a range of interactions, which are synergy, opposition, enhancement, protection, and balance. In utilising the property of synergy, herbs and mineral products with complementary actions are combined to enhance their effectiveness.

Some substances used in Ayurvedic medicine are toxic in their original form, for example, poisonous herbs (aconite) or metals (lead, mercury, arsenic, antimony). The substance may be detoxified to a safe therapeutic level by a specific purification process (*shodhana*). Sometimes the property of opposition is utilised when a herb or mineral that is too prominent for the use intended is counterbalanced by adding another ingredient with the opposite action or the protective properties of another ingredient are invoked by adding mild laxatives or diuretics that promote elimination.

Enhancement occurs when substances that promote the action of the principal herb by increasing its activity or its absorption are added to a formulation. By using these properties, a state of balance occurs when opposing actions of different portions of a formula are considered to act together. Furthermore, each formula has a preferred vehicle (*anupana*) that promotes efficient absorption and minimises adverse effects. Traditional methods of preparing Ayurvedic medicines are based on the principles of extraction, concentration, and purification. Water is the major vehicle used to deliver the medication but milk, oil, or fermented juice, are also used. Distilled spirits were not used but medicinal wine (*asava-arishta*) is sometimes used. The order in which substances are added during preparation, using specific vessels at different stages of preparation and the duration of time preparations should be stirred, incubated or shaken, are specified. Once extraction is completed, the final product is administered as a liquid, powder, or a pill orally, by inhalation, enema or nasal insertion (*snehana* or *nasna*).

10.5 Maintaining Good Health

Ayurveda emphasises health maintenance as opposed to disease prevention. Establishing a daily routine of good habits (*svasthavartha*) is recommended following the underlying principle of moderation. Health is maintained by avoiding excess but Ayurvedic practitioners recognise that moderation and good habits must be inculcated. Maintenance of health depends on enjoying everything in life at the appropriate moment, in appropriate amounts while rejecting excess in any form. The process of increasing desirable lifestyle and qualities, reducing negative aspects, introducing absent qualities is referred to as *sanskara* (doing well/good).

Sanskara is a ritual of regular repeated activity, which maintains an individual in society. Neglect of such routines is said to risk descent into individual and, if unchecked in society, to cultural chaos.

Mental and spiritual health

The principles of Ayurveda hold that a close relationship exists between mind and body. The concept of desire (*kamaya*) for longevity (*ayusha*), *ayushakamaya* recognises that *ayusha*, though translated as life span, does not indicate length of life alone. The Ayurvedic concept of longevity is a life lived well irrespective of its length. There is no longevity without satisfaction, which is only possible when mind and body are in harmony. The prominence (*adi*) of passion (*raga*) may be detrimental. *Ragadi*, a state of uncontrolled passion, drags the mind away from balance. The balance of *raga* leading either to healthy enjoyment or disease is a matter of degree and there is a fine line between satiation and excess.

The effects of *ragadi* on the mind are *autsukya* (unease), *moha* (confusion, folly, infatuation) or *arati* (discontent). Health cannot exist when the two essential components of a being are in disharmony. Three goals are set in order to achieve harmony: *dharma* (destiny or path), *artha* (resources) and *sukha* (happiness) where mental and spiritual health is intertwined and cannot be separated.

Classical Ayurvedic texts do not include religious practices and blessings, as is the case in the monasteries of Europe where it was not uncommon for texts to be preserved in places of religious worship such as monasteries. Hence Ayurveda is associated with the beliefs and practices of Hinduism or Buddhism in the different parts of the world in which it flourished. It is, therefore, not uncommon for local religious practices of a prayer to be incorporated into Ayurvedic practice. Wearing of a prayer or blessing written on a thin metal scroll encased in a cylinder of gold or silver and worn on a gold chain or bracelet is common in South Asia.

Acupressure (Marma)

Although not prominent in classical texts as a stand-alone Ayurvedic treatment, massage is becoming increasingly popular in Europe and Australasia. 'Marmasthans' are special energy points in the body. The ancient practice of acupressure was probably transported to China where it evolved into acupuncture. It is still widely practised in India and Sri Lanka. The word *chakra* is Sanskrit and means *wheel*. *Prana* or the life force moves through the *Chakras* to produce different states of health or illness. Ayurvedic Indian massage is used as part of a management plan to achieve balance and integrate these forces.

Yoga

Yoga is derived from the Sanskrit word *yug* meaning to join. It is a technique used to control breathing, physical exercise and meditation with the aim of producing mental social, spiritual and physical well-being. Yoga exercises consist of an initial phase where the person concentrates on breathing to relax their bodies and calm their minds. Breathing techniques are followed by a sequence of difficult exercises of progressing complexity. The last phase consists of meditation and concludes with chanting a mantra such as Om shanthi (let there be peace). Transcendental meditation is a popular form of yoga, which focuses on repeating a phrase or mantra.

10.6 Ayurveda and Diabetes

Pathogenesis and clinical features

The ancient word for diabetes is *Madumehaya*, 'madhu' meaning sweet or honey and 'meha' excessive urination. In Ayurvedic understanding, diabetes is one of many urinary disorders (*meha*) that are accompanied by a predisease state or *prameha*. The aetiology, symptoms, pathology, prognosis, and management of diabetes were described in detail in the manuscript *Yogarathnakaraya,*which was translated by the Scottish physician Christie, in 1811 (Muller 1985). Christie obtained a copy of the manuscript from an indigenous diabetes practitioner while he was working in Ceylon in 1805. The manuscript defined *Madumehaya* as the disease in which the patient passes urine characterised as astringent, sweet, and rough. Experts believe the manuscript was based on the *Charaka samhitha* and *Susrutha ayurvedaya*.

The surgeon Susrutha used the term *kshaudrameha* for diabetes and stated that the urine resembles honey (*ksaudra*) and acquires a sweet taste. Another term for *Madumehaya* is *dhatupaka janya vikruti*, which indicates that diabetes was regarded as a disorder of metabolism (*dhatupaka*) associated with a change for the worse (*vikuti*) of inherited (*janya*) characteristics. This definition is not dissimilar to the modern understanding of type 2 diabetes.

Madumehaya is classified as a group of *prameha*. Depending on the main imbalance of the *dosha* involved, the characteristics are further classified as *kaphaja*, *pittaja* and *vataja* from the three *doshas kapha, pitta*, and *vata*. *Madumehaya* is considered to be a *vataja prameha* that is, a result of disordered *vatta* (Muller 1985). The quality of urine is described as excessive (*atyartha*), sweet (*madhura*), cold (*sita*) and tasting like sugar cane juice (*iksu rasa*). In health, urine should be clear (*accha*), abundant but not excessive (*bahu*), and odourless (*nirgandha*).

The aetiology of *Madumehaya* is considered to be multifactorial due to a combination of tendencies inherited at birth and subsequent derangements of *doshas* or directly from abnormalities in the body tissues such as fat (*medas*), muscle (*mansa*), and lymphatics (*vasa*). In particular, the Ayurvedic texts refer to a form of 'evil fat' or *dushtamedha* as being an integral component of the *vataja pramrehas*. This may well be similar to the visceral fat now known to be associated with the impaired glucose metabolism and type 2 diabetes. An imbalance in these tissues was attributed to external and environmental factors such as excessive sleep, excessive appetite especially for sweet food, lack of physical exercise, excessive sexual intercourse, suppressing natural urges, uneven body postures, and other behaviours in addition to the inherent individual *prakirti*. Ayurvedic practitioners describe diabetes as being more prevalent among city dwellers (*nagarikas*) and the affluent (pers. comm. with REALFASL). A common belief is that the affluent urbanites indulge in excesses (*abhisyandi*), which causes diseases in people who have too much of everything (Svoboda 1995).

Vagbhata sought to answer a question that plagues modern public health medicine: why do people who know how to remain healthy permit themselves to become ill? He ascribes their actions to *pragnaaparadha*, a 'crime against wisdom'. In addition to a selfish fixation of the mind on satisfying senses (*tamas*) or actions (*rajas*), Vagbhata recognises that a harmful lifestyle may be forced on an individual by society, the season, and climate. He also distinguishes between environmental influences on health, which can be avoided and those that cannot. The role of poor public health governance is also implicated as cause of disease because 'an evil ruler sickens the nations' workplaces, schools, homes and even the land itself'.

Ayurvedic classification of diabetes

Two types of *vataja pramehas* are described for diabetes. *Sahaja*, which is thought to be due to a defect inherited from a parent. These patients are described as being thin and having more serious disease. The second type, *apathyanimittaja*, is acquired later in life and ascribed to poor lifestyle such as overindulging in food or sweets. These two descriptions reflect the modern classification of type 1 and type 2 diabetes.

Symptoms

Susrutha describe the symptoms of diabetes as a honey or sugar cane-like sweetness of urine (*iksu rasa*), thirst, tiredness, obesity, looseness of limbs, non-relishing of food, burning sensation of the skin, epileptic fits, insomnia, numbness of body, and constipation (Muller 1985). Charaka wrote that chronic *pramehas*, of which *Madumehaya* is one type, gives rise to boils and abscesses, and indicated the sweetness of urine, which attracts flies or ants, was sufficient to make the diagnosis of *Madumehaya* although Christie in 1811 marvelled 'that the Indian physicians had described sweetness in taste long before the time of Willis' (Muller 1985). Willis and Christie's comments refer to the discovery that the urine of people with diabetes tasted sweet by Thomas Willis who is better known for his description of the blood supply of the brain at a much later date.

Principles of Ayurvedic diabetes management

The specific management plan differs according to the type of *madhumeha* present and whether the patient is obese or lean. Management of obese patients with diabetes begins with a cleansing. However, lean people with diabetes are considered too frail to undertake radical cleansing and are prescribed milder cleansing procedures. Both groups are then treated with specific herbal therapy and diet (Lad 1999).

In the words of Charaka:

> This much is evident to us all, namely that we treat a disease-ridden man with disease removing measures, and the depleted man with impletion. We nourish the emaciated and we starve the corpulent and fat. In our hands, administered in this manner, the pharmacopoeia shows itself to the best of its excellence.
>
> (Charaka Sutrasthana, trans. Svoboda 1995)

Cleansing (*shodhana*) therapy commences by applying medicated aromatic oils to the body followed by emetic therapy, which treats excess *kapha*, and then purgation to treat excess *pitta*. Fasting, physical exercise and herbal medicines are used to reduce the excess *doshas* and restore balance among *dhatus*. Dehydration and diuresis clearly pose a hazard in older people, those on diuretics and those with borderline renal dysfunction. Likewise, fasting places those treated with insulin and oral hypoglycaemic agents at risk of hypoglycaemia.

The word 'fasting', however, may not mean a total fast but abstinence from foods deemed unfavourable to the person and particular disease state. An appropriate diet is determined by examining qualities of the food, which can be altered by the preparation method, combinations, the capacity of the eater, and the rules of eating. The quality of food, as in the case of medicines, is described in terms of: *rasa* (taste), *guna* (physical properties), *veerya* (potency), *vipaka* (effectiveness), and *prabhava* (efficacy). The capacity is determined by an individual's ability to digest, which in turn, is determined by their *agni*. The amount of food prescribed is in keeping in what can be safely eaten. The rules of eating include eating in a congenial place and unhurriedly, refraining from eating when one is not hungry, not failing to eat when one is hungry and refraining from food when one is emotionally agitated. The prescribed diet also varies according to age, body constitution, season, and environment, as well as the socio-economic status of the patient.

Exercise is regarded as an important adjunct to the primary diabetes treatment. When exercise is contraindicated or difficult, patients are advised to assume specific yoga positions. Yoga is considered to benefit mind and body with the least physical stress. Various techniques of massage at ayurvedic (*marmasthans*) life force points and yoga are currently used but do not appear to have been described in classical treatises.

Developing the concepts of self-care

Maintaining good health through a daily routine of good habits (*svasthavartha*) is not limited to diabetes. It is offered as a general advice on lifestyle to everybody.

An underlying Ayurvedic principle is that individuals are responsible for their self- care and moderation by resisting temptation. The process of creating good habits (*samskara*) is said to restore and maintain health. Neglect by members of a community will lead both the individual and society into chaos. This, and comments about the duty of rulers to create healthy environments, are not out of place in a current pandemic of lifestyle-related disorders such as obesity and diabetes.

10.7 Research Studies on Ayurvedic Herbal Remedies

No studies recorded in bibiliographic databases appear to have tested Ayurveda as a whole system. However, Ayurvedic herbs have varying degrees of glucose-lowering activity in experimental trials. Some of the plants studied in relation to diabetes are: *Gymnema sylvestre, Momordica charantia, Salacia reticulata,* and *Pterocarpus marsupium,* see Chapters 9 and 11.

- *Salacia reticulata*: *Vairi* or *Pitica* (Indian vernacular), *kotala himbatu* (Sinhala). In animal studies oral administration of an aqueous decoction of *Salacia reticulata* root bark to rats fasted overnight caused 30 per cent reduction in glucose levels (Karunanayake *et al.* 1984). Natural α-glycosidase inhibitors such as kotalanol and salacinol have been isolated from the roots and stems of the plant. These have an action similar to acarbose, which is used to manage type 2 diabetes (Yoshikawa *et al.* 1998). A recent randomised double-blind cross-over trial in humans showed *Salacia reticulata* reduces sulphonylureas doses and HBA1c (Jayawardena *et al.* 2005).
- *Momordica charantia*: *Karela* (Hindi), *Karawila* (Sinhala) and bitter gourd (English). Karunanayake *et al.* (1990) demonstrated the glucose-lowering activity of *M. charantia* in laboratory animals. Welihinda and Karunayake (1986) demonstrated that *M. charantia* stimulated insulin release from beta cells isolated from obese hyperglycemic. Welihinda and Karunayake (1985) also demonstrated blood glucose-lowering activity of *M. charantia* in a clinical study without a control group.
- Animal studies have been performed using extracts of many other plants (Grover 2002). At a conference organised by the Central Council of Research in Ayurveda and Siddha to prioritise research on the most promising Ayurvedic herbs, 190 single plant medicines were identified for further study (Dev 1999). Thus, out of an estimated 250,000 plants, less than 1 per cent have been screened pharmacologically and very few in regard to diabetes (Grover 2002).
- Although not described in detail in the major classical treatises on managing diabetes, yoga involves rhythmic exercise-like movements and meditation that can lead to improved blood glucose contol (Jain 1993; Singh 2004). Yoga has also been shown to reduce vascular risk factors (Bijlani *et al.* 2005) and hypertension in small non-randomised studies (Raub 2003). In the USA, however, CAM use including yoga is associated with more frequent visits to both emergency care and primary care practitioners among people with diabetes (Garrow 2006).

10.8 The evidence base for Ayurvedic medicines

Like most traditional and folk remedies, Ayurvedic methods of treatment have not been subjected to rigorous scientific analysis. Ayurveda, possibly because it originated in religious texts, has been accepted on faith. However, modern medical practice assumes all new treatments have no effect and tries to disprove this hypothesis.

Many human trials that have been undertaken had methodological flaws. These include lack of placebo-controlled double-blind clinical trials, small sample size, inadequate description of the method, inadequate statistical analysis and short duration, all of which reduce the validity and value of many studies. There is a need for better designed studies with an adequate number of subjects to have the power to demonstrate clinical effects. Studies comparing the effects of interventions against placebos that cannot be distinguished from the trial medicine in terms of taste, colour, or smell, have not been documented. In the available studies the methods used to select patients and assign them to study groups are often poorly described and the results do not include statistical analysis. Many studies were not long enough to determine a clinical effect. For example, HbA_{1c}, the most valid intermediate clinical measure of glucose control, requires a study duration of at least three months.

Based on the current data, there is some evidence of glucose-lowering effects in animal studies but no convincing clinical trials providing evidence that Ayurvedic herbal medicnes are effective or satisfy the criteria for safety and efficacy required by agents to be licensed as pharmaceutical products. However, lack of evidence should not be viewed as lack of effectiveness. Criticism of the validity and weight of evidence supporting Ayurveda is often met with a suspicion that they are attempts at 'marginalizing, unorthodox medical claims and findings' (Grover *et al.* 2002) or suppression of a rival form of medicine (pers. comm. with REALFASL).

10.9 Adverse Effects of Ayurveda

Except in a few centres the practice of the classical or *suddha* form of Ayurveda has not been preserved. The physician originally formulated Ayurvedic remedies. Few pharmacies in South Asia manufacture medicines according to traditional principles. Although many Ayurvedic medicines are now manufactured in factories, there is no satisfactory method of evaluating and maintaining uniform standards. A hybrid form of medicine oscillating between extremes of classical Ayurveda and using modern conventional medicines by practitioners not trained in their use or authorised to prescribe is emerging.

In South Asia, this occurs with no apparent enforcement of existing government regulation on prescribing modern medicines. In Sri Lanka aspiration of oily nasal insufflation of nashnayas has been reported to cause aspiration pneumonia in infants and long-term use of herbal remedies has been implicated in renal failure (pers.

comm.). The dangers of unregulated herbal remedies are not confined to South Asia. Wood described a man who attained excellent glycaemic control using herbal medicine obtained in India. On closer examination, samples of blood were found to contain chlorpropamide in a therapeutic concentration and chlorpropamide was also found in one of the medicine balls obtained in India (Wood *et al*. 2004).

There is increasing concern that such cases will have an adverse effect on surveillance programmes in developed countries (Woodward 2005). Hence the concept that Ayurvedic physicians deal in innocuous herbal preparations, herbal oils, massage and acupressure and that their practice has an impact only in rural Asia is not applicable today. There is widespread recognition of the need for regulation (Rousseau and Schachter 2003) and licensing (Ashcroft and Po 1999) of an increasingly popular system of health care.

Unfortunately the nature of Ayurveda and its approach to health may not be compatible with the methods of a randomised controlled trial required to provide evidence of efficacy and safety required for licensing as a medicationl. The Ayurvedic approach uses lifestyle modification, herbal medicines and other treatment modalities in different proportions for the same disease in different people. A situation in which two people with the same disease state could receive two different treatment regimens does not lend itself to evaluation using a randomised clinical trial.

In addition, the classical Ayurvedic methods of preparing herbal medicines are complex and minor variations in the preparation method can make a significant difference in the efficacy and safety of the resultant product. It is worth remembering that many medicines commonly used in modern conventional medicine such as aspirin, antimalarials, and digitalis originated from plant sources. Unlike conventional medicines, whole herbs or whole plant extracts are used in Ayurvedic medicines, rather than isolated active ingredients, which makes standardisation difficult. Many practitioners are reluctant to disclose the method by which a herb is prepared, particularly where the formula is inherited as a secret formula passed down from father to son. This secrecy makes independent verification and replication of results by other researchers difficult.

Lack of funding, research infrastructure and an academic base also hamper the generation of research-based evidence. Further research into alternative systems of medicine such as Ayurveda is needed to help identify safe and effective practice. Ayurveda diagnostic and management techniques follow a well-documented process. The ideal study should, therefore, integrate Ayurvedic diagnosis and assessment methods into their design, but studies should be conducted as randomised double-blind clinical trials with appropriate statistical analysis.

If health professionals are to be in a position to advise the increasing number of people seeking alternative remedies using valid evidence-based advice, such research should receive priority in the allocation of research funding. The availability of such data will facilitate the integration of different medical systems and is a preferable alternative to leaving such integration to market forces and consumer demand as it is at present, see Chapter 4.

References

Ashcroft D, Po A. Herbal remedies: issues in licensing and economic evaluation. *Pharmacoeconomics* 1999; **16**(4): 321–328.

Astin J. Why patients use alternative medicine. *Journal of American Medical Association* 1999; **14**: 1548–1553.

Bijlani R, Vempati R, Yadav R, Ray R, Gupta V, Sharma R, Mehta N, Mahapatra S. A brief but comprehensive lifestyle education program based on yoga reduces risk factors for cardiovascular disease and diabetes mellitus. *Journal of Alternative and Complementary Medicine* 2005; **11**(2): 267–274.

Dev S. Ancient-modern concordance in Ayurvedic plants: some examples. *Environmental Health Perspectives* 1999; **107**(10): 783–789.

Egede LE, Zheng D, Xiaobou Y, Silverstein MD. The prevalence and pattern of complementary and alternative medicine use in individuals with diabetes. *Diabetes Care* 2002; **25**: 324–329.

Eisenberg D, David R, Ettner S. Trends in alternative medicine use in the United States 1990–1997. *Journal of American Medical Association* 1998; **280**: 1569–1575.

Fisher P, Ward A. Complementary medicine in Europe. *British Medical Journal* 1994; **309**: 107–111.

Garrow D, Egede L. Association between complementary and alternative medicine use, preventive care practices, and use of conventional medical services among adults with diabetes. *Diabetes Care* 2006; **29**(1): 15–19.

Grover J, Yadav S, Vats V. Medicinal plants of India with anti-diabetic potential. *Journal of Ethnopharmacology* 2002; **81**(1): 81–100.

Hardy M, Coulter I, Venuturupalli S, Roth E A, Favreau I, Morton S, Shekelle P. *Ayurvedic Interventions for Diabetes Mellitus: A Systematic Review.* Evidence Report/Technology Assessment No. 41 (Prepared by Southern California Evidence-based Practice Center/RAND under Contract No. 290-97-0001). AHRQ Publication No. 01-E040.

Jain S, Uppal A, Bhatnagar S, Talukdar B. A study of response pattern of non-insulin dependent diabetics to yoga therapy. *Diabetes Research in Clinical Practice* 1993; **19**(1): 69–74.

Jayawardena M, de Alwis N, Hettigoda V, Fernando D.A double blind randomized placebo controlled crossover study of a herbal preparation containing Salacia reticulata in the treatment of type 2 diabetes. *Journal Ethnopharmacology* 2005; **97**(2): 215–218.

Karunanayake E, Jeevathayaparan S, Tennekoon K. Effect of *Momordica charantia* fruit juice on streptozotocin-induced diabetes in rats. *Journal of Ethnopharmacology* 1990; **30**(2): 199–204.

Karunanayake E, Welihinda J, Sirimanne S, Sinnadorai G. Oral hypoglycemic activity of some medicinal plants of Sri Lanka. *Journal of Ethnopharmacology* 1984; **11**(2): 223–231.

Lad V. *Ayurveda: The Science of Self-Healing*, 2nd edn. Wilmot, WI: Lotus Press, 1985.

Lad V. An introduction to Ayurveda. *Alternative Therapies in Health and Medicine* 1995; **1**(3): 57–63.

Lad V. Ayurvedic medicine. In: Jonas WB and Levin JS, (eds), *Essentials of Complementary and Alternative Medicine*. New York: Lippincott Williams & Wilkins, 1999, pp. 200–215.

Leese G, Gill G, Houghton G. Prevalence of complementary medicine usage within a diabetes clinic. *Practical Diabetes International* 1997; **14**: 207–208.

Mills S. Regulation in complementary and alternative medicine. *British Medical Journal* 2001; **322**: 158–160.

Muller R. The urinary flux of the ancient Indians (prameha) (with special reference to Carakasamhita). In: Von Engelhardt, D (ed.), *Diabetes its Medical and Cultural History*. Berlin: Springer Verlag, 1985; pp. 160–200.

Porter R. *The Greatest Benefit to Mankind: A Medical History of Humanity.* New York: WW Norton & Co, 1997.

Raub J. Psychophysiologic effects of hath yoga on musculoskeletal and cardiopulmonary function: a literature review. *Journal Alternative and Complementary Medicine* 2003; **8**: 797.

Rousseaux C, Schachter H. Regulatory issues concerning the safety, efficacy and quality of herbal remedies: birth defects. *Res B Dev Reprod Toxicol* 2003; **68**(6): 505–510.

Ryan E, Pick M, Marceau C. Use of alternative medicines in diabetes mellitus. *Diabetic Medicine* 2001; **218**: 242–245.

Singh S, Malhotra V, Singh K, Madhu S, Tandon O. Role of yoga in modifying certain cardiovascular functions in type 2 diabetic patients. *Journal Association Physicians India* 2004; **52**: 203–206.

Svoboda R. Theory and practice of Ayurvedic medicine In: Van Alpen J, Aris A (eds), *Oriental Medicine*. London: Serindia Publications, 1995; p. 67–97.

Welihinda J, Arvidson G, Gylfe E, Hellman B, Karlsson E. The insulin-releasing activity of the tropical plant *Momordica charantia*. *Acta Biologica et Medica Germanica* 1982; **41**(12): 1229–1240

Welihinda J, Jarunanayake EH, Sherriff MH, Jayasinghe KS. Effect of *mormordica charantia* on the glucose tolerance in maturity onset diabetes *Journal of Ethnopharmacology* 1985; **13**: 227–228.

Welihinda J, Karunanayake EH. Extra-pancreatic effects of *Momordica charantia* in rats. *Journal of Ethnopharmacology* 1986; **17**(3): 247–255.

Wood DM, Athwal S, Panahloo A. The advantages and disadvantages of a 'herbal' medicine in a patient with diabetes mellitus: a case report. *Diabet Med.* 2004; **21**(6): 625–627.

Woodward KN. The potential impact of the use of homeopathic and herbal remedies on monitoring the safety of prescription products. *Hum Exp Toxicol.* 2005; **24**(5): 219–233.

Wujastyk D. Medicine in India. In: Van Alpen J, Aris A (eds), *Oriental Medicine* London: Serindia Publications, 1995, pp. 19–37.

Yoshikawa M, Murakami T, Yashiro K, Matsuda H. Kotalanol, a potent alpha-glucosidase inhibitor with thiosugar sulfonium sulfate structure, from antidiabetic Ayurvedic medicine *Salacia reticulata*. *Chemical and Pharmaceutical Bulletin (Tokyo)* 1998; **46**(8): 1339–1340.

11 Chinese Medicine Treatment of Diabetes

Kylie A. O'Brien and Charlie Changli Xue

11.1 Introduction

Diabetes has long been treated with Chinese medicine as the clinical entity '*xiao ke*', which translates as 'thirsting and wasting disorder'. The two major modalities used in Chinese medicine are herbal medicines and acupuncture. The way Chinese medicine practitioners manage diseases such as diabetes is very different from the way practitioners in other systems of medicine operate. Understanding Chinese medicine requires knowledge of the underlying philosophy, the features of the medicine, and the key theories that guide practice.

This chapter provides an overview of the Chinese medicine management of diabetes. It begins with a description of some of the key features of Chinese medicine, the key theories that guide clinical practice and the diagnostic methods used, and gives a general description of the two main treatment modalities: Chinese herbal medicine and acupuncture. The remainder of the chapter describes how diabetes is understood in Chinese medicine and how it is managed with Chinese herbal medicine and acupuncture and discusses the scientific evidence for these modalities.

11.2 What Is Chinese Medicine?

Chinese medicine is a unique medical system with a history that dates back over four thousand years (Cai *et al.* 1995). The theoretical system began to form during the second half of the fifth century BC (Cai *et al.* 1995). The main modalities of Chinese medicine are Chinese herbal medicine and acupuncture. Others include:

- Chinese massage (*tuina*);
- cupping (the application of glass cups to areas of the body);
- exercise therapy such as *tai qi* and *qi gong*;
- diet therapy;
- moxibustion.

Complementary Therapies and the Management of Diabetes and Vascular Disease   Editor Trish Dunning
© 2006 John Wiley & Sons, Ltd.

In China, Chinese medicine is well integrated with conventional medicine. In fact, the World Health Organization (WHO) cited China as the only country with a truly integrated system in its *Traditional Medicine Strategy* (WHO 2002). Like conventional medicine, Chinese medical practitioners specialise in specific areas including:

- internal medicine
- acupuncture and moxibustion
- surgery
- orthopaedics
- gynaecology and obstetrics
- paediatrics
- ophthalmology
- gastroenterology.

Chinese medicine consists of diverse practices and schools of thought. Nowadays, biomedical knowledge is integrated with Chinese medicine knowledge. Nevertheless, key philosophies and theories unique to Chinese medicine underpin and guide Chinese medical practice.

Unique features of Chinese medicine

Chinese medicine is a sophisticated medical system that describes the body in an essentially energetic model. Central to the model is the existence of a concept called *Qi*, which is comprehensively described in Zhang and Rose's text *A Brief History of Qi* (2001). *Qi* is a complex concept. At a basic level, *qi* can be envisaged as a subtle and rarefied form of energy, which is responsible for human life and forms the material basis of the body and determines its physiological functioning (Cai *et al*. 1995.

Qi flows through the body in a system of channels or 'meridians'. There are several types of *qi* within the body, for example, *wei* or defensive *qi* that protects the body from invasion by outside pathogens and *ying* and nutrient *qi* that promotes growth and development and supports organ and tissue functions. In addition, each organ has its own *qi*, for example *Lung qi* and *Heart qi*. *Qi* is manipulated during acupuncture treatment. Historically, the concept of *qi* did not solely belong to medicine: it permeated the arts, literature and many other areas of life that were subsumed into Chinese medicine (Zhang and Rose 2001).

A philosophy of holism, which recognises the interdependence of humans and nature, underpins Chinese medicine (Cai *et al*. 1995). Extending from the holistic philosophy is the concept that the body functions as an organic whole. Although all the organ systems and tissues have their own unique functions within the body, they exist in an interdependent relationship with each other. The connections between organs, tissues and body parts occur through a system of meridians (Cheng *et al*. 1999). Briefly, meridians are pathways throughout the body through which the vital substance called 'qi' circulates. As a result, illness in a particular organ system can affect other systems. Therefore, Chinese medicine practitioners take into account the primary organ/s involved as well as the other organs that might be affected because of their interdependent relationships. Another dimension of the holistic philosophy is the belief that the mind and body are not separate and emotions can impact on the body and vice versa.

The concept of balance is fundamental to many complementary and alternative medicine systems and is central to Chinese medicine. Health and illness are understood and couched in very different terms from conventional medicine. Chinese medicine conceptualises health (balance) and illness (imbalance) as being fundamentally related to two opposing yet complementary forces, Yin and Yang. Changes due to illness are further described as functional and material changes in vital substances of the body and functional disturbances of the meridians and the internal or *zang-fu* organ systems. The concept of an '*organ*' in Chinese medicine is conceptually broader than in conventional medicine. In Chinese medicine, organs represent functional systems. For example, *zang-fu* organs are understood to exist in interdependent relationships with other *zang-fu* organs and their functions are described in terms of vital substances such as '*qi*' and '*blood*'.

Another unique feature of Chinese medicine is the subcategorisation of diseases, disorders or symptoms into diagnostic subcategories referred to as Chinese medicine (CM) syndromes. A CM syndrome is essentially an *underlying pattern of disharmony* within the body that reflects a summary of the pathology of the disorder at a particular point in time and is understood according to Chinese medicine theory. A CM syndrome is characterised by particular signs and symptoms that reflect the underlying pathogenesis, location, aetiology and nature of the disease as well as the relationship between the body's defence system and the pathogen (Cai *et al.* 1995). A person may present with more than one syndrome, and syndromes may change over time as the condition deteriorates or improves. Chinese medicine management focuses on the disease/disorder and is specific for the underlying CM syndrome.

Herbal medicine and acupuncture treatment of a particular CM syndrome are quite different from another CM syndrome in terms of the herbs or acupuncture points chosen. Treatment with acupuncture or Chinese herbal medicine is individualised, taking into account factors such as age, constitution, the season at the time, and for women the stage of menstrual cycle. Typically, a disease or disorder may have three to six CM syndromes. The prescription and herbs used are continually adjusted according to the individual's symptoms.

Chinese medicine also focuses on preventing illness. Chinese medicine diagnosis provides a means by which subtle energetic changes within the body that could lead to internal imbalances can be detected and preventative strategies instituted. Chinese herbal medicine, acupuncture, exercise therapy, Chinese massage and diet therapy are utilised as preventive strategies as well as to treat imbalances.

Finally, Chinese medicine is underpinned by unique and quite complex theories that describe the physiological functioning of the body and pathogenesis of illness. These theories and concepts are described in terminology heavily borrowed from everyday language. However, in modern practice, Chinese medicine does not operate in isolation from conventional medicine and biomedical knowledge is integrated with Chinese medicine knowledge although it has its own understanding of the aetiology of illness.

11.3   Key Theories that Guide Chinese Medicine Practice

Five key theories guide Chinese medicine practice:

1. Yin Yang theory
2. Five Phase theory
3. Zang-Fu theory
4. Meridian theory
5. Qi, Blood and Body Fluids.

Aetiology

In Chinese medicine, the body's ability to fight disease is believed to depend on the strength of the *antipathogenic qi*. Antipathogenic *qi* is a concept that includes the individual's ability to resist disease and the functional activities of their body (Cai *et al.* 1995). Antipathogenic *qi* encompasses the defence system, including the immune system, the skin as a barrier, and maintaining a positive mental and emotional state.

Pathogenic factors or causative agents of illness can be external climatic factors including wind, cold, dampness, fire, dryness, and summer heat. These climatic factors correspond to normal seasonal changes, however, they can become pathogenic if they occur abruptly, out of season, or with excessive force when the body is weak in relation to the external factor and fails to adapt (Cai *et al.* 1995). The characteristics of the climatic factor are used to describe the clinical manifestations it causes. For example, dampness has the characteristics of stickiness and turbidity. Examples of dampness within the body include nasal and vaginal discharges.

In addition to external factors that cause illness, there are internal causative factors that include malfunctioning of the *zang-fu* organs. Excessive or prolonged emotions are capable of disturbing the functions of the *zang-fu* organs and are also considered to be internal causes of illness. Other causes of illness include trauma, insufficient or excessive exercise and inadequate or inappropriate diet. Inappropriate diet is considered to be a very important causative agent in illness and diet therapy is a central management strategy in Chinese medicine.

Vital substances of the body

According to Chinese medicine theory, several vital substances make up the material body including *qi* and blood. In Chinese medicine, the term 'blood' is conceptually broader than in conventional medicine. In Chinese medicine, blood is one of the carriers of *qi* and has a 'nourishing' function. It nourishes the *zang-fu* organs, muscles, hair and skin (Cai *et al.* 1995).

Yin Yang theory

Yin Yang is the most important theory that guides Chinese medicine concepts of the aetiology, pathogenesis, diagnosis of imbalance and how treatment principles are applied to deciding whether to prescribe acupuncture or Chinese herbal medicine. The Yin Yang theory emerged during the Yin and Zhou Dynasties prior to 221 BC (O'Brien and Xue 2003a). The theory most likely originated from peasants observing the cycle of day and night as they watched the changing shadows and light across the mountains as the sun moved across the sky (Maciocia 2005). They designated the sunny side of the mountain Yang, and the shady side, Yin. As the sun moved, the light and warmth shifted to the opposite side of the mountain and Yang became Yin and vice versa. The essential tenet of Yin Yang theory developed from these observations and describes Yin and Yang as complementary but opposite states of the same cycle. Yang corresponded to light, sun, brightness and activity and Yin corresponded to dark, moon, shade and rest (Maciocia 2005). Further relationships subsequently developed and the theory began to be applied in medicine.

The complementary aspects of Yin Yang were later applied to body parts, constitutional patterns, physiological processes and clinical signs and symptoms in order to guide diagnosis of health or ill health. For example, a weak voice, pale skin and cold limbs are all Yin signs, whereas a strong voice, red complexion and warm limbs are all Yang signs. Acute disorders with rapid onset and changes are in general considered Yang, whereas chronic illnesses such as diabetes are considered Yin. In a healthy body, Yin and Yang are in a state of dynamic balance. If either Yin or Yang is excessive or deficient in relation to the other, internal disharmony and eventually ill health can occur.

Pathogenesis can also be described in terms of Yin and Yang, for example, the kidney Yin might be deficient. Typical symptoms and signs of kidney Yin deficiency can include dry skin, low back pain, a sensation of heat in the palms and soles of the feet, scanty and dark urine, thirst, a radial pulse that feels thread-like, weak and rapid on palpation, night sweating and a tongue that is redder than average with little tongue fur or coating. Treatment is designed to restore the balance of Yin and Yang.

Five Phase theory

Five Phase theory developed through observations of elements in nature, particularly fire, earth, water, wood and metal. These elements were seen as symbolising the behaviour of phenomena in nature and the phases of life. The characteristics of the elements in nature were used analogically to describe phenomena within the body. For example, the nature of fire is to flare upwards, therefore, fire became the symbol of anything associated with heat and a flaring action (Cai *et al.* 1995). A series of correspondences among colours, sounds, climate, tastes, body organs, related sense organs and emotions were compiled. For example, the liver was associated with the element wood, its related sense organ is the eye, and it is related to the season of spring, the colour green, the emotion of anger and a sour taste. A headache of sudden onset associated with red eyes might be seen as being caused by liver fire blazing upwards because a branch of the liver meridian goes to the eyes and head.

Thus, a model was developed on the basis of the interrelationships between the five elements and applied in medicine to explain the normal physiological functioning of the body and the pathological changes that occur in disease. Each element and its related organ exist within interdependent relationships with other elements/organs according to particular rules set out in Five Phase theory. The relationship between the five elements implies that when there is pathology in one organ system, other organ systems are involved or could become involved. Therefore, treatment may be directed at the primary *zang-fu* organ system involved as well as other organs that could already be affected or could become involved.

Zang-fu theory

Zang-fu theory is the main theory of the interdependent relationships among the internal organ systems, which are collectively known as *zang-fu organs*, through observing their external manifestations (Cai *et al.* 1995). The concept of 'organ' described in Zang-fu theory is different from that understood by conventional practitioners, although conventional understanding is largely incorporated into Chinese medicine. For example one of the main functions of the liver *zang-fu* organ is to ensure *qi* flows smoothly around the body and to 'harmonise' the emotions. It is also responsible for regulating the circulating blood volume and, in women, regulating the menstrual cycle. The *zang* organs are solid and include the heart, liver, lung, kidney, spleen and the pericardium. The *fu* organs are 'hollow' and primarily involve the digestive and urinary systems.

Each *zang* organ has a paired *fu* organ and a related sense organ connected by the meridian system. For example, the paired *fu* organ of the kidney is the bladder, the related sense organs are the ears, and the condition of the kidney is reflected in the head hair. Thus, Zang-fu theory describes the relationship between particular *zang-fu* organs and how particular illness patterns of disharmony involving pairs of organs or several organs occur. Underlying patterns of disharmony or Chinese medicine syndromes of a disease or condition are typically described according to Zang-fu theory.

Meridian theory

The meridian system consists of pathways in which *qi* and blood circulate. The meridian system connects the *zang* and *fu* organs, body tissues, sense organs and every part of the body (Cai *et al.* 1995). There are 14 major body meridians. Each meridian follows a particular path along the body surface and internal branches connect with the associated *zang-fu* organ, its paired *zang* or *fu* organ and related sense organ. Specific points called 'acupoints' or 'acupuncture points' occur along each meridian and are believed to be points where the *qi* is particularly concentrated.

Each acupoint has a particular Chinese name, however, a system of numbering the points has been developed and helps Westerners understand the system. Each acupoint is named according to the meridian it is associated with and its numerical sequence on the meridian. For example, the acupoint 'tai xi' is also known as 'kidney 3' because it is the third acupoint on the kidney meridian.

Each acupoint has a number of specific functions as well as general functions related to the meridian itself. For example, the acupoint *Neiguan* (pericardium 6) is used to treat nausea, but may, like other points on the meridian, be used to treat pain on the medial side of the arm (Deadman *et al.* 1998).

Meridian theory can be used to assist in diagnosing disorders. For example, palpating a tender point or a change in the appearance of the skin along a particular meridian can provide clues about which meridian or zang-fu organ is involved. Treatment with acupuncture involves stimulating particular acupuncture points according to a prescription tailored to the individual to address the CM syndrome and other individual factors.

Eight Guiding Principles

The Eight Guiding Principles summarise the basic characteristics of the underlying CM syndrome/s and are usually used in conjunction with Zang-fu theory in order to arrive at a specific Chinese medicine syndrome diagnosis. The Eight Guiding Principles classify Chinese medicine syndromes on the basis of four pairs of opposing principles. The principles describe the location of the disorder, either as interior or exterior, the nature of disorder as being cold or hot, and one of 'excess' or 'deficiency':

- An *'excess syndrome'* is one in which the pathogen is strong and the antipathogenic *qi* is also strong. These are usually acute disorders.
- A *'deficiency syndrome'* is one in which the antipathogenic *qi* is weakened and describes chronic conditions such as diabetes.
- An *'exterior syndrome'* is one in which a battle between the exterior pathogen and the antipathogenic *qi* is waged on a superficial or exterior level, for example a common cold.
- An *'interior syndrome'* is one in which the pathogenic factor is located within the body. Usually the zang-fu organs are involved.
- A *'heat syndrome'* is characterised by signs or symptoms of heat such as fever, redness, swelling, or a red complexion.
- A *'cold syndrome'* is characterised by cold symptoms or signs, for example, cold extremities.

Yin and Yang are overarching summary principles. Cold, deficiency and interior syndromes are Yin syndromes, and heat, excess and exterior syndromes are Yang syndromes.

11.4 Diagnostic Methods

Chinese medicine practitioners use four main diagnostic methods that engage their senses and yield diagnostic information. These are: inquiry, inspection, auscultation/olfaction and palpation, and are similar to the assessment practices of conventional practitioners. However, they are applied differently.

Inquiry

Inquiry involves taking a detailed history from the individual, including the primary complaint, as well as bodily functioning. Some of the information the Chinese practitioner probes for may seem unusual to conventional practitioners, however, it is logical within the Chinese medicine system. For example, questions may be asked about the character of the stools or urine, preference for particular flavours of foods, presence of a particular taste in the mouth, occurrence of sweating during the day or at night, that give the Chinese medicine practitioner clues to the nature of the underlying condition, as understood according to Chinese medicine theory. To give a specific example, stools that are sticky in consistency and difficult to evacuate indicate 'internal dampness' whereas loose stools or diarrhoea indicate malfunctioning of the 'spleen' *zang-fu* organ. Another example is the presence of night sweats that indicate 'Yin deficiency' whereas sweating during the day with very little exertion indicates 'qi deficiency'.

Inspection

Inspection involves visually observing the patient including their complexion and the condition of their skin, physical stature, movement, the head hair, and particularly observing the tongue, which is referred to as 'tongue diagnosis'. Tongue diagnosis is one of the more peculiar diagnostic techniques of Chinese medicine and involves observing characteristics of the tongue and the character of any coating on the tongue.

Auscultation and olfaction

Auscultation and olfaction involve using the senses of hearing and smell to gather diagnostic information. For example, a weak cough is typical of a deficiency condition whereas a strong barking cough is typical of an excess condition.

Palpation

Palpation includes palpating body parts of the body as necessary and pulse diagnosis, which involves palpating the radial arterial pulse at both wrists and is different from taking the pulse in conventional medicine. Within Chinese medicine, the location and nature of the disorder and in particular the condition of the zang-fu organs can be ascertained by palpating the radial pulse at three adjacent positions of each wrist beginning at the styloid process. Chinese medicine generally describes

28 different pulses, one of which is normal, and the others indicate pathology. Each pulse has particular characteristics that are diagnostically significant.

Formulating a diagnosis and treatment principles

After the practitioner gathers the relevant diagnostic data, they analyse it according to the Chinese medicine theories described in the preceding sections, in particular Zang-fu theory and the Eight Guiding Principles. Other theories are used simultaneously including the Yin Yang and Five Phase Theories. The *pattern* of signs and symptoms that emerges, not just individual signs and symptoms, help the practitioner formulate a diagnosis and identify the underlying pattern of disharmony and the particular CM syndrome present. In many cases, diagnosis includes a conventional diagnosis, particularly in modern Chinese medical practice and reflects the integration of the two systems.

The CM syndrome includes the name of the *zang-fu* organ involved and a descriptor of the disharmony that occurs. For example, a syndrome of 'kidney Yin deficiency' identifies the kidney organ as the primary organ involved and a deficiency of the Yin aspect as the principal pathological process. In clinical practice, more than one CM syndrome can be present, and syndromes often change over time as the condition improves or deteriorates.

Treatment principles derive directly from the diagnosis. For example, when the CM syndrome kidney Yin deficiency is diagnosed, the practitioner aims to tone the kidney Yin. Chinese medicine aims to treat both the root cause of the disorder, the *ben* and the secondary manifestations or branches, the *biao*. The manner in which the treatment is delivered and the particular treatment is used depends on the underlying disease processes and imbalance. For example, in an acute disease it may be more important to deal with the *biao* first, then the *ben* when the acute situation resolves. For example, a new diagnosis of diabetes presenting in ketoacidosis (*biao*) requires fluid and insulin replacement initially and then education and an ongoing management plan (*ben*).

11.5 Chinese Herbal Medicine

The term 'Chinese herb' includes substances of plant, mineral and animal origin. Examples of mineral herbs include abalone shell, pearl and haematite. Examples of animal herbs include cicada moulting, flying squirrel faeces and earthworms. Countries such as Australia are signatory to the Convention for the International Treatise on Endangered Species (CITES) that prohibits the use of exotic and endangered animal products such as tiger bone. In addition, the Modernised Chinese Medicine International Association (MCMIA) aims to establish standardised preparations of Chinese herbal medicines by using modern biochemical techniques such as high performance gas and liquid chromatography and gene chips. Standardisation is important to make it possible to assess the efficacy and potential toxicity of herbs, identify likely herb – herb and herb – medicine interactions and enable more optimal outcome monitoring.

Each Chinese herb is described in terms of its taste and temperature characteristic. For example, herbs may be cool, cold, warm, hot or neutral in their temperature characteristic. The taste characteristics of herbs are bitter, sour, sweet, bland, spicy or salty. The taste and temperature characteristics partly determine the therapeutic functions of the herb. For example, salty taste is associated with or has an affinity with the kidney zang-fu organ, therefore, salty tasting herbs are prescribed to target the kidney. Sweet herbs are nourishing and harmonising and are often used to tonify *qi* or blood or restore yin or yang balance. Cool or cold herbs are used to treat hot conditions, whereas warm or hot herbs are used to treat cold CM syndromes.

In addition, herbs have a particular directional tendency. For example, many of the lighter flower herbs have an upward moving tendency and are used to treat conditions of the head. The therapeutic function is also partly a function of the ability of the herb to 'enter' certain meridians and target specific zang-fu organs. Herbs are categorised primarily according to their main therapeutic function according to Chinese medicine theory. Most herbs have three or four different functions. Examples of categories of herbs include those that: cool blood; tonify *qi*; tonify yin; invigorate blood; and drain dampness.

The pharmacological actions of Chinese herbs have been well researched. Different categories of Chinese herbs often have similar properties to conventional medicines. Many of the herbs in the Chinese medicine category 'Herbs that Drain Dampness' have similar actions to conventional diuretic medicines (Bensky and Gamble 1993). Likewise, herbs in the category 'Herbs that Clear Heat and Relieve Toxicity' have anti-inflammatory and antipyretic properties; others have anti-cancer properties (Bensky and Gamble 1993).

Unlike other herbal medicine traditions, herbs in Chinese medicine are rarely prescribed singly. A typical Chinese medicinal formula or prescription consists of between two and 12 different herbs and is formulated to address the disease or disorder and its underlying Chinese medicine syndrome. As a result of combining herbs into medicinal formulae, multiple signs and symptoms can be treated simultaneously. Often, when raw herbs or herbal extracts are used, the prescription can be tailored to the individual to treat secondary complaints and take into account individual factors including age and constitution. Other forms of Chinese herbal medicines include proprietary formulations such as pills and tablets that have fixed doses of particular herbs.

A medicinal formula is structured according to particular 'guidelines'. These guidelines include avoiding particular combinations of herbs that could cause adverse events and also refers to the manner in which medicinal formulas are structured in order to elicit a therapeutic action. The components of a medicinal formula are described according to the court hierarchy that existed in Imperial China and as such is likely to reflect Confucianism (Zhang and Rose 1995). In general, the main therapeutic action is provided by the Chief herb/s, usually one or two herbs. The Minister or Deputy herbs support the main therapeutic action of the Chief herb/s. The Assistant or Adjutant herbs treat secondary signs and symptoms and assist the Chief and Deputy herbs. The Guide or Envoy herbs, usually one or two herbs, guide the other herbs into a particular area of the body or meridian and harmonise the herbs in the formula to minimise any potential adverse effects that could occur when herbs are combined (Bensky and Gamble 1993). Herbal prescribing for diabetes is described later in the chapter.

Not all Chinese herbs are safe and adverse reactions can occur, including skin reactions, gastrointestinal symptoms, increased blood pressure, hypokalaemia and renal and hepatic toxicity (De Smet 2002; Pittler and Ernst 2003). A number of herbs are toxic and care must be taken to use the herbs correctly or in some cases, avoid them completely. The toxicity of herbs ranges from mild to moderate to strong. The cautions and contraindications of individual herbs are set out in standard *Materia Medica*. Categories of herbs have general cautions or contraindications for particular Chinese medicine syndromes. For example, if a patient has an excess heat syndrome, herbs from the category of 'Warm the Interior' should not be used because they are warm or hot in terms of their temperature characteristic. Herbs that are draining in nature or those that 'invigorate blood' are contraindicated in pregnant women, as are herbs known to be toxic in pregnancy. In general, herbs that have harsh properties or toxic herbs must be used with caution, particularly in weak patients.

Certain herbs are processed in order to minimise their toxicity or alter their therapeutic function. For example, frying a herb in wine can improve its ability to 'invigorate blood' and remove 'blood stagnation', which is perceived to be part of the pathogenesis of many different diseases and disorders including angina, various pain syndromes, tumours, dysmenorrhoea and stroke, to name but a few. Frying a herb with salt, the flavour associated with the kidney zang-fu organ according to Five Phase theory enhances the ability of the herb to target the action of the herb on the kidney.

Quality and safety of herbal medicines in both the raw state and in proprietary forms remain an important issue. Attention has been drawn to the problem of adulteration of Chinese herbal medicines with Western pharmaceutical substances such as corticosteroids and dexamethasone, substitution with other herbs, and contamination with pesticides and heavy metals (Ernst 1998, 2002, 2004; D'Arcy 1999). Huang *et al.* (1997) found 24 per cent of 2,609 samples of Chinese proprietary medicines collected in Taiwan were contaminated with at least one adulterant. Ko (1998) found 32 per cent of 260 Chinese herbal products from herbal stores in California contained heavy metals or undeclared pharmaceuticals.

There is evidence that a number of Chinese herbs might interact with conventional medicines, therefore care needs to be taken (Braun 2000; Chan and Cheung 2000; De Smet 2002; Izzo 2004). The Chinese herb Dan Shen (*Radix salviae miltiorrhizae*) adversely interacts with warfarin and prolongs prothrombin time and partial thromboplastin time (Chan and Cheung 2000). However, there is a lack of specific evidence about interactions between the majority of Chinese herbs and conventional medicines.

11.6 Acupuncture and Moxibustion

Acupuncture is the therapeutic use of fine needles to stimulate particular points on the surface of the skin, called acupuncture points or acupoints, in order to elicit a therapeutic effect (O'Brien and Xue 2003b). Usually the needle penetrates the skin although the needle does not necessarily penetrate the skin in some acupuncture systems such as the Japanese Toyohari system. In addition, laser acupoint stimulation is a modern invention in which a laser is used to stimulate the acupoints. Acupuncture is practised according to diverse schools of thought. Acupuncture can be used to treat many disorders including musculoskeletal pain, rheumatoid conditions, gastrointestinal conditions, gynaecological disorders, and cardiovascular conditions. Acupuncture is increasingly being subjected to clinical trials to establish efficacy as well as clarify the mechanism of action.

As mentioned previously, each acupuncture point has a number of specific functions. The choice of acupuncture points depends on the condition and underlying syndrome involved. As a rule, the choice of acupuncture points is guided by Chinese medicine theory. Acupoints can be distal, local or adjacent to a particular region of the body being treated. Distal acupoints are generally below the knees or elbows and are often used to treat conditions on the trunk or head. The needling technique determines the therapeutic action. Many different techniques are used to manipulate the acupuncture needle and different techniques elicit different effects on the body.

There are different types of acupuncture, for example, scalp acupuncture, which is particularly used to treat neurological conditions. Ear acupuncture involves stimulating points on the ear with either small seeds, magnets or directly with an acupuncture needle. The ear reflects a 'map' of the body in the shape of an inverted foetus. The ear map is a similar concept to the body maps on the hands and feet used in reflexology, see Chapter 13. Electroacupuncture involves electrically stimulating acupoints.

Moxibustion is a technique of applying heat to the body in the form of a smouldering herb or mixture of herbs called moxa or moxa wool. Most commonly, the moxa wool in stick form is held above the surface of the body and ignited so that it smoulders to warm particular areas or acupoints. Alternatively, the moxa is placed on the end of the acupuncture needle and left to smoulder. Care is taken to protect the skin from any ash that falls by placing a simple protective guard over the skin surrounding the needle. Moxa is often used to treat 'cold' conditions in order to warm the meridians and improve the circulation of *qi* and blood.

11.7 How is Diabetes Understood in Chinese Medicine?

Diabetes was recognised in ancient China as the condition '*xiao ke*', '*xiao ke zheng*' or '*xiao dan zheng*', which in Chinese means 'thirsting and wasting disorder' (Li *et al.* 2004). Several of the main symptoms and signs of diabetes such as polydipsia, polyuria and polyphagia, as well as other related symptoms and signs also fall under other Chinese medicine clinical entities including the following:

- *duo shi* (profuse eating);
- *duo yin* (profuse eating);
- *duo niao* (profuse urination);
- *fei pang* (obesity);
- *qing mang* (clear-eyed blindness);
- *chuang yang* (sores);
- *yang mei* (impotence);
- *ma mu* (numbeness and tingling) (Flaws and Sionneau 2001).

Aetiology and pathogenesis

In Chinese medicine, the main pathogenesis of diabetes is considered to be the consumption or deficiency of *Yin fluid* and generation of endogenous dryness heat (Li *et al.* 2004). In the early stages of diabetes Yin deficiency predominates. With time, both Yin deficiency and dry heat coexist. In the later stages Yin deficiency again predominates (Li *et al.* 2004).

The aetiology of diabetes includes incorrect diet, particularly excess consumption of greasy foods and alcohol that may damage the digestive system and create internal heat. Other factors include congenital weakness of the five *zang* organs, particularly the kidney, excessive emotional strain that can cause the liver *qi* to become stagnant and create internal heat, and excessive sexual activities that can impair the kidney *zang* organ (Xie and Liao 1993; Chen 1994). Dietary and other factors play important roles in the development of type 2 diabetes, although an underlying weakness of the zang-fu organs, particularly the kidney may also be present (Chen 1998).

In Chinese medicine, the body is divided into three main areas: the 'triple jiao' or 'san jiao'.

1. the 'upper jiao', which contains the heart and lung zang organs;
2. the 'middle jiao', which contains the spleen and stomach, which are both involved in digestion in Chinese medicine;
3. the 'lower jiao', which contains the liver and kidney *zang* organs.

If the Yin deficiency is predominantly associated with upper jiao, lung dryness and lung Yin deficiency can occur (Xie and Liao 1993; Chen 1994). A key symptom in this case is polydipsia. In Chinese medicine the lung is involved in water distribution around the body. If the middle jiao is involved, 'stomach heat' or 'stomach fire' is usually present (Xie and Liao 1993; Chen 1994). Polyphagia is the major symptom of 'stomach Yin' deficiency. When the lower jiao is involved, 'kidney Yin deficiency' may occur resulting in the major sign, polyuria (Xie and Liao 1993; Chen 1994). In many cases all three 'jiaos' are involved, as is often the case with diabetes.

Due to the interdependent relationships among the body organ systems, more than one organ system is often affected simultaneously. The spleen *zang* organ, whose function is to convert nutrients into *qi* that circulates around the body as a function of digestion, is often involved. That is, the *Spleen qi* is deficient

(Flaws and Sionneau 2001). Complex clinical syndromes can arise, for example where kidney Yin deficiency can lead to kidney Yang deficiency. Impaired blood circulation, referred to as 'blood stagnation' occurs as a complication of most diabetes CM syndromes (Flaws and Sionneau 2001).

Diabetes and Chinese medicine syndromes

Many different Chinese medicine (CM) syndromes can be associated with diabetes. The main ones are:

- 'lung Yin deficiency';
- 'excess stomach heat';
- 'stomach Yin deficiency';
- 'kidney Yin deficiency'.

However, other zang-fu organs can be involved in pathogenesis including the heart, liver and spleen. For example, if the liver *qi* does not flow as it should, the CM syndrome, 'liver Qi Stagnation', can develop. A deficiency of the heart *qi* may lead to disturbance in blood circulation and heart function resulting in the CM syndrome 'Heart Blood Obstruction' (Chen 1994). This may manifest with the symptom of chest pain and, in Western biomedical terms, the condition of angina. In severe cases, it manifests as a heart attack.

Management principles

Management principles are applied according to the CM syndrome/s present. As a general principle Yin is nourished or 'tonified' and internal heat is cleared. Blood stagnation generally complicates most diabetes CM syndromes, therefore, management is directed towards improving blood circulation, which might include using herbs that have circulation-improving actions.

As discussed previously, in keeping with holistic philosophy underpinning Chinese medicine, practitioners aim to treat the whole person by addressing the root cause and the secondary manifestations of any diseases/disorders present. Diet therapy forms an important part of treatment including recommending the patient avoid particular types of foods that can cause internal heat and damage the *Yin fluids* of the body such as hot and spicy foods and alcohol. In contrast, other foods generally tonify the Yin particularly the kidney, stomach and lung Yin and may be included in the diet as a therapeutic measure.

11.8   Chinese Herbal Medicine in the Treatment of Diabetes

Managing diabetes with Chinese herbal medicine aims to correct the underlying pattern of disharmony or CM syndrome. Specific combinations of herbs are chosen according to Chinese medicine theory, that is, according to the underlying Chinese medicine syndrome or pattern of disharmony present, and knowledge of the pharmacological actions of the herbs. Yin deficiency is predominant in diabetes, thus herbs that tonify or nourish Yin are typically recommended. These herbs differ in their ability to target specific organs, for example, certain herbs tonify lung and stomach Yin while others tonify liver and kidney Yin.

Commonly used herbs include: Radix Ginseng (Chinese *ren shen*, classified as a 'Qi tonifying herb'), Poria (Chinese *fuling*, a herb that tonifies the spleen *qi*), *Radix Rehmanniae* (Chinese *sheng di huang*, a herb that particularly tonifies kidney Yin), *Radix rehmanniae praeparata* (Chinese *shu di huang*, a herb that 'nourishes blood') *Rhizoma coptidis* (Chinese *huang lian*, a herb that clears stomach heat and 'tonifies stomach Yin'), *Radix salviae miltiorrhizae* (Chinese *dan shen*, classified as a 'blood invigorating herb') and *Panax notoginseng* (Chinese *san qi*, a herb that promotes blood circulation) (Li *et al.* 1994).

Many commonly used Chinese herbs have proven glucose-lowering activity in animals and humans (Li *et al.* 2004; Liu *et al.* 2002) and there is a great deal of information about the pharmacology and mechanism of action of Chinese herbs. From a conventional perspective these include:

- regulating glucose metabolism by a number of mechanisms such as inhibiting glucose absorption from the gut, improving insulin sensitivity in target tissues, regulating insulin receptors and increasing insulin secretion;
- reducing cholesterol;
- eliminating free radicals (Li *et al.* 2004; Liu *et al.* 2002).

The active constituents and chemical structure of many Chinese herbs have been isolated. The bioactive compounds most likely to be responsible for the glucose lowering actions include polysaccharides, terpenoids, flavonoids, sterols and alkaloids (Li *et al.* 2004). For example, Radix Ginseng (*ren shen*) contains a number of active principles including saponins that promote insulin secretion and lower blood glucose by enhancing insulin sensitivity, and directly or indirectly regulating the enzymes involved in glucose metabolism (Li *et al.* 2004).

A potential problem in taking what could be considered a reductionist approach to Chinese herbal medicine by attempting to isolate active constituents is that, in clinical practice, the *combination* of herbs produces the therapeutic effect rather than isolated compounds. Chinese prescriptions rarely involve single herbs. The synergy among herbs and the quenching properties of their chemical constituents are likely to be an important determinant of efficacy. Herbs may have many active constituents and the possible synergies among the various herbs in a medicinal formula are potentially enormous. Synergystic actions create potential problems in pharmacological research.

Specific Chinese herbs are combined to address complex clinical patterns, are tailored to the individual and address the underlying root cause as well as secondary manifestations of disease/imbalance. The formulae are usually altered over time as the underlying pattern of disharmony, symptoms and signs change.

The efficacy of medicinal formula in the treatment of diabetes has been assessed in many studies but much of the available research is methodologically flawed. A Cochrane Review of Chinese herbal medicines used to manage type 2 diabetes identified 66 randomised clinical trials involving, 8302 patients who met the inclusion criteria. Ten studies compared Chinese herbal medicinal formulae with a placebo and 25 compared medicinal formulae with glucose-lowering conventional medicines (Liu *et al.* 2002). Six medicinal formulae demonstrated improvements in blood glucose control over placebo. The reviewers concluded that, on the basis of positive results, some herbs possess glucose-lowering effects. A meta-analysis of three clinical studies of one medicinal formula, *Xiaozhen Pian* indicates further research into its glucose lowering potential is warranted (Liu *et al.* 2002). Fifteen studies demonstrated additional benefits of combining Chinese herbal preparations with conventional glucose-lowering medicines compared with conventional medicines alone (Liu *et al.* 2002).

The herbal medicines used in the studies cited in the review appeared to be safe, however, safety data were not reported in the majority of studies (Liu *et al.* 2002). Lui *et al.* (2002) concluded that there were several limitations to the studies they reviewed that made it difficult to arrive at clinical recommendations. The limitations include small sample sizes (underpowered), lack of blinding, short duration of the study and the fact that in the majority of the studies the herbal formulae were tailored to individual patients and their underlying Chinese medicine syndrome, which made it impossible to make accurate comparisons. In addition, there was lack of follow-up in the majority of studies, therefore, the long-term effects are not known. The majority (90 per cent) of the trials involved Chinese patients and the applicability to other populations cannot be assumed. Only one medicinal formula was tested in more than one study. The authors recommended that future research into the effectiveness and safety of Chinese medicines should include stratifying the herbal prescriptions according to Chinese medicine syndromes (Liu *et al.* 2002).

11.9 Treating Diabetes with Acupuncture and Moxibustion

Acupuncture is not a primary therapeutic method of treating diabetes in Chinese medicine: herbal medicine is the main therapeutic method. However, acupuncture is commonly used as a supplementary treatment to manage diabetes-related symptoms such a peripheral neuropathy and nausea associated with gastric stasis, and may also be used to manage concomitant diseases such as arthritis. Acupuncture is particularly useful for easing symptoms of neurological complications (Abuaisha *et al.* 1998). Acupuncture prescriptions are individualised, that is, a set of acupuncture points (acupoints) are chosen according to the Chinese medicine syndrome/s diagnosed, taking into account any additional (secondary) signs and symptoms present. Generally a course of acupuncture treatments is required and the acupoints chosen may vary from appointment to appointment as the condition changes.

Acupuncture points and prescriptions

Acupuncture treatment of people with diabetes is guided by the same underlying principles as Chinese herbal medicine, that is, to restore the functions of the three major organs concerned, the lung, stomach and kidney, because dysfunction of these organs is seen as the root cause of the disease and, in Western biomedical terms, the resultant hyperglycaemia. Thus, the acupoints are usually selected from the lung, stomach and kidney meridians. Acupoints might also be selected from related meridians such as the large intestine, spleen and the bladder meridians because these are the paired meridians of the lung, stomach and kidney organs respectively, and are connected via the meridian system (Wang 2000).

The key pathogenesis of diabetes is *qi* and yin deficiency; therefore, key acupoints are commonly selected from the bladder, spleen and stomach meridians. The spleen and stomach are paired zang-fu organs involved in producing *qi*. Clinically, the 'backshu points' on the bladder meridian, especially the points associated with the lung, spleen, stomach and kidney, are considered to have the most potent therapeutic effects for primary yin and *qi* deficiency. The backshu points are located on either side of the thoracic and lumbar areas of the spine.

Therefore, the following points are used as the primary acupuncture points for improving yin and *qi* deficiency in diabetes:

- Yi Shu (Extra point)
- Ge Shu (Bladder 17)
- Fei Shu (Bladder 13)
- Pi Shu (Bladder 20)
- Shen Shu (Bladder 23)
- Zhu San Li (Stomach 36)
- San Yin Jiao (Spleen 6)
- Di Ji (Spleen 8)
- Chi Ze (Lung 5)
- Yang Chi (San Jiao 4)
- Qi Chi (Large Intestine 11)
- Tai Xi (Kidney 6).

These acupoints might be needled in different sequences using different needling techniques to achieve the desired therapeutic outcomes. In clinical practice, needling any one acupoint can produce different therapeutic outcomes depending on the needling techniques applied. For example, a tonification technique is applied to correct a 'deficiency syndrome' and a reduction technique is applied to manage an 'excess syndrome'. As previously indicated, patients may present with a combined deficiency and excess syndrome depending on metabolic abnormalities present at particular stages of the disease. Therefore, the acupoints are used in different sequences (order) and/or with different needling techniques depending on the individual underlying imbalance.

Supplementary acupuncture points may be added depending on the Chinese medicine syndrome/s and complications present. For example, when a patient presents with a predominantly: lung deficiency syndrome (Upper Jiao), the Tai Yuan (Lung 9) and Shao Fu (Heart 8) points might be added to strengthen the therapeutic effect of the prescription. If the patient has a stomach syndrome (Middle Jiao), the acupoints Wei Shu (Bladder 21) and Nei Ting (Stomach 44) may be used. And with a kidney deficiency syndrome (Lower Jiao), the following points can be added: Gan Shu (Bladder 18) and Tai Chong (Liver 3). Other points might be selected to treat specific symptoms in addition to the points that address the Chinese medicine syndrome/s. For example, the acupoints Lian Quan (Conception Vessel 23) and Cheng Jiang (Conception Vessel 24) are normally used to treat extreme thirst.

Other acupuncture methods such as auricular acupuncture and plum blossom needles are also commonly used to manage symptoms. In auricular acupuncture the body morphology is mapped out on the surface of the ear. Ear acupoints that relate to the zang-fu organs involved in diabetes may be chosen. Other points might be chosen to treat diabetes-related comorbidities such as hypertension. Plum blossom needling uses a hammer-like instrument, which has needles attached to the head that is struck against the skin to treat pain associated with diabetes.

Adhering to infection control guidelines and appropriately disposing of used needles is extremely important when undertaking acupuncture. People with diabetes complications may be particularly at risk of infection if their blood glucose is not well controlled and their immune system is impaired. Using disposable acupuncture needles is recommended.

Clinical research evidence of acupuncture and diabetes

Despite the long history of clinical application of acupuncture and other related stimulating methods such as auricular acupuncture and 'plum blossom' needling, there is very little scientific evidence of the efficacy of acupuncture in the management of diabetes and its related complications.

Despite a thorough literature search using a number of databases on acupuncture, only three publications addressing acupuncture and diabetes were identified: Chen (1987), Chen et al. (1994), and Feng et al. (1997). Of these, only one reported a clinical study of the efficacy of acupuncture in treating diabetes (Chen et al. 1994). The other two used a combination of acupuncture and Chinese herbal medicine.

Chen et al. (1994) studied 60 patients who were randomly assigned to either an acupuncture treatment (n = 38) or control group (n = 22). Both groups included a mix of type I and type 2 diabetes. Subjects in the acupuncture group received acupuncture treatment according to a Chinese medicine diagnosis and the control group received a Chinese proprietary medicine routinely used to treat diabetes in China. After one month of treatment, both groups showed significant improvement in symptom scores using a three point scoring system, significant reduction of blood glucose levels ($p < 0.01$) and a significant reduction in insulin requirements ($p < 0.05$). However, there were no between-group differences.

Chen et al. concluded that acupuncture was effective for diabetes particularly if it was combined with moxibustion when it was useful in preventing diabetes complications, although details of how moxibustion was included were not provided. There are reports of burns to neuropathic legs following moxibustion, which suggest neuropathy may represent a contraindication to moxibustion. The usefulness of a proprietary Chinese herbal medicine as a control could be questioned since the efficacy of the proprietary medicine, if it is established over the placebo, is not reported. More quality research is needed to establish the effectiveness of acupuncture and its role in managing diabetes and diabetes complications. In addition, the effectiveness of acupuncture in improving mental health and quality of life needs to be explored.

Diet and exercise

Although diet and exercise therapy are important management strategies for many diseases and conditions of the body, research into their effectiveness in disease management including diabetes is lacking. Tai chi and qi gong are both forms of gentle bodily movements, usually performed in a sequence, that incorporate regular breathing techniques and stretching to stimulate the flow of *qi* around the body. Both have been described as a kind of meditation in motion, having benefits in calming the mind and emotions as well as exercising the physical body. Tai chi and qi gong may enhance quality of life including pain management and mental health of people with diabetes.

Diet therapy, the judicial use and avoidance of particular foods, deserves further attention. The usefulness of diet therapy as an adjunctive treatment in the management of diabetes including blood glucose levels, though logical within the system of Chinese medicine, has not been conclusively established using scientific research methods.

11.10 Summary

Chinese medicine adopts a unique approach to understanding humans, health and illness. There is a long history of treating diabetes with Chinese herbal medicine and acupuncture. The methods of treatment are understood within the context of the philosophies underpinning Chinese medicine and several theories of Chinese medicine. Increasingly, conventional research methods are being applied to Chinese medicine treatment of diseases such as diabetes. The pharmacological actions of many Chinese herbs have been elucidated and a number have demonstrated glucose-lowering properties. Similarly, acupuncture may alleviate some of the symptoms and signs associated with diabetes including the pain of peripheral neuropathy.

However, it is important to be aware that the efficacy of Chinese herbal medicines and acupuncture may be a result of the manner in which Chinese medicine is practised. The recognition and treatment of underlying Chinese medicine syndromes or patterns of disharmony of diseases/disorders and the individualisation of the herbal or acupuncture prescription are important features of Chinese medicine. Attempts to utilise Chinese herbs or acupuncture outside of a traditional framework where the treatment is not guided by traditional Chinese medicine theory, may not necessarily be efficacious.

Both conventional and Chinese medicine seeks the same goal: to improve health. They approach it in different ways. Well-designed research has the potential to improve current knowledge about diabetes. A collaborative interdisciplinary approach undertaken from the perspective of both medical systems could generate information that may contribute to both medical systems and health care generally.

References

Abuaisha B, Costanzi J, Boulton A. Acupuncture for the treatment of chronic painful peripheral diabetic neuropathy: a long-term study. *Diabetic Research and Clinical Practice* 1998; **39**(2): 115–121.

Bensky D, Gamble A. *Chinese Herbal Medicine: Materia Medica*. Revised Edition. Washington, DC: Eastland Press, 1993.

Braun L. Herb – drug interaction guide. *Australian Family Physician* 2000; **29**(12): 1155–1156.

Cai J, Chao G, Chen D, Chen K, Chen X, Cheng X, *et al.* (eds) *Advanced Textbook on Traditional Chinese Medicine and Pharmacology* (Vol. I – *History, Basic Theory and Diagnostics*). Beijing, China: New World Press, 1995.

Chan K, Cheung L. *Interactions between Chinese Herbal Medicinal Products and Orthodox Drugs*. Australia; Harwood Academic Publishers, 2000.

Chen D, Gong D, Zhai Y. Clinical and experimental studies in treating diabetes mellitus by acupuncture. *Journal of Traditional Chinese Medicine* 1994; **14**(3): 163–166.

Chen J. A hemorrheological study on the effect of acupuncture in treating diabetes mellitus. *Journal of Traditional Chinese Medicine* 1987; **7**(2): 95–100.

Chen J. *Treatment of Diabetes with Traditional Chinese Medicine*. Jinan, China: Shandong Science and Technology Press, 1994.

Chen K. (ed.) *Practical Integrative Western and Chinese Medicine: Internal Medicine*. Beijing, China: Joint Publishing House of Beijing Medical University and China Union Medical University, 1998.

Cheng X, Deng L, Cheng Y (eds). *Chinese Acupuncture and Moxibustion*. Rev. edn. Beijing, China: Foreign Languages Press, 1999.

D'Arcy P. Traditional Chinese medicines: safety hazards. *Adverse Drug Reaction Toxicological Review* 1999; **18**(2): 53–60.

Deadman P, Al-Khafaji M, Baker K (eds) *A Manual of Acupuncture*, Journal of Chinese Medical Publication, 1998.

De Smet P. Herbal remedies. *New England Journal of Medicine*. 2002; **347**(25): 2046–2056.

Ernst E. Harmless herbs? *American Journal of Medicine* 1998; **104**: 170–178.

Ernst E. Adulteration of Chinese herbal medicines with synthetic drugs: a systematic review. *Journal of Internal Medicine* 2002; **252**: 107–113.

Ernst E. Risks of herbal medicinal products. *Pharmacoepidemiology and Drug Safety*. 2004; **13**: 77–771.

Feng M, Li Y, Pang B, Wang Z, Wang S. Acupuncture combined with application of Xiaoke plaster for treatment of 309 cases of diabetes mellitus. *Journal of Traditional Chinese Medicine* 1997; **17**(4): 247–249.

Flaws B, Sionneau. *The Treatment of Modern Western Medical Diseases with Chinese Medicine: A Textbook and Clinical Manual*. Boulder, CO: Blue Poppy Press, 2001.

Huang W, Wen K-C, Hsiao M-L. Adulteration by synthetic therapeutic substances of traditional Chinese medicines in Taiwan. *Journal of Clinical Pharmacology* 1997; **37**: 334–350.

Izzo A. Herb – drug interactions: an overview of the clinical evidence. *Fund and Clinical Pharmacology* 2004; **19**: 1–16.

Ko R. Adulterants in Asian patent medicines. *New England Journal of Medicine* 1998; **339**: 847.

Li W, Zheng H, Bukuru J, De Kimpe N. Natural medicines used in the traditional Chinese medical system for therapy of diabetes mellitus. *Journal of Ethnopharmacology* 2004; **92**: 1–21.

Liu J, Zhang M, Wang W, Grimsgaard S. Chinese herbal medicines for type 2 diabetes. The Cochrane Database of Systematic Reviews Issue 3. 2002; The Cochrane Collaboration. Available at URL: http: www.thecochranelibrary.com (accessed July 2005).

Maciocia G. *The Foundations of Chinese Medicine: A Comprehensive Text for Acupuncturists and Herbalists*, 2nd edn. Philadelphia, MA: Elsevier Churchill Livingstone, 2005.

O'Brien K, Xue C. The principles used in Chinese Medicine. In: Leung P, Xue C, Cheng Y (eds) *A Comprehensive Guide to Chinese Medicine*. Singapore: World Scientific Ltd, 2003a, pp. 47–84.

O'Brien K, Xue C. Acupuncture. In: Robson T. (ed.), *An Introduction to Complementary Medicine*. Crows Nest, Australia: Allen & Unwin, 2003b.

Pittler M, Ernst E. Systematic review: hepatotoxic events associated with herbal medicinal products. *Alimentary Pharmacology and Therapeutics* 2003; **18**(5): 451–471.

Wang L. *Clinical Acupuncture*. Shanghai, China: Shanghai University of Traditional Chinese Medicine Press, (in Chinese), 2000.

World Health Organization. *Traditional Medicine Strategy 2001–2005*. Geneva: World Health Organization, 2002.

Xie Z, Liao J. *Traditional Chinese Internal Medicine*. Beijing, China: Foreign Languages Press, 1993.

Zhang Y, Rose K. *Who Can Ride the Dragon? An Exploration of the Cultural Roots of Traditional Chinese Medicine*. Brookline, MA: Paradigm Publications, 1995.

Zhang Y, Rose K. *A Brief History of Qi*. Brookline, MA: Paradigm Publications, 2001.

12 Australian Aboriginal Traditional Healing Practices

Heather McDonald

12.1 Introduction

> These days – since sugar – people are rather weak; we're just about dying now, from sugar. Our blood's no good now, it's deteriorated, gone dark; aged us prematurely, made our bodies slack. Our blood, our general condition, has gone downhill.
>
> (Anmatyerr woman, in Devitt and McMasters 1998)

Australian Indigenous people's diets and health were optimal at the time of colonisation. Explorers and travellers recognised the superb physical development, strength and stamina of Aboriginal people. Observers spoke of their quickness of sight and agility of limb, their skills in hunting, tracking and food gathering, and their ability to endure fatigue and privation (De Vries 1952, in Fallon and Enig 1999). Hunter-gatherer life is anti-obesity, anti-diabetes and anti-vascular disease. A nutrient-dense hunter-gatherer diet fits all the requirements for the prevention and treatment of diabetes (O'Dea 1994). Agricultural development, on the other hand, is linked to decreasing average height, increasing obesity and a decline in overall health (Wadley and Martin 2000) in all cultures.

Early health records show that Aboriginal people were fit, lean, and did not suffer from any diet-related chronic diseases (Cumpston 1928). Cardiovascular diseases were rare in Aboriginal communities before the 1960s and diabetes was rare before the 1970s (Moodie 1981; O'Dea 1991).

Compilations of Aboriginal herbal treatments reflect health issues common in hunter-gatherer societies. Many indigenous plants were available to treat common ailments such as accidental trauma, snake, bites, insect bites and illnesses such as respiratory, gastrointestinal and skin diseases (Lassak and McCarthy 2001). Lassak and McCarthy list the medicinal plants in Aboriginal pharmacopoeias.

Complementary Therapies and the Management of Diabetes and Vascular Disease   Editor Trish Dunning
© 2006 John Wiley & Sons, Ltd.

They only credit two plants with glucose-lowering properties, *Goodenia ovata* (constituents unknown) and *Scoparia dulcis*, which contains amellin, which has glucose-lowering properties but does not appear to have been used by Aboriginal people to manage diabetes (Lassak and McCarthy 2001).

Anmatyerr women of Central Australia talk about their love of sweet plants and fat grubs and animals in Green (2003). They indicated that animals eat particular plants and insects to make themselves fat, and people choose fat animals to eat. When these food preferences coincided with energy-dense, nutrient-poor rations on pastoral and mission stations, metabolic disturbances began to occur and eventually led to the current epidemic of diabetes and vascular disease. Unemployment and sedentary lifestyles resulting from post-industrial work practices contribute to the increasing incidence of chronic diseases in Aboriginal Australia.

As a result of colonisation, dispossession of land and livelihood and loss of control over their own destiny, Australian Indigenous people experience poor physical and mental health with morbidity and mortality rates many times the national average. Indigenous people have the highest prevalence of diabetes in Australia and an excess of avoidable complications and premature death (Australian Institute of Health and Welfare and Australian Bureau of Statistics 2003). Death rates for cardiovascular disease are three times the national average and death rates for diabetes are eight times the national average (Ring and Brown 2002).

Post-industrial societies are today learning from hunter-gatherer peoples such as the Inuit of the circumpolar region. Diabetes was virtually unknown in Nunavik Inuit peoples, and Greenland Inuit have significantly lower rates of cardiovascular disease than the people of Denmark. The traditional Inuit diet includes several grams of omega 3 fatty acids daily (Leaf and Weber 1988; Connor 2000; Dewailly *et al.* 2001). Hunter-gatherer diets are advocated today as therapeutic diets for people at risk of diabetes and vascular disease (Eaton *et al.* 1988; Washington 1994; Cordain *et al.* 2002).

12.2 Aboriginal Concepts of Health and Illness

To be understood, traditional healing practices need to be discussed within the context of Aboriginal cosmologies and ontologies. In Aboriginal Australian traditions, the cosmos and its life forms are composed of ancestral substances and energies. During their original cosmogonic journeys the ancestors left their bodily substances in the land. In the Eagle Dreaming story of the Gija people, the ancestral eagle flew over the Warmun hills with kangaroo fat in its beak, dropping pieces on the way (Patrick Mung Mung, in Bahr 2001). Life forms are consubstantial with and permeable to the living environment. Urine, sweat, blood, milk and semen flow through or stagnate in bodies and the land.

In relational cultures such as Australian Aboriginal cultures, the cosmos and its life forms are interconnected. In Western atomistic models of human agency, individuals act in isolation from others, and moral agents are limited only by their own values and capacities (Donchin 1995). In relational models of human agency, relationship with others always mediates individual actions and obligations. In Aboriginal cultures, relationship is prior to individual bodies and atoms (Edge 2000; Edge and Suryani 2002). The human body is not viewed an individuated body-object as it is in conventional biomedicine. Rather it is seen as a relational body-self, that is, a body that always exists in and is always defined by social relationship. In Aboriginal cultures, health and illness are relational-moral concepts (McDonald 2001). These concepts do not refer to relationship versus culture, but to relational cultures.

In northern and central Australia, a healthy body is clean and cool, which allows an optimum flow of life-energies. Fresh air blows in and out of the airways infusing the body and enlivening its faculties so that one can watch, listen and understand. Life energies flow through the bloodstream and disperse to all parts of the body to nourish and strengthen it. In early Aboriginal traditions, body organs were not collections of specialised tissue that perform specific functions in the body; rather, they were containers and channels through which the life energies flowed. In Gija and Jaru ontologies, the body's life force (*birlirr*) draws the wind into the *giningi* (respiratory organs and channels) and breathes the wind through the *jiluwa* (network of channels for body fluids and life energies). The wind pushes the blood along the *jiluwa* just as the wind pushes the water along a watercourse (McDonald 2001 and 2003). Other health traditions such as Chinese medicine and Ayurveda also refer to energy flow in the body, see Chapters 8, 10 and 11.

Blood is considered to be a particularly potent substance. In traditional ontologies blood is a source of life that originates in and flows like spring water from the ancestral uterus (Berndt 1951; Strehlow 1970). In human bodies, the ancestral blood is replenished by eating meat. Old people say animal food is the best medicine for them because meat replenishes human blood, strengthens the body, revives the spirit and enlivens the senses. When people are weak and sick, they cook kangaroo in the ground and drink the warm blood. People and animals have ancestral blood in their veins. The quality of blood is an important factor in Aboriginal understandings of health. Blood should be bright red in colour. It should be not too thick and not too thin. It should flow steadily, not too fast and not too slow, through the bloodstream. It should be cool and it should not dry up (Wiminydji and Peile 1978; Devitt and McMasters 1998; McDonald 2003).

Sickness is generally perceived as coming from malignant outside forces or antisocial actions. For example, sickness can come from war zones where people's actions create a moral imbalance and obstruct the flow of reciprocity, which is also a relational in the interconnected world. The moral blockage manifests as an accumulation of rubbish in the body, which obstructs the flow of life energies. In this context 'rubbish' refers to any object that has become useless and no longer able to perform its proper function in the social body or the human body (Young 2002). Foreign objects intrude into the body in various ways. In the past, Aboriginal people believed this occurred through ancestral intervention or sorcery. Today, 'whitefella substances' such as alcohol and tobacco have taken on the characteristics of rubbish in the body. Alcohol and tobacco mix with the blood, making it dirty and thick so that it is unable to flow properly. The thick mixture blocks the heart and respiratory organs and makes the person breathless (McDonald 2003).

Diabetes can have a similar effect. Old people in the Kimberley say that cane sugar is really whitefella food, not Aboriginal food. White people grow it and they can eat it without ill effect, whereas cane sugar is too strong for Aboriginal people. It makes them weak (with diabetes) as illustrated in this explanation by a Gija woman: 'Sugar mixes with the blood. Both mix up and get thick. Too much sugar stops the blood flowing properly.' Cane sugar acts like sorcery in the body and congeals the blood, blocks the organs and channels, and can eat the organs away altogether (McDonald 2003). In contrast, bush honey is regarded as Aboriginal food that makes people strong and energetic.

It is helpful to view diabetes and vascular disease as coming from outside forces such as the effects of colonisation and to speak in terms of tools to overcome these effects when designing Aboriginal health programs (Heffernan 1995). Cultural understandings such as Aboriginal concepts of strength and weakness, heat and coolness, flow and blockage, and cultural images of good lives and strong bodies can be developed to promote a sense of control over the disease. Indigenous health programmes need to be designed in collaboration with community members and developed within a framework of self-determination, community capacity building, and community control.

Aboriginal traditional healers, referred to as 'clever people' by many Aboriginal groups, do more than heal bodies. They play a central role and are frequently moral arbiters in an interconnected world where social relationship is the criterion against which individual behaviour is judged. They can see and visit the spirit world, which is normally invisible to ordinary people. They seek and manipulate ancestral powers in order to offset the influence of malign outside forces. Aboriginal healing practice emphasises the relationship between the person receiving treatment and the healer (Havecker 2002). In addition, the individual must believe they will get well.

In order to heal people of life-threatening illnesses, traditional healers need to have stronger powers than the human or spirit agencies that caused the illness. Ancestral powers are local or regional powers, not universalised powers. Therefore, clever people must travel to the sources of ancestral powers to access power for healing. Ceremonial leaders also use ancestral powers in their regional travelling ceremonies, and on these occasions, ancestral powers travel with the cult leaders beyond their original locations. Thus, ancestral powers are localised not universalised powers. Because they are localised, healers have to travel to them to access them. That is healers cannot just put up their hands and grasp universal powers out of the air. This represents a significant difference from Reiki, which is universalised.

Healers begin by investigating the causes of illness and redressing moral imbalances. Traditional healers remove sickness or moral blockages in bodies and in the cosmos to restore the normal flow of ancestral powers. They seek to reconcile people engaged in antagonistic relationships in order to restore a moral balance and flow of reciprocity (McDonald 2001). Sometimes healers are accused of using their powers for malevolent purposes because they traffic in powers beyond the ordinary person. Aboriginal concepts of strength and weakness need to be taken seriously in health education programmes. East Kimberley people believe that cane sugar is too strong for their bodies and traditional healers say they cannot cure people of diabetes. But some Aboriginal people claim that they are stronger than whitefella substances such as tobacco and therefore cigarettes cannot harm them (McDonald 2003).

12.3 Traditional Healing Practices

Minor illnesses

Traditional healing practices include bush medicines, healing waters, healing songs, ceremonies, and consultations with traditional healers. Songs contain ancestral words that are carried on sound waves that vibrate through the social body and the human body. The country is a rich source of healing substances. Bush medicines and healing pools that contain ancestral powers are used for preventive and curative purposes. Ceremonies are performed to increase the health of the country and the people. The healing power that emanates from special performances spreads out to influence everything within its social range. Women's healing ceremonies consist of painting designs on sick people's bodies, singing healing songs, and massaging people with fat and red ochre to infuse their bodies with strength (Berndt 1950; Bell 1983).

Australia has a wide range of pharmacologically active plants and herbs (Healers of Arnhem Land, Lassak and McCarthy 2001). Aboriginal women traditionally prepared and administered herbal medicines and other treatments (Reid 1978; Malbunka 2003; Green 2003). Bush medicines were mainly used for symptoms of colds and flu, toothache, fever, eye problems, gastrointestinal disorders, joint and muscle pain, bone fractures, snake bites, skin infections and burns. In Central Australia, plants used on wounds have been found to contain proteolytic enzymes. The Bauhinia root (*Lysiphyllum cunninghamii*) is as effective as conventional medicines in treating boils, sores and scabies (McLean *et al.* 1996). *Spilanthes acmella*, a native daisy used to treat toothache, contains spilanthol, a local anaesthetic (Devanesen 2000).

In the Kimberley the konkerberry shrub (*Carissa lanceolata*) is regarded as a bush medicine *par excellence*. Aboriginal people smoked the leaves for diarrhoeal and respiratory complaints and made wood pulp infusions for respiratory problems. Wood smoke was used to repel mosquitos. A general tonic was made from infusions of crushed bark, leaves and twigs. The sap was used as a liniment for rheumatism and the roots were ground up and soaked to wash skin sores (Reid 1977).

Modern research supports some of these traditional uses. For example, the leaves of the konkerberry shrub contain triterpenes and the roots contain carissone (Lassak and McCarthy 2001). The leaves and stem contain cardiac glycosides, which are cardiac stimulants used in conventional medicine to strengthen cardiac contractions and regulate heart rhythm (Reid 1977). Lindsay *et al.* (2000) carried out a phytochemical analysis of *Carissa lanceolata* and isolated three antibacterial agents – eudesmanes carissone, dehydrocarissone and carindone – from the wood of the plant in an effort to identify novel antibacterial compounds. All three constituents were found to be biologically active against *Staphylococcus aureus, Escherichia coli* and *Pseudomonas aeruginosa*.

Aboriginal people believe their ancestors put the bush medicine in the ground for them to use. They claim that plants in their particular region have special potency and work more rapidly for anyone, not just for themselves, than bush medicines from other regions (Devansen and Henshall 1982).

Aboriginal people smoke the body to remove rubbish and infuse medicine into the body. Strong smelling leaves are believed to contain strong medicine. Smoking involves digging a shallow depression in a dry creek bed, placing branches of bush medicine trees in the hollow and setting it on fire. When the fire is burning well, smaller branches with leaves are splashed with water and placed on the fire for a few seconds, then rubbed over the patient's body. Babies and children are held over the smoke. People with respiratory complaints put their head covered by a towel or blanket into the smoke and steam and inhale deeply, see Figure 12.1.

The medicine in the leaves enters the body through the nose, ears and the pores of the skin. The smoke takes the path of the breath and blood through the body, clearing out rubbish, drying up secretions, and infusing the body with ancestral medicine. Today, when Kimberley people suffer from conditions that do not respond to conventional medicine, they will go into the bush (away from the European gaze) to perform smoking treatments. Kimberley people say:

> You can feel the *jiluwa* [blood vessels] working, feel the blood flowing [during a smoking treatment]. I was heavy before . . . now I'm fresh and light. We can feel the medicine going into us. When we take *gardiya* [whitefella] tablets, we don't feel anything.
>
> (Gija woman, in McDonald 2003)

Animal fat and plant oils were used as internal and external medicines. Bush gum and fat from the goanna, a large lizard, were taken orally to settle stomach complaints. Animal fat was used to treat dry skin, cracks, rashes and sores and to keep the body cool on long journeys. Liniments were made from goanna fat mixed with other ingredients. In cases of severe bodily depletion, fat was mixed with red ochre and applied to infuse the body with strength. In northern Australia, conventional medicine has been incorporated into Aboriginal health systems at the same level as bush medicine, that is, to treat the symptoms of illness (Devanesen 2000).

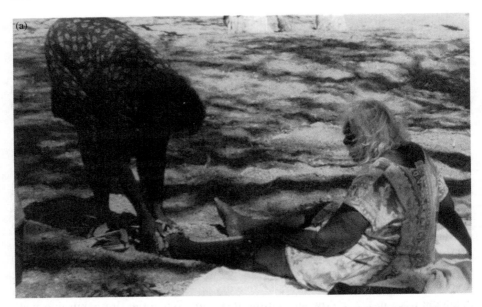

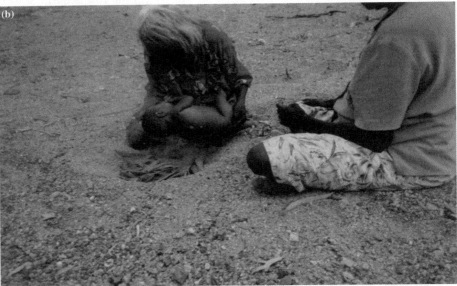

Figure 12.1 Two examples of Australian Aboriginal smoking treatments for (a) arthritis in an older woman and (b) a new baby from the East Kimberley region of Australia.

Aboriginal people interpret conventional explanations of diseases within a larger moral framework and use conventional medicine to alleviate symptoms. Indigenous people's pharmacopoeias can extend indefinitely to include extra-traditional elements from herbal to biomedical preparations. Patients with vascular disease believe their blood has become dirty and thick, blocking the heart and respiratory organs. They take conventional medicine to melt the congealed blood.

People with diabetes take conventional medicine to render the sugar weak and clear it out of the blood (McDonald 2003).

Serious illnesses

Minor or short-lived illnesses do not require the specialist knowledge of traditional healers. However, when the person does not respond to ordinary medicines, the illness worsens, or the patient's condition becomes life-threatening, they consult a traditional healer. Healers possess power-knowledge beyond that of ordinary people and are called on to investigate the relational-moral causes of a patient's illness. Traditional healers gain their knowledge and credentials by working with experienced healers, dreaming experiences and attending to the quality of their own body-life.

The healer's body is a conduit for healing life forces. Healers prepare themselves for the task of healing through ritual practices and dietary restrictions, not by studying books for many years in large, imposing buildings. During a healer's initiation in some regions, pearl shells are inserted into his body to augment his senses. Shells are placed in his ears, for example, so that he can hear and understand communications in the animal and spirit worlds and in more distant human worlds. Women in most areas are believed to be capable of obtaining and manipulating healing powers, but not to the same extent as men (Berndt 1982; McDonald 2001).

In northern and central Australia, unknown and potentially malign powers are believed to exist on the peripheries of people's countries and in more distant places. However, pitting one's wits against unknown elements is part of the human and ancestral condition. People, who expose themselves to dangerous powers and do not die, become powerful and dangerous themselves. To be strong and dangerous is to be able to break ancestral taboos without fear of retribution. Traditional healers who travel widely to engage with dangerous powers are believed to be potent and dangerous.

Ancestral powers can be used for good and bad purposes. For this reason, traditional healing takes place in the public domain rather than in enclosed architectural spaces. An important cultural factor in Aboriginal healing processes is not privacy or patient confidentiality, but community witnessing. Healing events require witnesses to ensure that the healer performs their task correctly and does not harm the patient. If things go wrong and the patient is harmed, the witnesses will be implicated in the blame because they did not intervene to save the patient. Both healer and witnesses are required and both are part of the healing performance (Sansom 1980; McDonald 2004). At Warburton Ranges in the southern Western Desert:

> People all come in at once and crowd into the clinic. I thought, "Hang on a minute, there is a waiting room." No-one wanted to leave and wait in the waiting room. So I saw them one by one while they all sat together.
>
> (Nurse practitioner, in Cramer 2005)

Intercultural health services are being established in some Fourth World contexts today. An intercultural approach promotes empathy, respect, and synergies to attain results that could not be achieved independently. Treatment and preventive programmes are inclusive of clients' perspectives on health and healing (Garcia 2002). In northern and central Australia, rather than focussing solely on individual consultations, health professionals can develop treatment regimes, diabetes education, and chronic disease management programmes within group sessions. People with diabetes can form their own support groups that meet to think about diabetes, its effects on community life, and ways to combat its life-threatening complications. Occupational and cultural therapies and physical activities can be developed within these groups. Indigenous health programmes need to be carried out within a framework of self-determination, self-governance and community control.

Quartz crystals, which capture and reflect light, are used in healing traditions around the world. Many cultures believe clear crystals absorb qualities from the surrounding environment. In northern Australia rainmakers soak quartz crystals in cold water before using them in rainmaking ceremonies. Traditional healers use quartz crystals to see inside sick bodies, absorb foreign material, and cool the blood (Reid 1983; Tonkinson 1982). After clearing the rubbish out of a sick body, the healer may infuse the patient with healing power from his underarm sweat or from medicinal plants. Potent spirits of the dead, who travel further and see more clearly than human healers, assist traditional healers in their practices. For Aboriginal people in northern and central Australia, traditional healers have strong powers to divine the causes of illness, redress moral imbalances, and clear the rubbish out of sick bodies. Conventional doctors have strong medicines to alleviate the symptoms of illness (Reid 1983; McDonald 2001 and 2003).

For these reasons, sick people consult traditional healers as well as attend conventional medical clinics. Aboriginal people say that Western medicine does not clear all the obstructing debris out of a sick body. They argue that traditional healers should be employed to clear the rubbish out of a sick body and their healing can be supported by conventional medicine (McDonald 2003). Conventional health professionals and community members can explore Aboriginal understandings of healing and the perceived benefits of conventional medicine to treat chronic diseases in intercultural health programmes. There is an urgent need for Aboriginal and non-Aboriginal health professionals, researchers, and community members to work together to develop better medication management programmes for Aboriginal people in northern and central Australia and this includes diabetes medicine regimens (Kowanko et al. 2003).

Chronic illnesses

Traditionally, when people got sick, bush medicines or a traditional healer restored their health. Sometimes the person could not be cured and died. The notion of chronic diseases that cannot be cured is foreign to Indigenous people. Traditional remedies, when effective, were believed to produce almost immediate and lasting, results (Heffernan 1995). Healing narratives usually end with 'And the person became well and never suffered again'. Aboriginal people who survived the infectious diseases of the industrial era are now falling prey to the chronic diseases of post-industrialism. They have become victims of unemployment and purposelessness, with the bloated bodies of obesity, diabetes and vascular disease; the broken bodies of trauma and self-inflicted injury; and the wasted bodies of substance misuse (McDonald 2001). Today Aboriginal people become ill and cannot be cured, but as a result of conventional medical care they do not die but live on as chronically ill people (Devitt and McMasters 1998).

O'Dea's study of ten Kimberley Aborigines who reverted to a hunter-gatherer lifestyle for seven weeks revealed a low-energy intake (1200kcal/person/day), and weight loss (average 8 kg). Fasting glucose fell from 11.6 ± 1.2 mM to 6.6 ± 0.8 mM and fasting insulin fell from 23 ± 2 mU/L to 12 ± 1 mU/L. Fasting plasma triglycerides fell from 4.0 ± 0.5 mM to 1.2 ± 0.1 mM (O'Dea 1984).

During the pastoral era in northern Australia (1880s–1960s), Aboriginal people were able to supplement station rations with nutrient-rich bush foods that were still relatively easy to locate. Today, Aboriginal community stores provide approximately 95 per cent of all food consumed in communities (Lee et al. 1994: 212). Despite two decades of research into the nutritional adequacy of community stores in northern Australia, most stores continue to stock large quantities of white flour, white bread, white sugar, fatty cuts of meat, highly processed foods, and sugar-sweetened soft drinks. There is also considerable pressure on young Aboriginal people to conform to a global fast food culture (Kouris-Blazos and Wahlqvist 2000).

Some communities have developed critiques of and are generating the capacity to take control of community stores. In Central Australia, Nganampa Health Council, NPY Women's Council, and Anangu Pitjantjatjara Council developed the Mai Wiru Regional Stores policy, stating that community stores must be an extension of health services rather than commercial enterprises. Food and other essentials must be priced within the budget of Indigenous people and the healthiest food must be easily accessible in the store. Some Anangu Pitjantjatjara community stores are now entirely run by local Aboriginal people as non-profit organisations, selling healthy food at low prices (Flick 2001).

The Fred Hollows Foundation, in response to an Aboriginal request, established their Remote Community Stores Program in the late 1990s to develop food and nutrition policies, effective governing committees, retail management skills, and strategies to improve access to affordable healthy food for Jawoyn community stores in the Katherine region of the Northern Territory. The Program developed partnerships with major supermarket chains, which are training local Aboriginal people to manage their community stores. In 2004, the Minister for Indigenous Affairs gave a $1.5 million grant to enable the Hollows Foundation Remote Community Stores Program to expand their work to other communities (Vanstone 2004).

As a result of colonisation and its trail of introduced diseases, traditional healing practices have become sidelined by powerful conventional treatments.

Aboriginal healers were relegated from being central to peripheral actors in their own communities. In the 1950s, traditional healers were reviled as 'menacing' presences with 'flat, calculating stares' who hovered on the fringes of hospitals and nursing stations interfering with hygienic practices and nursing care (Gartrell 1957). In urban situations, Aboriginal spiritual healers have emerged, whose practices differ from those of traditional healers. They have adopted concepts and practices from other philosophical traditions, and privilege the spiritual realm over the physical. In the 1970s, political changes at the national level led to changes in health policy and practice in urban, rural and remote communities. A report on Aboriginal health in 1979 recommended that:

> Aboriginal cultural beliefs and practices which affect their health and their use of health services such as their fear of hospitalisation, their attitudes to pain and surgery, the role of traditional healers and the differing needs and roles of Aboriginal men and women, be fully taken into account in the design and implementation of health care programs.
>
> (Commonwealth of Australia 1979, in Devanesen 2000)

Traditional healers, where they still practise, find they do not have the power knowledge to heal people of diseases that emanate from Western industrial and post-industrial practices. Healers say that they cannot cure people of drug or alcohol addiction, which comes from Western culture, as illustrated in the following quotes.

> If people have problems with their bones being misaligned, I can manipulate them back into place and take the pain away.
>
> (Sam Watson, in Ngaanyatjarra Pitjantjatjara Yankunytjatjara Women's Council 2003)

> There are some problems that *ngangkari* [traditional healer] can't help with. For example, *ngangkari* can't stop people who want to sniff petrol or drink alcohol.
>
> (Andy Tjilari and Rupert Peter, in NPY Women's Council 2003)

In the past, patients and healers shared common understandings of health, illness and appropriate treatment, which is no longer the case. Conventional doctors refer to micro-level bodily functions that can be measured by scientific instruments. Traditional healers and their patients speak in terms of macro-level bodily functions, fluids and life energies, reciprocity and balance, flow and blockage. Body organs are associated not only with physiological processes but with cognition, volition and emotions. Spirit or life force is associated with the physiological processes of breathing and blood flow as well as perception, consciousness, speech, emotions and desires. An Aboriginal participant in a Port Lincoln medicines survey came to the conclusion that Aboriginal and white people have different bodies and therefore need different medicines: 'I don't believe in it [conventional medicine], but that's my belief, that our body structure's different . . . you know they are treating us like white people which is wrong' (Kowanko *et al.* 2003).

Kimberley people believe good medicine should clear the rubbish out of a sick body, revive the spirit, and make the person walk again. Good medicine is strong medicine but it should not be too strong for sick bodies. When the body is weak, it may not be able to tolerate strong medicine. Aboriginal people frequently complain that medicine prescribed by conventional doctors for diabetes and vascular disease is too strong for them. As a result, their body loses condition, their blood dries up and their spirit becomes sluggish. When the body is weak and sick, weak or diluted medicine should be given until the body builds up its strength again. When people feel that conventional medicine is too strong for them, they may stop taking it for a while to give their bodies a rest. Others only take conventional medicine when they feel weak and sick. They stop taking it when they feel strong (McDonald 2003).

Aboriginal people do not accept a hierarchical, authoritarian relationship between doctor and patient. In the provider–patient relationship Aboriginal people see themselves as having a choice (McDonald 2003). At Warburton Ranges, conventional health professionals interpret these behaviours as non-compliance and dependence on white people:

> People are shocking in their compliance with treatment regimes. They are just not willing to comply for whatever reason . . . There is still the expectation that the clinic will fix it, we will give them an injection to fix it . . . We are still here to pick up the pieces.
>
> (Cramer 2005)

Self-management of chronic illness, however, is a new concept to Aboriginal people. In an analysis of diabetes care in 27 northern Australian communities, glycaemic control was poor. The mean HbA_{1C} level was 8.9 per cent, good glycaemic control was defined as $HbA_{1C} < 7$ per cent. Only 4 per cent of Aboriginal patients compared with 58 per cent of non-Aboriginal patients self-monitored blood glucose (McDermott *et al.* 2004). Aboriginal people had a higher prevalence of hypertension and albuminuria than the non-Aboriginal cohort in the 2002 National Association of Diabetes Centres Study of 2077 adults with diabetes from 24 diabetes centres around Australia. The level of glycaemic control relates to the progression of renal disease and high rates of albuminuria are associated with rapid progression to end-stage renal disease. However, non-adherence to long-term therapy is not confined to Indigenous patients. Adherence to long-term treatment regimes for chronic illness is less than 50 per cent in developed countries (McDermott *et al.* 2004).

If diabetes education is taken out of a narrow biomedical framework, which focuses on micro-level bodily functions, it will become more accessible to Aboriginal people. Diabetes can be discussed within a larger sociopolitical framework, for example, its origins in agricultural practices and its intensification in industrial and post-industrial practices. Health programmes can be developed within a framework of community empowerment to explore the relationship between globalisation and the increasing incidence of chronic diseases in economically deprived regions. Healthy eating programmes are undermined by the global food industry, which monopolises food production, distribution, and retail markets (Morelli 2003). Food marketing is frequently targeted at children and local food outlets sell highly processed food cooked with cheap bad fats (Hawkes 2002). Community empowerment programmes can explore ways to offset the negative impact of globalisation on Aboriginal community life.

12.4 Traditional Healing Practices as Complementary Medicine

Industrial and post-industrial practices have led to unemployment, sedentism and cultural stress in Aboriginal communities. The 1970s homelands movement in Northern and Central Australia, which dispersed large multi-language communities, alleviated social and emotional stress for some Aboriginal families. Since the 1970s, also, rural health centres recognise to varying degrees, co-operate with and sometimes employ traditional healers (Devanesen 2000). The Northern Territory Department of Health recognises the value of traditional healing practices as complementary therapies and stated that: 'traditional medicine is a complementary and vital part of Aboriginal health care, and its value is recognised and supported' (Northern Territory Department of Health 1982, in Devanesen 2000).

Traditional healers have been reintroduced to health services in specific capacities, for example, in social and emotional well-being programmes, to help manage the social and emotional effects of chronic illnesses and to assist with quality of life issues. Chronic stress, which results in raised blood glucose levels, insulin resistance, and abdominal obesity can contribute to diabetes and vascular disease (Brotman and Girod 2002). Symptoms of hyperglycaemia include fatigue and lethargy, fluid retention, and visual changes. Hypoglycaemic episodes cause people to feel shaky, jittery, anxious, sweaty, confused and irritable. Side effects of oral hypoglycaemic agents include weakness, muscle cramps, and fluid retention (Cowan 2004). Chronic diseases drain people's life-energies and depress their spirits. Aboriginal people with multiple chronic diseases are often afraid to leave dysfunctional central communities for family homelands. Family members become dislocated from community life when they are relocated to regional towns for specialised treatment.

The complications of diabetes include heart disease and circulatory problems, neurological disease, kidney disease, retinal disorders leading to blindness, neuropathy resulting in numbness, tingling, pain and burning in the extremities, foot ulcers leading to gangrene, and high risk of infection and amputation (Leonard *et al.* 2002; Maple-Brown *et al.* 2004). Diabetes is frequently complicated by conditions such as depression, which reduces quality of life (McDermott *et al.* 2004). Treatment of stress and depression is important in the management of diabetes, and traditional healers can play a significant role, especially in rural and remote areas.

In April 2000, *ngangkari* (traditional healer/s, southern Central Australia and Western Desert regions) and their supporters from the Ngaanyatjarra Pitjantjatjara Yankunytjatjara (NPY) Lands attended the first *ngangkari* meeting in the Northern Territory. They compiled a book of stories in order to encourage greater collaboration between non-Aboriginal health professionals and traditional healers (NPY Women's Council 2003). The NPY Women's Council employs two *ngangkari* healers through its Regional Social and Emotional Well-Being Centre. The Koonibba Aboriginal Health Service at Ceduna employs a *ngangkari* healer. The Puntukurnu Aboriginal Medical Service in the Pilbara employs a *maparn* (traditional healer, northern Central Australia and Western Desert regions) as an Aboriginal Health Worker.

Ngangkari who work for NPY Women's Council say that, while they do not specifically aim to treat diabetes and cannot cure people of diabetes, they can help patients in other ways. People may be suffering from traditional afflictions, which may or may not contribute to their chronic condition. Traditional healers carry out non-invasive treatments, which do not diminish the spirit or deplete the body's life energies. They aim to reduce blockages and enhance blood flow by massage and smoking treatments. They work to redress moral imbalances, relieve stress, and make patients feel happier and more balanced by a healing process called 'making level' (Andy Tjilari and Rupert Peter, pers. comm.).

[Conventional] doctors treat people with serious illnesses. Yet that sick person's spirit may still harbour something that will continue to affect their recovery. So the *ngangkari* can help cure the patient on this level.

(Andy Tiljari, in NPY Women's Council 2003)

The *ngangkari* balances up the sick person to make him totally better.

(Rupert Peter, in NYP Women's Council 2003)

In relational cultures, where all life forms coexist in an interconnected world, the notion of balance is important. Humans must strive to live in a relationship of balance with other powers and agencies in the world. People's life energy is diminished by negative events occurring in the world, whether physical, social or moral. There are obvious similarities here to healing traditions such as Chinese Medicine and Ayurvedic medicine, see Chapters 10 and 11. However, as Braun, noted in Chapter 9, Chinese and Ayurvedic medicines are complex health-care systems with formal methods of diagnosis and treatment. Such processes require literacy, recording procedures, systemisation and other disciplinary techniques that were developed in militarised city-state societies. Traditional Aboriginal cultures were oral cultures, and in northern and central Australia a culture of oral transmission of knowledge continues to exist within the wider Western culture of literacy.

Devitt and McMasters (1998) found that Central Australian patients with end stage renal disease incorporate traditional healing practices into their care on a regular basis. Traditional healing practices are not seen as alternatives to their clinical treatment regime, but as complementary therapies. Relatives of a town-based haemodialysis patient sent her a bundle of the medicinal plant, *karrinyarra* (*Cymbogon ambiguus*) and a chunk of red ochre with the message 'so you can . . . rub it on you at night time, when you get back from the [dialysis] machine'. *Cymbogon ambiguus* is a Central Australian medicinal plant whose crushed leaves produce a strong scent (Latz 1995).

The town-based patient chopped up the leaves and twigs of the medicinal plant, boiled them in water, and added them to a mixture of red ochre and fat. She poured the prepared ointment into containers to use at home. Devitt and McMasters also found that many patients with end stage renal disease consulted *ngangkari* healers at some point during their illness. When people feel particularly ill they may return to their own community to consult a *ngangkari* (Devitt and McMasters 1998).

Northern Australian people continue to maintain and enhance their health through traditional healing practices. Traditional healers provide important protective and resilience factors that support social and emotional well-being. They reinforce the values, relationships and responsibilities of kin, land and ancestral resources for personal and communal health. They provide people with spiritual resources when they are faced with significant life problems. A young man from Kukatja country manages his chronic illness by visiting a *maparn* healer in the morning and the medical clinic in the afternoon: 'one in the morning and one in the afternoon, like tablets, you know'. Both systems were seen as important sources of help that could assist him to manage his illness. 'But' he added, 'I believe more in *maparn*' (McCoy 2004).

Adverse events occur when Aboriginal people with chronic diseases use traditional healing practices (or other complementary therapies) as alternatives to conventional treatment. Aboriginal patients, and traditional healers, may not be aware that the relational-moral aetiology of diet-related chronic diseases is global (requiring global solutions) rather than local or regional. Aboriginal people may consult traditional healers to look for moral solutions at the local or regional level. If Aboriginal patients feel that conventional medications are making them weak and ill, they may stop taking them and cease attending the health clinic, choosing to consult a traditional healer or other complementary healer instead. For this reason, registration of Aboriginal patients with chronic diseases, and adequate follow-up procedures, are as important as it is with communicable diseases.

12.5 Summary

In Aboriginal Australia today, metabolic diseases such as diabetes and vascular disease have reached epidemic proportions. Aboriginal people suffer from multiple early onset chronic diseases, which are incomprehensible in their complexity. The biomedical model of illness tends to ignore relational-moral causality such as the effects of economic globalism, world trade agreements, and neoliberal politics on people's health. In rural and remote Australia traditional healers provide motivational resources to help restore Aboriginal people's sense of purpose and support their social and emotional well-being. Aboriginal and non-Aboriginal health professionals, researchers, and community representatives must also work together to develop health programmes that are inclusive of traditional and contemporary Aboriginal healing practices.

To be effective, health initiatives must engage with Aboriginal people's cultural values and social imperatives. Medical treatment tends to be tailored to the requirements of self-motivating individuals. Chronic disease self-management programs are articulated in terms of future-oriented, goal-directed individuals who adhere to an ethic of delayed gratification. Aboriginal people live in relational cultures, demonstrate relational autonomy, and adhere to a temporal system in which the rewards of immediate consumption outweigh future adverse health outcomes. Aboriginal and non-Aboriginal health professionals and researchers need to work together to develop common conceptual frameworks around health and illness within which medical practitioners and patients can negotiate comprehensible treatment regimes, chronic disease management programmes and prevention strategies.

References

Australian Institute of Health and Welfare and Australian Bureau of Statistics. *The Health and Welfare of Australia's Aboriginal and Torres Strait Islander Peoples*, Catalogue No. 4704.0. Canberra: Australian Institute of Health and Welfare and Australian Bureau of Statistics, 2003.

Bahr E. (ed.) *The Unseen in Scene*. Aboriginal Art Galerie Bahr, Speyer, Leverkusen: Kulturabteilung Bayer, 2001.

Bell D. *Daughters of the Dreaming*. Melbourne: McPhee Gribble, 1983.

Berndt C. Women's changing ceremonies in northern Australia. *L'Homme* 1950; **1**: 1–87.

Berndt R. *Kunapipi: A Study of an Australian Aboriginal Religious Cult*. Melbourne: F.W. Cheshire, 1951.

Berndt C. Sickness and health in Western Arnhem Land: a traditional perspective. In: Reid, J. (ed.), *Body, Land and Spirit: Health and Healing in Aboriginal Society*. St Lucia: University of Queensland Press, 1982.

Brotman D, Girod P. The metabolic syndrome: a tug-of-war with no winner. *Cleveland Clinic Journal of Medicine* 2002; **69**(12): 990–994.

Connor W. Importance of omega-3 fatty acids in health and disease. *American Journal of Clinical Nutrition* 2000; **71**: 171–175.

Cordain L, Watkins B, Kehler M, Rogers L, Li Y. Fatty acid analysis of wild ruminant tissues: evolutionary implications for reducing diet-related chronic disease. *European Journal of Clinical Nutrition* 2002; **56**: 181–191.

Cowan T. *Treating Diabetes: Practical Advice for Combating a Modern Epidemic*. Washington, DC: The Western Price Foundation, 2004.

Cramer J. *Sounding the Alarm: Remote Area Nurses and Aboriginals at Risk*. Perth: University of Western Australia Press, 2005.

Cumpston J. *Health and Disease in Australia: A History*. Introduced and edited by M.J. Lewis, 1989. Canberra: AGPS, 1928.

Devanesen D. Traditional Aboriginal medicine practice in the Northern Territory, paper presented at the International Symposium on Traditional Medicine, Awaji Island, Japan, 11–13 September, 2000.

Devansen D. and Henshall T. A study of plant medicines in Central Australia. *Transactions of the Menzies Foundation* 1982; **4**: 161–166.

Devitt J, McMasters A. *Living on Medicine: A Cultural Study of End-stage Renal Disease among Aboriginal People*. Alice Springs: IAD Press, 1998.

Dewailly E. n-3 fatty acids and cardiovascular disease risk factors among the Inuit of Nunavik. *The American Journal of Clinical Nutrition* 2001; **74**(4): 464–473.

Donchin A. Reworking autonomy: toward a feminist perspective. *Cambridge Quarterly of Healthcare Ethics* 1995; **4**: 44–55.

Eaton S, Shostak M, Konner M. *The Paleolithic Prescription: A Program of Diet, Exercise and a Design for Living*. New York: Harper & Row, 1988.

Edge H. Extraordinary claims in a cross-cultural context. Paper presented to the Third Symposium of the Bial Foundation, *Aquem e Alem do Cerebro, Vivencias Exceptionais*, Porto, Portugal, 2000, pp. 159–180.

Edge H, Suryani L. A cross-cultural analysis of volition. *Florida Philosophical Review* 2002; **2**(2): 56–72.

Fallon S, Enig M. Australian Aborigines: living off the fat of the land. *Price-Pottenger Nutrition Foundation Health Journal* 1999; **22**(2): 574–581.

Flick B. *Development of a Consultation Strategy for Aboriginal and Torres Strait Islander Peoples in Australia*. Report on Aboriginal and Torres Strait Islanders Consultation, Darwin and Alice Springs, 2001.

Garcia H. An intercultural approach: a tool for enhancing the quality of health services, Direction of Traditional Medicine and Intercultural Development, Secretario de Salud, Mexico. Trans. J. Gapella, Canberra: John Curtin School of Medical Research, 2002.

Gartrell M. *Dear Primitive: A Nurse among the Aborigines*. Sydney: Angus and Robertson, 1957.

Green J. (compiler) *Anmatyerr Ayey Arnang-akert: Anmatyerr Plant Stories by the Women from Laramba (Napperby) Community*. Alice Springs: IAD Press, 2003.

Havecker, C. Understanding Aboriginal culture. *Cosmos Periodicals*. Brisbane, 2002.

Hawkes, C. Marketing activities of global soft drink and fast food companies in emerging markets: a review. In: *Globalization, Diets and Non-communicable Diseases*. Geneva: World Health Organization, 2002.

Heffernan M. Diabetes and Aboriginal peoples: the Haida Gwaii diabetes project in a global perspective. In: Stephenson, PH *et al*. *A Persistent Spirit: Towards Understanding Aboriginal Health in British Columbia*. British Columbia: University of Victoria, 1995, pp. 261–296.

Kouris-Blazos A, Wahlqvist M. Indigenous Australian food culture on cattle stations prior to the 1960s and food intake of older Aborigines in a community studied in 1988. *Asia Pacific Journal of Clinical Nutrition* 2000; **9**(3): 224–231.

Kowanko I, de Crespigny C, Murray H. *Better Medication Management for Aboriginal People with Mental Health Disorders and their Carers: Report on Research Conducted in the Port Lincoln Region*. A collaborative project of the Flinders University School of Nursing and Midwifery and the Aboriginal Drug and Alcohol Council SA, 2003.

Lassak E, McCarthy T. *Australian Medicinal Plants*, Sydney: Reed New Holland, 2001.

Latz P. *Bushfires and Bushtucker: Aboriginal Plant Use in Central Australia*. Alice Springs: IAD Press, 1995.

Leaf A, Weber P. Medical progress: cardiovascular effects of n-3 fatty acids. *New England Journal of Medicine* 1988; **318**(9): 549–557.

Lee A, O'Dea K, Matthews J. Apparent dietary intake in remote Aboriginal communities. *Australian Journal of Public Health* 1994; **18**(2): 190–197.

Leonard D, McDermott R, O'Dea K. Obesity, diabetes and associated cardiovascular risk factors among Torres Strait Islander people. *Australian and New Zealand Journal of Public Health* 2002; **26**: 144–149.

Lindsay E, Berry Y, Jamie E, Bremner J. Antibacterial compounds from *Carissa lanceolata* R.Br. *Phytochemistry* 2000; **55**: 403–406.

Malbunka M. *When I Was Little Like You*. Sydney: Allen & Unwin, 2003.

Maple-Brown L, Brimblecombe J, Chisholm D, O'Dea K. Diabetes care and complications in a remote primary health care setting. *Diabetes Research and Clinical Practice* 2004; **64**(2): 77–83.

McCoy B. 'I believe more in *maparn*': the contested site of desert health. Paper presented to AIATSIS Conference, Indigenous Studies: Sharing the Cultural and Theoretical Space, 22–25 November, Canberra, 2004.

McDermott R, Tulip F, Schmidt B. Diabetes care in remote Australian Indigenous communities. *Medical Journal of Australia* 2004; **180**: 512–516.

McDonald H. *Blood, Bones and Spirit: Aboriginal Christianity in an East Kimberley Town*, Melbourne: Melbourne University Press, 2001.

McDonald H. East Kimberley concepts of health and illness: A contribution to intercultural health programs in northern Australia. Paper presented to AIATSIS Seminar Series, Health and Society: An Australian Indigenous Context, 27 October, Canberra, 2003.

McDonald H. Culture in health research and practice. Paper presented at the Social Determinants of Health Workshop, Cooperative Research Centre for Aboriginal Health, 5–6 July, Adelaide, 2004.

McLean M, Dow W, Bathern R. A study of the comparison between traditional Aboriginal medicines and Western preparations in the treatment and healing of boils, sores and scabies, Unpublished paper, 1996.

Moodie P. Australian Aborigines. In: Trowell HC, Burkitt DP (eds), *Western Diseases: Their Emergence and Prevention*. London: Edward Arnold, 1981, pp. 154–167.

Morelli C. The politics of food. *International Socialism Journal* 2003; **101**.

Ngaanyatjarra Pitjantjatjara Yankunytjatjara (NPY) Women's Council *Ngangkari Work – Anangu Way: Traditional Healers of Central Australia*. Alice Springs: NPY Women's Council, 2003.

O'Dea K. Marked improvement in carbohydrate and lipid metabolism in diabetic Australian Aborigines after temporary reversion to traditional lifestyle. *Diabetes* 1984; **33**(6): 596–603.

O'Dea K. Traditional diet and food preferences of Australian Aboriginal hunter-gatherers. *Philosophical Transactions of the Royal Society of London, Series B*, 1991; **334**: 233–241.

O'Dea K. The therapeutic and preventive potential of the hunter-gatherer lifestyle: insights from Australian Aborigines. In: Temple NJ, Burkitt DP (eds), *Western Diseases: Their Dietary Prevention and Reversibility*. Totowa, NJ: Humana Press, 1994, pp. 349–380.

Reid E. *The Records of Western Australian Plants used by Aboriginals as Medicinal Agents*. South Bentley, WA: Western Australian Institute of Technology, 1977.

Reid J. The role of the *marrnggitj* in contemporary health care. *Oceania* 1978; 49: 96–109.

Reid J. *Sorcerers and Healing Spirits: Continuity and Change in an Aboriginal Medical System*. Canberra: ANU Press, 1983.

Ring I, Brown N. Indigenous health: chronically inadequate responses to damning statistics. *Medical Journal of Australia*, 2002; **177**(11): 629–631.

Sansom B. *The Camp at Wallaby Cross: Aboriginal Fringe Dwellers in Darwin*. Canberra: Australian Institute of Aboriginal Studies, 1980.

Strehlow T. *Songs of Central Australia*. Sydney: Angus and Robertson, 1970.

Tonkinson M. The *mabarn* and the hospital: the selection of treatment in a remote Aboriginal community. In: Reid J. (ed.), *Body, Land and Spirit*, St Lucia: University of Queensland Press, 1982.

Vanstone A. Better nutrition through better management of remote Indigenous stores. Office of Immigration and Multicultural and Indigenous Affairs Media Release, 12 June 2004. Available at: http://www.atsia.gov.au/media/media04/v04029.htm

Wadley G, Martin A. The origins of agriculture: a biological perspective and a new hypothesis. *Journal of the Australasian College of Nutritional and Environmental Medicine* 2000; **19**(1): 3–12.

Washington H. The back to the future diet: healthy diet habits of traditional cultures. *Harvard Health Letter*, 6 June 1994.

Wiminydji, Peile A. A desert Aborigine's view of health and nutrition. *Journal of Anthropological Research* 1978; **34**(4): 497–523.

Young D. The colour of rubbish: a short paper about how things become 'rubbishy' on the Anangu Pitjantjatjara Lands in Central Australia. Paper presented at Ninth International Conference on Hunter-Gatherer Societies, Edinburgh, Scotland, 2002.

13 Massage and Reflexology

Paula Mullins

13.1 Introduction

'Massage' is defined as: 'Any skilled form of touch applied with sensitivity and compassion by professionally trained massage therapists with the specific intent of increasing comfort, complementing the medical treatment, improving clinical outcomes and promoting wholeness' (Gibson 1992). Massage has been used therapeutically for many thousands of years and is a key modality in medical traditions such as Ayurveda, Unami and Chinese medicine. There is evidence of the therapeutic use of massage in China more than 5000 years ago (Watson 1997) and Hippocrates is credited with saying: 'The physician must be experienced in many things but assuredly in rubbing for rubbing can bind a joint that is loose and loosen a joint that is too rigid' (Calvert 2002).

In Victorian times massage was a key aspect of diabetes management strategies along with relaxation, opium and mild exercise (Elson 1998). This treatment eventually lost favour as newer therapies were developed and the increasing interest in 'scientific' activities. Nightingale in her *Notes on Nursing* suggested that the need for touch in care actually increased as the use of technology increased (Naisbitts 1984). Technology and research have changed the way diabetes care is delivered and have improved outcomes. They have also increased expectations that the person with diabetes will participate in their care and undertake significant self-management, which increases the burden of having to cope with the disease. Modern diabetes management consists of psychological and spiritual care and stress management, as well as diet, activity and medicines to achieve metabolic control.

Massage is often combined with essential oils (aromatherapy) and may be directed at a defined area of the body or to the whole body, see Chapter 6. Many different types of massage are used depending on the indication for the massage, for example, gentle lymphatic drainage massage strokes are used to move the lymph in order to reduce oedema and remove toxins; rhythmic relaxation massage strokes reduce stress and promote sleep, and more vigorous sports massage strokes relieve muscle tension. The various forms of massage and touch therapies are outlined in Table 13.1.

Complementary Therapies and the Management of Diabetes and Vascular Disease   Editor Trish Dunning
© 2006 John Wiley & Sons, Ltd.

Table 13.1 Overview of the main types of massage and touch therapies and a brief description of each type. More details about touch therapies can be found in Chapter 8. Some types of massage are vigorous while others are more light and gentle depending on the degree of pressure used. The pressure may need to be adjusted in particular circumstance.

Massage type	Brief description
Swedish or Relaxation massage	Long gliding strokes (effleurage) or kneading strokes (petrissage) are combined with friction, vibration and tapping (tapotement) to induce relaxation and improve circulation.
Esalen massage	Esalen massage was developed in California and blends the long, flowing strokes of Swedish massage with light, rocking joint manipulations and deep tissue massage if indicated.
Bowen Therapy	A gentle technique developed in Australia that aims to improve joint flexibility, promote muscle relaxation and balance the energy systems in the body. Bowen therapists aim to trigger a response form the body rather than physically altering the body. It does not aim to 'fix health problems' but to achieve a harmonious state to help the body heal itself. The mechanisms of action are not known. It is postulated that manipulating soft tissue triggers a response in the sensory nerve endings that results in changes in the nervous system, which induce relaxation.
Compassionate Touch	Compassionate Touch combines gentle touch, communication skills such as listening and reflective feedback as part of a system of focussed attention and was developed specifically for use with older people.
Therapeutic Touch (TT)	TT practitioners believe energy extends beyond the skin into an energy field that surrounds and penetrates the body (the aura). The aim of TT is to rebalance energy blockages in the aura. TT practitioners do not actually touch the body; they work with their hands in the aura to stimulate the individual's innate healing powers. It can be very useful if actual touch is contraindicated or the person dislikes being touched.
Holistic Touch	Is an energy-based therapy that considers as a sacred art. It consists of a collection of non-invasive modalities where healing is achieved through the centred heart and is therefore a spiritual process.
Acupressure (see Chapter 11)	Is a component of Chinese Medicine. Pressure is applied to points along the energy channels or meridians to activate the *chi* or life force or eliminate excess chi to restore balance. Acupressure can be firm or light and either stimulating or relaxing depending on the points used and the pressure.
Shiatsu. Similar therapies are: Jin Shin Jyutsu® Reiki	Shiatsu is similar to acupressure and originated in Japan. Pressure is applied using the fingers, hands, elbows and knees to balance the *ki* (Japanese form of *chi*). There are different forms of Shiatsu. Some focus on meridians, some on the muscular system, breathing practise and Buddhist philosophy. Reiki may or may not involve actual touch. It aims to strengthen the individual's natural life force by balancing the energy field. Reiki has been adopted in such modalities as the Radiance Technique and Mariel.

Craniosacral therapy	Practitioners use gentle pressure to align the bones and soft tissue of the head, vertebral column and sacrum to balance the flow of cerebrospinal fluid. The main application is to relieve headache, neck and back pain and assist with balance and stress management
Lomi Lomi	Hawaiian shaman as originally performed Lomi Lomi as a spiritual modality. Deep pressure is applied with the elbows and forearms but gentle strokes, pressure point therapy, walking on the individual's back and rhythmical rocking movements are also used. It is used to stimulate the innate life force or mana.
Trigger point therapy	Trigger point therapy encompasses a range of modalities that aim to treat sore areas, which are felt as 'knots' in the muscle. They are known as trigger points because they can cause pain to radiate to other areas. Therapies include myotherapy.
Reflexology	A specific massage technique usually performed on the hands or more commonly the feet. The underlying philosophy is that every part of the body is associated with a specific point on the feet or hands, the reflex point, and lies within a specific longitudinal zone. Stimulating the points can affect the reciprocal part of the body to improve homeostasis and induce relaxation.
Lymphatic drainage	Lymphatic drainage is a specific type of massage where the practitioner uses very light, slow, repetitious strokes to move the lymph to excrete excess toxins and fluids. It is very effective in managing post surgical limb oedema and relieving pain.
Polarity therapy massage	The aim of polarity therapy is to balance the positive and negative poles of electrical energy in the body. The energy is believed to flow in five vertical currents and horizontal zones and outside the body. The aim is to remove blockages to restore energy flow or dissipate excess energy using gentle pressure above and below the blockage.
Myofacial release	Aims to reduce tension in connective tissue and fascia supporting muscle, bones and organs to correct alignment and reduce pain and spasm by restoring alignment. A sustained pressure is used to apply long, slow gliding strokes with the fingers, hands and forearms.
Syncardial massage	Syncardial massage is given using Fuch's apparatus, which works on the principle that when a cuff is placed around an extremity and inflated at the moment when the pulse wave passes beneath the cuff, the applied pressure aids arterial contraction and the output and blood flow are increased.

When delivering a massage the therapist ensures:

- The patient knows what to expect from the massage.
- If essential oils are used, they are therapeutically appropriate and chosen according to the principles of Quality Use of Essential Oils (QUEO) (Dunning 2005) and the condition being treated, see Chapter 6.
- They are knowledgeable and competent to perform the massage and to use essential oils therapeutically if relevant.
- The privacy and comfort of the patient.
- Where possible, the environment is conductive to achieving the massage goals, for example, by selecting an appropriate temperature, music, and lighting.
- The massage type, pressure and duration of the massage suit the patient.

- The position of the patient does not increase or cause discomfort and is appropriate to any underlying health condition especially in acute care settings.
- Hand contact is maintained with the person receiving the massage as much as possible.
- The outcomes are relevant to the massage goals and are monitored.
- The massage, essential oils if used and other relevant information are documented and communicated to relevant carers.

Although there is a great deal of research into the effects of massage, sample sizes are often small, the research methods differ among studies, the type of massage used is often not specified, and the measurement tools are not described or are not validated (Vickers 1996; MacDonald 2005). There is, however, some evidence to support positive effects such as reducing nausea, cortisol levels, pain and anxiety, improving sleep, and reducing hospital length of stay. Less compelling evidence exists for improvements in depression, pressure area care and other vital signs (Vickers 1996).

13.2 Massage Diagnosis and Care Processes

Consultation sheets completed by the therapist before the massage begins provide important information and a record of the initial communication between the client and the therapist. The record includes information about the client's health, both past and present, and medications and is the basis on which the massage therapist decides how the treatment should progress.

Having completed the history and assessment, the therapist informs the client what to expect from the treatment and sets a realistic aim/goal for the treatment, and indicates the number of treatments likely to be needed to achieve the goal. The clients should be told how to prepare for a massage, for example, whether they need to undress, how to get on the couch and any special precautions including the possible risk of hypoglycaemia. The therapist also needs to explain what to expect during the massage and how it will be carried out. Massage, just like any other treatment, aims to achieve certain results. The therapist assesses the condition of the client and uses the assessment and history to develop a treatment plan and the outcomes to be achieved, which must be realistic. Progress is monitored by assessing relevant changes between treatments.

The therapist continuously reassesses the client's condition, symptoms and changes in the original problems as well as how they feel after each treatment. The rhythm, the speed and the direction of the strokes are adjusted as necessary to prevent adverse events and achieve maximum benefit. The wishes of the client are key issues when deciding these issues. The slower, smoother and more continuous the strokes are, the more relaxing and soothing the treatment. The more rapid the strokes are, the more stimulating the effect. Whatever the massage method and style, the client eventually feels a change taking place. This usually happens around the fourth or fifth week in a course of weekly treatments.

13.3 Massage and Diabetes

There are many potential benefits of massage for people with diabetes particularly relaxation massage such as physical and emotional comfort and small reductions in blood glucose (1–2 mmol/L) (Rose 2005). Living with diabetes is inherently stressful. Fluctuating blood glucose levels cause significant short- and long-term complications, see Chapter 1. The practical demands of balancing food intake with insulin or oral medications, monitoring blood glucose and regulating exercise, as well as undertaking usual life activities, can be a daunting task for many people. Worry about developing diabetes complications or anxiety relating to work or interpersonal relations, can add to the stress of self-care. Massage can reduce stress and improve well-being, which has secondary effect on blood glucose and lipid levels, and therefore may play a role in preventing complications.

Andersson *et al.* (2004) carried out a pilot study of 11 women with type 2 diabetes to determine the short-term effects of tactile massage on blood glucose, stress hormones and well-being. The women had an hour whole body massage each week for 10 weeks and continued their usual diabetes treatment. A small but significant reduction in HbA_{1c} occurred, but there were no significant changes in hormone levels. There are a number of confounding factors in the study, which are acknowledged by the authors but the results suggest massage may complement usual diabetes care.

Field (Field *et al.* 1992) provided 30-minute back massage daily for five days to 52 hospitalised depressed and adjustment disorder children and adolescents and compared them to a control group who viewed relaxing videotapes. The massaged subjects were less depressed and anxious. Lower salivary cortisol levels were recorded after massage in depressed subjects. Nurses rated the subjects as less anxious and more cooperative and reported better sleep patterns. The study did not specifically address diabetes but depression is a significant problem in diabetes and the findings may be relevant to adolescents with diabetes and depression or anxiety. In another study Field *et al.* (1997) demonstrated reduction in blood glucose levels and reduced anxiety in children whose parents gave them regular massages. The parents also reported feeling more relaxed, which helped them cope with their child's diabetes.

Massage increases the circulation of blood and lymph, which helps eliminate toxins from the body (Price and Price 1999). Circulation is often impaired in people with diabetes, which can reduce the delivery of oxygen and nourishment to the tissues and the removal of waste products from the tissues. Although not specifically tested in people with diabetes, massage may have a complementary role in foot care to help support the circulation to the feet. Khanman (2005) undertook a small study involving 15 people with type 2 diabetes in Thailand. Foot massages were given on three consecutive days and lasted for an hour each session. Foot numbness was assessed before and at 15 and again 30 minutes after each massage using pinprick and visual analogue scales. Short-term improvements in numbness were recorded. There are a number of inherent flaws in Khanman's study but it does suggest further research is warranted.

If diabetic neuropathy is present, the massage strokes should be gentle. Gentle strokes help alleviate the numbness, irritation or tingling and reduce pain, which are common neuropathic symptoms. People with diabetes are prone to connective tissue damage as a result of long-term hyperglycaemia, which reduces mobility and elasticity of the myofascial system. Tissue glycosolation results in stiffness in muscles, tendons and ligaments, as well as a reduced range of motion in the joints. Massage helps facilitate greater joint mobility and increases the range of movement, particularly if it is combined with stretching and regular exercise, making activity easier and less painful.

Syncardial massage, see Table 13.1, may improve blood flow in people with peripheral neuropathy. Voltonen and Lilius (1973) treated 38 people with diabetes with syncardial massage every second day for four weeks and reported 'improved symptoms' in 50 per cent of patients. Syncardial massage is uncommon and may not be practical on a day-to-day basis. In addition, the study is old, is poorly reported and has not been repeated.

Dillon (1983) observed that eight lean, well-controlled patients with type 1 diabetes, using their usual dosages of regular and intermediate-acting insulins, who massaged their insulin injection sites with an electric vibrator for three minutes 15 minutes after injecting had higher blood insulin levels and lower glucose levels 15 minutes after the start of massage, which lasted for 29 minutes. Serum glucose levels fell and were 8.3 per cent lower 30 minutes after massage and 44 minutes post-injection compared to the control day when participants did not massage their injection sites and the change was significant ($p < 0.05$). At 45 minutes post-massage, the difference in glucose levels was even more striking ($4.2\,\text{mmol/L} \pm 6$) when compared to the control day ($4.9\text{mmol/L} \pm 4$). Eight of these patients and 18 others were followed up for two years. They massaged their injection sites for three minutes at each meal. After three to six months, the mean Hb_{A_1} for the 26 patients fell from 10.5 per cent ± 1.73 to 8.5 per cent ± 1.69 per cent (normal Hb_{A_1} was 8.2 per cent according to the laboratory assay used).

After 12–18 months of injection-site massage, eight had normal Hb_{A_1} levels, and the remaining 18 patients had mean Hb_{A_1} levels of 8.41 per cent ± 1.58 per cent, which was a significant improvement from baseline ($p < 0.001$). Dillon proposed that injection-site massage could increase the bioavailability of insulin in the post-prandial state. This is an old study and the significance is difficult to interpret. It is unlikely people with diabetes massage their injection sites at all, let alone with an electric vibrator. However, it suggests that massage over an insulin injection site immediately after an injection may improve insulin uptake.

Klauser et al. (1992) undertook nine 20-minute abdominal massage treatments in people suffering from constipation and a control group and compared stool frequency and colon transit time with baseline. They found a modest increase in stool frequency from 0.59 stools per day to 0.68 after abdominal massage. The transit time reduced from 126 hours to 111 hours compared with no change in the control group but the change was not statistically significant. People with diabetes and autonomic neuropathy often suffer erratic blood glucose levels and abdominal discomfort due to gastroparesis. Anecdotally, abdominal massage relives such discomfort but good quality evidence for a beneficial effect is lacking.

13.4 Massage and Cardiovascular Disease

There is some evidence to support a role for massage in managing cardiovascular disease and its management. For example, massage may help reduce shoulder and neck pain following surgical procedures such as stents and angiograms and provide emotional comfort as people come to terms with a life-threatening complication. Short sessions are usually recommended considering the position of electrodes, oxygen therapy, IV lines and the medication regime (MacDonald 2005).

Stevenson (1994) undertook a randomised controlled trial of post-cardiac surgical patients (n = 100) who received (a) foot massage with a carrier oil; (b) foot massage with essential oils; or (c) a chat and no massage. Each group was treated for 20 minutes. Respiratory and heart rates and blood pressure and pain were measured as well as anxiety and tension using the Spielberger Score. Groups (a) and (b) showed minor, transient physical effects and a statistically significant reduction in the respiratory rate. Psychological changes were clinically and statistically significant during the treatment and lasted for at least two hours after the massage. It is not known whether Stevenson's subjects included people with diabetes but since heart disease is a major cause of morbidity and mortality in people with diabetes, the findings could reasonably be extrapolated to this population.

However, some authorities suggest vigorous back massage could put undue strain on a damaged heart (Tyler *et al.* 1990). Tyler *et al.* found venous oxygen saturation dropped from 67 per cent to 63 per cent and heart rate increased from 99 to 103 beats per minute after a 1-minute back rub in post-cardiac surgical patients, but returned to normal within 4 minutes. The clinical relevance of this finding is unclear and it is not clear whether Tyler *et al.*'s subjects included people with diabetes. People with diabetes may have atypical signs of cardiac disease and silent myocardial infarction could make such changes difficult to interpret. Therefore, massage therapists need to be aware of the indicators of cardiovascular disease, avoid vigorous or stimulating massage strokes and discuss the treatment with the individual's doctor before undertaking a massage.

Benefits of massage for people with diabetes

Despite the lack of quality evidence, there appear to be a number of benefits of massage that may apply to people with diabetes (Rankin-Box 2001). These benefits are shown in Table 13.2. In interpreting these potential benefits, it must be remembered that people with diabetes frequently take multiple medicines, which can have associated positive effects or adverse events that can make it difficult

Table 13.2 Some reported benefits of massage.

Effects	Potential benefits
Increases cellular metabolism.	Efficient use of energy. Detoxification. Improves healing. Improves skin tone and condition. May assist intracellular glucose utilisation.
Increases local circulation by dilating the peripheral blood vessels.	Improves distribution of nutrients, oxygen and medicines to tissues. Improves removal of waste products. Aids healing and tissue repair. Reduces blood pressure. May increase insulin uptake and play a role in controlling blood glucose levels.
Relieves psychological stress.	Stimulates endorphins and serotonin. Reduces muscle spasm. Improves sense of well-being. Induces relaxation.
Reduces muscular tension.	Improves muscle contractility and relaxation. Relieves cramps and pain. Improves circulation. Improves joint mobility.
Reduces oedema.	Improves circulation and lymph flow. Relieves local pain
Reduces pain.	Improves circulation. Improves removal of waste products. Reduces oedema. Reduces muscle spasm. Psychological effects on pain perception. Endorphin production.
Boost immune system.	Improved circulation. Endorphin production. Reduces stress. Improved immunity/resistance to infection.
Removal of lung secretions (specific massage strokes, physiotherapy)	Improved breathing. Clear lungs.
Energetic and spiritual effects to rebalance charkas, meridians, reflex zones.	Improved sense of well-being. Ease transitions.

to interpret whether the outcomes achieved are attributable to the massage, the medicine or a combination of both.

Precautions to consider when considering massage for people with diabetes

Massage is generally a safe therapy with few reported adverse events. Most people become relaxed and sometimes a little disorientated after receiving a massage, which can make it difficult for them to recognise hypoglycaemia. In addition, small reductions in blood glucose during massage have been recorded, which may be enough to contribute to hypoglycaemia. Therefore, it is important to monitor the blood glucose before and after the massage treatment and to time the massage appropriately with respect to food consumption and hypoglycaemic medicine doses.

Likewise postural hypotension is possible when changing positions from a lying or sitting position especially if the person has autonomic neuropathy, or is old. Appropriate care during position changes can avoid unwanted consequences of postural hypotension such as light-headedness or falls.

People with diabetes who are unwell with an intercurrent illness, a diabetes-related complication, receiving any form of treatment including those involving medical devices, and people taking complementary and/or conventional medicines may require extra monitoring and short duration, gentle massages. That is, the massage should be adapted to the individual's physical and mental status taking into account the pressure to be used, the site of any devices such as drain tubes, casts, IV lines, and the position the person can assume at the time (MacDonald 2005).

In addition, lotion may be a preferable lubricant to oil in bed-bound people because it absorbs into the skin without leaving a greasy residue, does not affect clothing or gloves worn by staff delivering the routine care and is less likely to spill (MacDonald 2005), which reduces the possibility of falls for both the patient and staff. Petroleum-based products are not recommended because they clog the skin and can inhibit elimination and uptake of topically applied medicines. However, in hypothermic states, for example, older people after severe hypoglycaemia or in the winter, thicker oils such as caster oil can be very warming.

Extra care is required for people with low platelet levels, fragile skin, neuropathy and oedema and those taking anti-coagulant medicines. In these circumstances pressure should be gentle and the massage of short duration to avoid causing bruising, bleeding and fatigue. Massage is generally contraindicated over surgical incisions, open wounds, tumours, petechiae and bruises. The position may be restricted by respiratory difficulties, cardiovascular disease or orthopaedic or surgical incisions. Great care should be taken to ensure privacy during the massage and to follow appropriate infection control procedures.

Contraindications to massage in people with diabetes

Many authors list contraindications to massage, for example MacDonald (2005), often in clinical guidelines, and frequently for specific speciality areas such as cancer, see Table 13.3. The frequently cited contraindications to massage apply equally to people with diabetes and include:

- the presence of acute systemic infection;
- acute episodes of diseases affecting the musculoskeletal system such as rheumatoid arthritis;
- using techniques likely to be inappropriately stimulating such as vigorous strokes to increase the circulation in ill or weak patients, for example, older people or during acute illness;
- vigorous massage when the skin is fragile or in the presence of osteoporosis or Charcot's arthropathy or where bruising is likely. In these cases lighter pressure or touch therapies should be used;

- presence of deep vein thrombosis or phlebitis;
- during a massage the therapist should avoid massaging over burns, tumours, broken skin and localised infections such as fungal infection on the feet (Vickers 1996).

Some massage therapists include hypertension, cancer, severe asthma and diabetes as contraindications to massage. However, no definitive research was identified to support massage being contraindicated in people with these conditions. With respect to diabetes, the major concern appears to be causing hypoglycaemia during long massages. However, massage may actually be a beneficial adjunct to conventional care in managing the blood glucose if the massage is of an appropriate duration and timing and offered in consultation with the individual's doctor.

Adverse events associated with massage

Specific adverse events associated with massage and people with diabetes are rare in the literature. Adverse events that are described in the general population are mild (Vickers 1996). However, when essential oils are used as part of the massage, allergies and other adverse events may occur, see Chapter 6. Adverse events are more likely if the person's position or the massage pressure is not adjusted to suit the individual, especially when the person is acutely ill, diabetes complications are present or they are taking medications such as anticoagulants, see Table 13.4.

Table 13.3 Contraindications and precautions when using massage. It is advisable to consult the nurse/doctor before undertaking massage in acute care settings.

Precaution/ Contraindication	Management
Broken skin Cuts/boils Injection sites	Cover the site, if small. Do not massage over the site.
Big bruises	Use very light pressure.
Inflammation and/or swelling	Use very light pressure.
Recent surgery	Do not massage over broken skin.
Recent fracture	Avoid fracture site.
Diabetes	Consider possibility of hypoglycaemia if a long massage and the person is on insulin or oral glucose lowering agents agents. Take care in presence of autonomic or peripheral neuropathy. Consider possibility of postural hypotension.
Varicose veins	Use very light pressure over varicose veins.
Cancer	There is no evidence that massage spreads cancer. Consider the type of massage used, massage pressure, the state of the skin, tiredness.
Recent alcohol intake or large meal	Time the massage appropriately.

Table 13.4 Categories of medicines people with diabetes could be taking and the potential adverse events associated with massage.

Medicine	Potential adverse events
Narcotics	Positioning is important to reduce the risk of falls. May not recognise hypoglycaemia.
Anticoagulants	Bruising. Bleeding. Light pressure and not massaging over bruises is important.
Insulin and oral glucose lowering agents	Hypoglycaemia. Therapists need to watch for signs of hypoglycaemia and ensure treatment is available. Monitor blood glucose. Take care to reduce the falls risk associated with hypoglycaemia.
Antihypertensive agents	Body wraps and hot packs can cause peripheral blood vessels to dilate and result in hypotension, especially postural hypotension if autonomic neuropathy is present and make increase the risk of falls. Long massages may be contraindicated.
Lipid-lowering agents.	May cause muscle pain, therefore, the massage may increase the discomfort. It may be necessary to use gentle massage strokes.

A potential adverse effect of massage is hypoglycaemia in people taking insulin or glucose lowering agents. The risk is extrapolated from massage studies using healthy volunteers. No study using massage in people with diabetes reports hypoglycaemia or other adverse effects. However, it is not clear from the reports whether adverse effects did not occur, or whether they did occur, but were not measured or not reported (Ezzo *et al.* 2001).

13.5 Reflexology

Reflexology is a focused pressure technique usually applied to the feet or hands. It is based on the theory that the reflexes and zones on parts of the body correspond to all organs, glands and other muscle parts. Stimulating the reflex areas assists the body to return to a state of homeostasis (Bisson 2005). Although reflexology has been known since ancient Egypt, Dr William Fitzgerald (1872–1942) an ear, nose and throat specialist from the United States is credited with developing modern reflexology, which he named 'zone therapy'. Fitzgerald found that pressure applied to the mouth, nose, throat, tongue, hands, feet and joints relieved pain. He also reported that reflexology relieved morning sickness and nausea from other causes, although his findings were not substantiated in controlled trials. Dr Shelby Riley worked closely with Fitzgerald and developed the zone theory further. In turn, Eunice Ingham, a physiotherapist, who worked with Riley, developed her own foot reflex theory in the early 1930s, including a chart depicting the areas of the feet that corresponded to specific parts of the body. Many reflexes overlap each other. Manipulating specific reflexes reduces stress and activates the parasympathetic nervous system.

The zones consist of ten longitudinal systems running from the head to the toes and fingers that organise the relationship among the parts, organs and glands of the body, each of which are represented in a particular zone. There are five zones on each side of the body. The reflexes pass within the zones and are three-dimensional in that they are the same on the back as they are on the front of the body. Reflexologists suggest that pressure applied to any part of the zone affects the entire zone. Usually working on the right foot treats the right side of the body and the left foot the left side, except disorders of the brain or central nervous system where points on the opposite foot are worked.

Reflexology also uses four horizontal zones to treat the parts of the body in a particular location or 'map', commonly the transverse pelvic line, transverse waistline, transverse diaphragm and the transverse neckline. The zones and reflexes are different from the acupuncture points and meridians used in Chinese medicine or Ayurveda.

Ingham (1938) and Goodwin (1988) considered that malfunction of any organ or part of the body results in tiny crystalline deposits of calcium and uric acid on the nerve endings of the feet. They indicated that gentle pressure facilitates the breakdown and elimination of these deposits to promote health and well-being. The process is referred to as detoxification and the signs that it is occurring are known as a 'healing crisis' because once the deposits are eliminated, healing can begin.

Reflexology treatment

Usually the reflexologist only uses his or her hands to work the points with specific 'caterpillar' and 'hook' massage strokes. However, in some Asian countries electrical or mechanical stimulation is used, which may be contraindicated on the feet of people with diabetes and peripheral neuropathy because of the possibility of causing trauma. A reflexology treatment usually lasts between 30 and 60 minutes and begins on the right foot commencing on the bottom of the foot at the heel, which is said to support the innate feedback loops that control temperature, blood pressure, respiratory and heart rates to maintain homeostasis.

Goodwin (1988) stated that the foot is treated by applying gentle pressure along each zone systematically until the entire foot has been covered, including the dorsum, sides and top of both feet. Initially, gentle massage and stroking movements are used followed by deep thumb and finger pressure. If there is an imbalance or blockage of energy in any of the zones or reflexes, the corresponding point on the foot may feel tender or painful. Even though the reflexologist may be specifically working on one organ, other organs in the same zone might be affected, for example, the eyes and kidneys lie in the same zone. Tension, congestion or some other imbalance affects the whole zone and it is possible to treat one part of the zone, such as the eye, to bring about a change in other specified parts of the body, for example, the kidneys (Barron 1990).

Bisson (2005) recommended using gentle pressure in people with cardiovascular disease to avoid undue strain on the heart and circulation particularly when the individual has a pacemaker or artificial heart valves. He suggested reflexology could relieve the symptoms of angina, regulate the heartbeat and 'treat hypertension and hypotension' but does not cite any references to support these benefits. He recommends avoiding working on any reflexes related to thrombosis when it is in an unstable condition.

It is possible that working on the pancreas and adrenal gland points could help manage blood glucose levels especially in people with type 2 diabetes, primarily by reducing stress (Boothe 1994). However, no objective evidence was found to support this contention. The other endocrine points and the digestive and lymphatic system might also be worked. Working on the sex organ points may be beneficial when sexual dysfunction is present but again, no evidence for a beneficial effect was found.

The feet of people with diabetes should be checked very carefully before commencing a reflexology treatment. Impaired circulation and nervous function may mean peripheral neuropathy is present with reduced sensation in the feet that can make it difficult for the person to tell if the pressure is too hard, especially those with or at risk of Charcot's arthropathy. If a reflexologist notices active infection, ulceration or trauma, they should refer the person to their doctor or a podiatrist before undertaking a reflexology treatment to ensure appropriate treatment is commenced.

Increased circulation following a reflexology treatment may cause the blood glucose levels to fluctuate. Therefore, blood glucose levels should be monitored before and after a reflexology treatment. Hypoglycaemia can occur and the therapist and person with diabetes must watch for any warning signs such as a rapid pulse, sweating and disorientation. Table 13.5 illustrates the purported risks and benefits of reflexology.

Evidence to support beneficial effects of reflexology in diabetes

Boothe (1994) stated that, although a number of articles describe how individual health-care professionals successfully combine reflexology in their areas of work,

Table 13.5 The risks and benefits of reflexology. Reflexology is generally a safe non-interventional therapy provided the therapists monitor the person, particularly those at risk of hypoglycaemia, hypotension and foot trauma. Note: Only anecdotal evidence was found to support these benefits.

Benefits	Risks
Relaxation, reduced stress. Improved circulation, especially locally. Reduced pain, for example peripheral neuropathy and the discomfort and nausea of gastroparesis	Fatigue, nausea, increased perspiration on the feet following a treatment that might increase the risk of tissue maceration and infection. Hypotension, hypoglycaemia. Increased risk of damage if Charcot's arthropathy is present

almost all of these texts refer to case histories and it is extremely difficult to find details of clinical trials especially concerning diabetes.

Despite wide-scale practice, reflexology remains under-researched and some reflexologists maintain that because the reflexology treatment is so closely tailored to the needs of individuals, large-scale trials are not feasible. Some small-scale studies pertaining to diabetes and vascular disease were identified but many contain methodological flaws. For example, Wang (1993) studied 32 people with diabetes randomised into two groups. One group was treated with glucose-lowering agents (GLA) and foot reflexology, the other group received GLA only. Fasting blood glucose levels, platelet aggregation, length and wet weight of the thrombus senility symptom scores and serum lipid peroxide were monitored for 30 days. These parameters were significantly reduced in the foot reflexology group ($p < 0.05$) but not in the GLA only group. Wang (1993) suggested that foot reflexology was an effective treatment for type 2 diabetes. However, due to the limited information provided, it was not possible to determine whether other factors such as changes in diet, exercise and medication could have influenced the glucose levels. In addition, the time and financial commitments needed for daily reflexology treatment may make it prohibitive for many people with diabetes.

Ying Ma (1998) observed the blood flow rate using a colour Doppler ultrasonic examination before and after foot reflexology in a treatment group of 20 people with type 2 diabetes and control group of 15 people without diabetes and no arterial disease affecting blood flow to the lower limbs. There was a significantly higher blood flow rate to the feet of people with type 2 diabetes after reflexology treatment than in the control group. Again, the significance of this finding is difficult to determine.

Frankel (1997) explored the physiological effects of reflexology in a pilot study to 'Identify if reflexology and foot massage affect the physiology of the body by measuring baroreceptor reflex sensitivity, blood pressure, and sinus arrhythmia.' Twenty volunteers were randomised to receive either reflexology or foot massage and four volunteers acted as controls. There was no difference between the reflexology and foot massage groups, although both responded treatment groups had a greater response than the controls. These results appear to indicate that reflexology is no different from foot massage but it is not possible to determine whether reflexology only produced a relaxation effect or whether there was a true effect. Frankel discussed the limitations of the study, including non-randomisation of the control group and the fact that he delivered and evaluated the treatments, which could have introduced researcher bias. Frankel suggested the study be repeated using a larger sample and full randomisation could address some of the limitations. However, Mackereth et al. (2000) suggest an alternative approach would be to employ some form of quasi-experimental design.

Dryden et al. (1999) offered hand and foot massage incorporating reflexology techniques to 18 patients in a study conducted over four months. A total of 61 treatments were administered. Initially the intention was to deliver a maximum of six treatments to every patient (98 treatments), however, the actual number of treatments received per person varied according to their length of stay on the ward and the availability of a practitioner at a time convenient to the patient. Twenty-seven hand and 34 foot massages were given. Thirty-seven men and 24 women took part; age range 17–68 years, mean 44.

The aim was to deliver treatments of 30-minutes duration. In practice, treatment times varied between 19 and 46 minutes, mean 30.8. Physiological findings of statistical significance were pre- and post-recordings of heart rate and systolic blood pressure. A typical bell-shaped distribution curve was identified that allowed for a two-tailed T-test to be performed using SPSS. Both showed post-treatment reductions. Highly significant was the difference in the heart rate after treatment from 90 bpm to 84 bpm ($p = 0.000$). Post-treatment recordings of systolic pressure were also significant, dropping from 127 mmhg to 122 mmhg ($p = 0.003$). Diastolic blood pressure and respiratory rate also showed some reduction; however, these were not statistically significant.

Adverse events associated with reflexology

Reflexology is safe and adverse events are rare (O' Mathuna 2003; Bisson 2005). The most commonly reported adverse effects are minor and include fatigue, increased parasymapathetic activity, headache, nausea, increased perspiration, and diarrhoea (Bisson 2005). Anecdotally, reflexologists indicate that reflexology can elicit a catharsis or a 'healing crisis' due to the breakdown and elimination of the crystalline deposits as part of the detoxification process, which usually lasts one to two days. Symptoms of the healing crisis include physical symptoms such as headaches, nausea, diarrhoea and feeling cold, and emotional effects such as unexplained crying and lowered mood. Good quality evidence to support these effects or the frequency with which they occur or their significance is lacking.

References

Acolet D, Modi N, Giannakoulopoulos X, Bond C, Weg W, Clow A, Glover V. Changes in plasma cortisol and catecholamine concentrations in response to massage in preterm infants. *Archives of Disease in Childhood* 1993; **68**: 29–31.

Andersson K, Wandell P, Tornkvist L. Tactile massage improves glycaemic control in women with type 2 diabetes: a pilot study. *Practical Diabetes International* 2004; **21**(3): 105–109.

Barron H. Towards better health with reflexology. *Nursing Standard* 1990; **4**: 32–33.

Bisson D. Reflexology. In: Frishman W, Weintraub M, Micozzi M. (eds) *Complementary and Integrative Therapies for Cardiovascular Disease*. Missouri: Elsevier Mosby, 2005, pp. 331–341.

Calvert R. *History of Massage*. Rochester: Healing Arts Press, 2002.

Dillon R. Improved serum insulin profiles individuals who massaged their insulin injection sites. *Diabetes Care* 1983; **6**(4): 399–401.

Dryden S, Holden S, Mackereth P. Just the ticket: the findings of a pilot complementary therapy service (part 11). *Complementary Therapy in Nursing and Midwifery* 1999; **5**: 15–18.

Dunning T. Applying a Quality Use of Medicines framework to using essential oils in nursing practice. *Complementary Therapies in Clinical Practice* 2005; **11**: 172–181.

Elson D, Meredith M. Therapy for type 2 diabetes mellitus. *World Medical Journal* 1998; **97**: 49–54.

Field T, Hernandez-Reif M, LaGreca A, Shak K, Schenberg K, Khun C. Massage lowers blood glucose levels in children with diabetes. *Diabetes Spectrum* 1997; **10**: 237–239.

Field T, Morrow C, Valdeon C, Larson S, Kuhn C, Schanberg S. Massage reduces anxiety in child and adolescent psychiatric patients. *Journal of the American Academy of Child and Adolescent Psychiatry* 1992; **31**(1): 125–131.

Frankel B. The effects of reflexology on baroreceptor reflex sensitivity, blood pressure and sinus arrhythmia. *Complementary Therapies* 1997; **5**: 80–84.

Gale E, Mackereth P. Touch/massage workshops – a pilot study. *Complementary Therapies in Medicine* 1994; **2**(2): 93–98.

Gibson K. *Developing a Hospital Based Massage Therapy Program*. Boulder CO: Carebased Technologies, 1992.

Goodwin H. Reflex zone therapy. Cited in Rankin-Box D (ed.), *Complementary Health Therapies: A Guide for Nurses and the Caring Professions*. London: Chapman and Hall, 1988.

Ingham E. *Stories the Feet Can Tell*. St Petersburg, FL: Ingham, 1938.

Khanman S. The effects of foot massage as a complementary nursing intervention on numbness in non-insulin dependent diabetes mellitus patients. Unpublished thesis, Faculty of Nursing, Mahidol University Thailand, 2005.

Klauser A, Flaschentrager J, Gehrke A, Muller-Lissner S. Abdominal wall massage – effect of colonic function in healthy volunteers and patients with chronic constipation. *Gastroenterology* 1992; **30**(4): 247–251.

MacDonald G. *Massage for the Hospital Patient and Medically Frail Client*. Philadelphia, PA: Lippincott, Williams and Wilkins, 2005.

Naisbitt W. *Megatrends*. New York: Warner Books, 1984.

O'Mathuna D. Reflexology for relaxation but not diagnosis. *Alternative Medicine Alert*, 2003, pp. 90–93.

Price S, Price L. *Aromatherapy for Health Professionals*, 2nd edn. Edinburgh: churchill Livingstone, 1999.

Rankin-Box D. *The Nurse's Handbook of Complementary Therapies*, 2nd edn. Edinburgh: Bailliere Tindall, 2001.

Rose M. Therapeutic massage: complementary care for diabetes. *Clearinghouse Publications* (accessed November 2005).

Stevenson C. The psychophysiological effects of aromatherapy massage following cardiac surgery. *Complementary Therapies in Medicine* 1994; **2**(1): 27–35.

Tyler D, Winslow E, Clark A, White K. Effects of a one minute back rub on mixed venous oxygen saturation and heart rate in critically ill patients. *Heart Lung* 1990; (**5** part 2): 562–565.

Vickers A. *Massage and Aromatherapy: A Guide for Health Professionals*. London: Chapman & Hall, 1996.

Voltonen E, Lilius H. Syncardial massage in diabetic and other neuropathies of lower extremities. *Diseases of the Nervous System* 1973; **34**(3): 192–194.

Wang X. Treating type II diabetes mellitus with foot reflexotherapy. First Teaching Hospital, Beijing Medical University, Chung Kul *Chung His 1 Chich Ho TSA Chin* (China) 1993; **13**(9): 517, 536–538.

Watson S. The effects of massage: an holistic approach to care. *Nursing Standard* 1997; **11**(47): 45–47.

Ying Ma. *Clinical Observation on Influence upon Arterial Blood Flow in the Lower Limbs of 20 Cases with Type II Diabetes Mellitus Treated by Foot Reflexology*. Beijing: China Reflexology Symposium Report, China Reflexology Association, 1998, pp. 97–99.

14 Naturopathy

Liza Oates

14.1 Introduction

Naturopaths often work in conjunction with conventional medical practitioners in order to achieve the best clinical outcomes for their patients. Naturopathy offers treatments derived from natural products that aim to correct imbalances in the body and restore the natural healing processes. Human beings have long used herbs and dietary modification to restore health, and all cultures possess a traditional system of medicine that recognises the value of these approaches. Evidence of the use of medicinal herbs dates back at least 60,000 years. One of Hippocrates' favourite epithets was 'Let food be your medicine and medicine be your food'. Modern naturopathy developed out of the 'nature cure' movement of the nineteenth century, which promoted the use of good food, clean water, sunlight, proper breathing and wild herbs to correct illness.

Naturopathy is not a distinct modality; rather, it is an umbrella term that describes a variety of modalities. However, the thing that most defines naturopathic practice is not the modalities used but the underlying philosophy. The American Association of Naturopathic Physicians (AANP) (2005) defines modern naturopathy as:

> a distinct system of primary health care — an art, science, philosophy and practice of diagnosis, treatment and prevention of illness. Naturopathic medicine is distinguished by the principles, which underlie and determine its practice. These principles are based upon the objective observation of the nature of health and disease, and are continually re-examined in the light of scientific advances. Methods used are consistent with these principles and are chosen upon the basis of patient individuality. Naturopathic physicians are primary health care practitioners, whose diverse techniques include modern and traditional, scientific and empirical methods.

The basic tenets of naturopathy include the following:

1. *Vis Medicatrix Naturae* (The healing power of nature). Naturopaths believe that given the correct circumstances, the body has an innate ability to heal

Complementary Therapies and the Management of Diabetes and Vascular Disease   Editor Trish Dunning
© 2006 John Wiley & Sons, Ltd.

itself. Therefore, therapies that support the vital force are used in an attempt to restore harmony to the whole person. Naturally, there are limitations to such an approach, for instance, when a condition has progressed beyond the individual's self-healing capacity. In such circumstances the naturopath generally plays a complementary role by maximising the benefits of other treatments and promoting the patient's quality of life.

2. *Primum Non Nocere* (First, do no harm), which in naturopathic practice includes the naturopath knowing their limitations and when to refer to or work in conjunction with another practitioner. It also includes avoiding treatments that interfere with the body's natural self-healing functions or have harmful side effects.
3. *Tolle Causam* (Treat the cause). The naturopath aims to identify the factors that contribute to ill health and treat the modifiable risk factors. Contributing factors vary from person to person and therefore treatment protocols also differ.
4. *Treat the whole person*, which involves addressing the mind and spirit as well as the physical body. It recognises the patient as a multifaceted being within a socio-economic construct. All of these factors need to be considered in order to treat the person rather than the disease.
5. *Docere* (Doctor as teacher). This involves empowering the patient to take responsibility for their health by providing advice specific to their needs and taking into account what they can realistically achieve and will adhere to.
6. *Prevention* (Prevention is the best cure). Naturopaths address possible factors that could impact on the person's future health.

In essence, the naturopath aims to address the individual causes of illness by focusing on the body, mind and spirit in order to restore natural healing processes. It is important that the factors requiring treatment are identified for each individual in order to select appropriate remedies from the range of naturopathic modalities to achieve the treatment aims of the individual. In the West, these modalities are most likely to include nutrition and herbal medicine but many naturopaths incorporate various other modalities into their practice. As a result, there is wide variation in the way naturopathy is practised. There is also significant variation among countries in the way it is regulated. For instance, in the United States, naturopaths are licensed in some states but not others, and in Germany naturopathy is practised by physicians as part of the mainstream medical system.

Naturopaths do not claim to 'cure diseases'. That is not to say, however, that naturopaths do not treat people who have diseases such as diabetes, but the naturopathic approach involves treating the person not the disease. In a case such as diabetes the naturopath generally takes a complementary approach, working in conjunction with other health professionals. Such partnerships can be highly successful because there are many similarities between naturopathy and conventional medicine with regard to understanding the causes and progression of diabetes and individualising the management plan. Naturopaths aim to support overall well-being and quality of life, help prevent the long-term complications of diabetes, address psychological and psychosocial needs, and minimise the requirements for medications.

14.2 The Naturopathic Consultation

A typical naturopathic consultation takes around one hour. In that time a comprehensive case history will be taken and the patient will be asked about their general health, test results such as blood glucose, insulin and lipid profiles, diet, lifestyle and environmental factors, and issues that could influence their ability to make recommended changes. The naturopath aims to obtain a clear picture of the relevant issues at the particular time as well as estimate future tendencies. Determining the person's experience of diabetes is part of the assessment.

The naturopath may undertake iris analysis (iridology) to assess the function of the various systems and organs in order to decide suitable treatment. Iridology generally involves examining the iris with a magnifying glass and torch. Iris analysis determines the integrity of systems and organs in the body by assessing the structure and colour of the iris, which reflects inherited weaknesses and functional problems. Iridology is not 'fortune telling'. It can provide information about inherent weaknesses that could contribute to disease onset or progression of ill health.

The naturopath also aims to identify the various causes of ill health and distinguish which causes can be removed or modified. The information is used to develop a list of management aims relevant to the particular person and prioritise them according to the degree of urgency. The most common treatment aims relating to diabetes are discussed later in the chapter but others are included depending on individual need. Once the treatment aims have been established, the naturopath considers the various treatment options that could be used to accomplish the aims.

An initial prescription will be developed in consultation with the patient. These might include one or all of the following: herbal formulations, nutritional supplements or flower essences, and dietary and lifestyle recommendations. The dietary and lifestyle recommendations need to be attainable, sustainable and enjoyable. If these factors are not considered, long-term, or even short-term compliance, is unlikely.

In most cases changes are introduced slowly, a few at a time, to enable the person to experience success in achieving their goals. The practitioner should avoid setting a patient up to feel like a failure by providing a comprehensive list of everything that needs to be done as if it needs to be done immediately. This may contribute to a sense of loss of control or be overwhelming and may lead to depression. It is also the naturopath's role to inspire, motivate and provide clear information to assist the patient to implement the recommendations. In this respect the role is very similar to that of conventional practitioners. An overview of a naturopathic consultation is shown in Table 14.1.

Choosing a naturopath

It should be noted that, at present, the naturopathic profession is not government regulated in many countries and, as such, educational standards vary. A four-year Bachelor degree is common for recent graduates but it is important to enquire about

Table 14.1 Overview of the main steps involved in a naturopathic consultation.

At an initial consultation the naturopath:

1. Gathers information: case history, test results, home blood glucose testing results, and iris analysis.
2. Forms a picture of the person: presenting symptoms and potential risk factors.
3. Identifies the individual factors: dietary, lifestyle, environmental, emotional and spiritual factors, and organ/system dysfunction.
4. Develops and prioritises treatment or management aims specific to the individual.
5. Considers treatment options, taking into consideration factors that could affect compliance such as financial restraints, beliefs and attitudes and considers the relevant cautions or contraindications to the various treatment modalities.
6. Negotiates with the patient to design an attainable, sustainable and enjoyable management plan to ensure long term compliance.

At later consultations the plan may be adjusted according to the person's progress or to address new issues.

the extent of training before recommending or referring a person to a naturopath. A well-trained naturopath has a good understanding of biomedicine as well as the naturopathic modalities. The major professional associations representing naturopathy can provide information about appropriately trained naturopaths in particular areas.

Self-prescribing

People with diabetes should be discouraged from self-prescribing naturopathic treatment. Although many naturopathic remedies might be extremely useful and may be readily available without consulting a health professional, they may not always be suitable for particular individuals or may interact with other medicines. A naturopath can help the individual determine the safest and most effective remedies and save them time and money.

14.3 General Management Aims

As previously discussed, the naturopath aims to identify and prioritise aspects of the management plan for the individual. Common treatment aims for a person with diabetes generally fall into one of two categories but there is considerable cross-over between the two:

1. Management – managing blood glucose regulation, cardiovascular risk factors, weight and other individual factors and reducing requirements for medications where possible within the context of the Quality Use of Medicines, see Chapter 4.
2. Prevention – preventing the initial onset or progression of diabetes and its acute and long-term complications.

Management

Reduce post-prandial hyperglycaemia

Studies indicate that an increase in blood glucose levels after eating contributes to the development of atherosclerosis and increases the incidence of cardiovascular disease (Dushay and Abrahamson 2005). Management options include: low Glycemic Index™ diet; fibre; oats; biotin; chromium; *Panax quinquefolius*.

Reduce fasting hyperglycaemia

Sustained hyperglycaemia affects virtually all cells. Cells that absorb glucose independently of insulin are particularly vulnerable to the accumulation of polyols such as sorbitol and glycosylation (including haemoglobin and serum albumin). These factors in combination with oxidative damage and dislipidaemia are largely responsible for many of the long-term complications associated with diabetes (Balado 1999).In addition, chronic hyperglycaemia can impair islet function and contribute to hyperglycaemia (Powers 2005). Management strategies include: low Glycemic Index™ diet; fibre; stress management; *Momordia charantia*; cinnamon; chromium; biotin; vanadium; *Codonopsis pilosula*; *Galega officinalis*; *Gymnema sylvestre*; *Panax ginseng*; *Trigonella foenum graecum*; *Vaccinium myrtillus*.

Blood glucose self-monitoring

Home blood glucose monitors are readily available. Regular blood glucose monitoring is essential to determine the effectiveness of the treatment, identify hypo or hyperglycaemia and institute early management such as dose adjustments, especially when insulin or oral glucose-lowering medications are used. HbA_{1C} is the standard method of assessing long-term glycaemic control and should be measured at least twice a year, or every three months in type 1 diabetes and those with poor glycaemic control or when therapy is altered (Powers 2005).

Manage cardiovascular risk factors

Many people with type 2 diabetes also have other cardiovascular risk factors such as high blood pressure, abdominal obesity, elevated triglycerides, lowered HDL cholesterol, elevated C-reactive protein (CRP), elevated homocystine and modestly increased LDL. The LDL tends to be small and dense and readily penetrates the vascular wall. These particles are easily oxidised initiating atherosclerotic processes (Dushay and Abrahamson 2005; Powers 2005). As a result, atherosclerosis is the most common complication of diabetes. The heart is the organ most susceptible to oxidative stress and responds to beneficial, targeted nutritional agents (Frishman *et al.* 2005).

Controlling blood pressure reduces the risk of both macrovascular and microvascular complications (Powers 2005). Therefore, as part of a comprehensive management plan it is important to regulate lipid profiles, specifically to increase

Table 14.2 Naturopathic treatment options that might be used in various combinations to reduce multifactorial cardiovascular risk factors.

Reduce lipids	Manage blood pressure	Reduce C-reactive protein	Reduce homocystine	Reduce oxidative tress
Low Glycemic Index™	Exercise	Omega 6 oils	Folate	Coenzyme Q10
diet	Stress management	Vitamin C	Vitamin B6	Lipoic acid
Fibre	Sodium restriction	Vitamin E	Vitamin B12	Niacin
Reduce saturated and trans fatty acids	Fish			Vitamin C
Exercise	Garlic and onions			Vitamin E
Stress management	Oats			Zinc
Cinnamon	Coenzyme Q10			*Scuttelaria baicalensis*
Fish	Magnesium			*Vaccinium myrtillus*
Garlic & onions	Omega 3 oils			*Vitis vinifera*
Oats	Vitamin C			
Chromium	Vitamin E			
Niacin	*Scuttelaria baicalensis*			
Omega 3 oils				
Vitamin E				
Panax ginseng				
Scuttelaria baicalensis				
Trigonella foenum graecum				
Vaccinium myrtillus				

HDL and reduce elevated triglyceride and LDL, reduce elevated blood pressure, C-reactive protein (CRP), homocystine and oxidative stress. Naturopathic treatment options are shown in Table 14.2.

Support weight loss and maintain a healthy weight

The onset of type 2 diabetes is often insidious and frequently occurs in association with obesity especially around the abdomen, which is known as central or visceral obesity. It appears to be a key factor in the Insulin Resistance Syndrome (IRS). Excess visceral fat affects insulin secretion and action through a range of mechanisms. As a result of insulin resistance, free fatty acids are formed and further impair glucose utilisation and islet function, and increase hepatic glucose production (Powers 2005; Dushay and Abrahamson 2005). Visceral fat also increases production of the enzyme 11-beta-HSD-1, which converts inactive cortisone to cortisol, which further promotes abdominal weight gain (Dushay and Abrahamson 2005).

Dietary and lifestyle interventions that reduced body weight by 5–7 per cent in people with impaired glucose tolerance have been shown to prevent or delay the progression to type 2 diabetes in 58 per cent compared to 31 per cent taking metformin (Powers 2005). Naturopathic management options include a diet high in fibre, exercise and *Gymnema sylvestre*.

Regulate insulin and improve insulin sensitivity

Type 2 diabetes is characterised by insulin resistance, impaired insulin secretion and increased hepatic glucose output (Powers 2005) see Chapter 1. Even in type 1 diabetes, insulin resistance can develop in response to stress and (Mitchell and Mitchell 2003). Therefore, improving insulin sensitivity is an important management strategy. Naturopathic management options include those herbs and supplements already listed, and those shown in Table 14.2

Correct nutritional deficiencies

Nutritional deficiencies can impair glucose regulation and increase the risk of long-term complications by contributing to oxidative stress. A number of key nutrients appear to be deficient in diabetes (Wilson and Gondy 1995; Huerta *et al.* 2005; Yokota 2005; Pham *et al.* 2005; Frishman *et al.* 2005 and Zhang *et al.* 2005), see Chapter 5.

In addition over 600 carotenoids and flavonoids are found in nature predominantly in fruit and vegetables. Beta carotene (in carrots) and lycopene (in tomatoes) are powerful antioxidants and lycopene is a precursor of vitamin E and may have a preventative role in reducing cardiovascular risk although further study is required (Frishman *et al.* 2005).

Reduce stress

Reducing stress, and improving the individual's ability to deal with prolonged stress is another important component of diabetes management. Mitchell and Mitchell (2003) hypothesised that chronic stress may be a contributing factor in the development of type 2 diabetes because it results in high levels of circulating cortisol and adrenalin. Cortisol release is stimulated by stress and is known to increase insulin resistance, promote abdominal weight gain, disrupt immune function, and trigger depression. Additionally, high blood glucose levels may amplify the cortisol response to psychosocial stress (Gonzalez-Bono *et al.* 2002) further contributing to the potential for negative effects. Cortisol may also stimulate appetite, especially for sweet foods, resulting in excessive eating and subsequent weight gain (Wolkowitz *et al.* 2001). In addition, adrenalin stimulates glycogenolysis (Mitchell and Mitchell 2003), which contributes to hyperglycaemia and insulin resistance.

In established diabetes, chronic stress may also result from day-to-day issues such as the demands of diabetes self-management tasks and the physical stress of sustained hyperglycaemia. Inability to manage stress and depression impacts on the person's ability to care for themselves adequately. Counselling strategies are described in Chapter 7. Naturopathic approaches to stress management also include promoting emotional and spiritual well-being; recommending regular exercise; using flower essences such as Rescue Remedy in acute stress situations; using herbal medicines such as *Codonopsis pilosula*.

Treat individual factors

In addition to managing the diabetic process, the naturopath also considers individual factors that directly or indirectly affect the individual's quality of life including the presence of the following:

- *Emotional factors and depression* There is a strong correlation between depression and diabetes (Wolkowitz *et al.* 2001). In addition, the perception of lack of control experienced by the person recently diagnosed with diabetes or those who develop complications may also contribute to depression.
- *Digestion* Gastric stasis can occur as a long-term complication of diabetes resulting in considerable discomfort and erratic blood glucose control. Good digestion is essential for the proper assimilation of nutrients and glucose metabolism.
- *Pain* Pain management may be required for conditions resulting from or in addition to diabetes, see Chapter 15.
- *Dysbiosis and thrush* The increased risk of infection in uncontrolled diabetes may require antibiotic therapy. As a result conditions such as thrush and intestinal dysbiosis may result. Candida infections are commonly observed in people with diabetes. (Powers 2005) and probiotics are commonly prescribed in such conditions.
- *Infections* People with uncontrolled diabetes have a higher incidence and severity of infection, possibly associated with abnormalities of cell-mediated immunity and altered phagocyte function associated with hyperglycaemia. (Powers 2005). Pneumonia, urinary tract infections and skin and soft tissue infections are common. Ensuring proper nutrition and supporting immunity should be considered as part of the management protocol.

Reduce requirements for medications

Type 1 diabetes

In type 1 diabetes, the primary aim of the naturopath is to support conventional therapy. Insulin should not be stopped in type 1 diabetes. The benefits of aggressive glycaemic control need to be weighed against the potential risks which include increased risk of hypoglycaemia, weight gain resulting in increased cardiovascular risk, economic and social costs (Powers 2005). Dietary changes, exercise and stress management might reduce insulin requirements. Blood glucose levels need to be monitored regularly to assess the efficacy of treatment and used to review insulin doses and dose frequency. A complementary naturopathic approach could include using the nutritional supplements already described and some herbs: *Galega officinalis*; *Gymnema sylvestre*; *Panax quinquefolius*; *Trigonella foenum graecum*; *Vaccinium myrtillus*.

Type 2 diabetes

Conventional medications commonly prescribed for type 2 diabetes were described in Chapter 1.

Patients should be closely monitored to determine changes in glycaemic control resulting from complementary treatment and medications and complementary therapies adjusted accordingly. Naturopaths should not recommend that patients stop taking conventional medicines but refer them to their doctor to reassess requirements for glucose-lowering medicines as glycaemic control improves. Naturopathic strategies include dietary modification; exercise; stress management; and the glucose lowering herbs listed on preceding pages.

Prevention

Risk factors for type 2 diabetes

The risk factors for type 2 diabetes are discussed in Chapter 1. Recognising risk factors that contribute to the development and progression of Type 2 diabetes is imperative in order to determine how aggressive management and prevention strategies need to be and to set management priorities for attention.

Prevent destruction of beta cells

Type 1 diabetes primarily affects children and adolescents and various theories exist to explain the initial onset. In type 1 diabetes there is complete or near complete destruction of the insulin-producing beta cells of the pancreas. As a result, people with type 1 diabetes need to inject exogenous insulin on a regular basis. Diabetes does not become overt until the majority of beta cells have been destroyed (~80 per cent). A 'honeymoon phase' where good glycaemic control can be achieved with little or no exogenous insulin often occurs in the first year (Powers 2005). Extending the honeymoon phase by protecting the remaining beta cells as long as possible may slow the progression of the disease.

The exact mechanism of injury to the beta cells is not known but appears to be accompanied by an inability of the body to regenerate damaged beta cells. Proposed triggers include viruses such as coxsackie and rubella and other infectious stimuli such as bovine milk proteins, nitrosourea compounds and free radicals (Powers 2005; Robertson *et al.* 2005; Lammi *et al.* 2005). An autoimmune mechanism has been proposed where antibodies to beta cells are present (Powers 2005; Dushay and Abrahamson 2005). A naturopathic approach to protecting beta cells consists of diet, exercise and stress management as well as supplemental: lipoic acid; niacin; magnesium; vitamin C; vitamin E; zinc.

Long-term complications

For more detailed information, see Chapter 1. Diabetes is the leading cause of adult blindness, end-stage renal disease and non-traumatic lower extremity amputation in the United States and the statistics are likely to be similar in other developed countries (Powers 2005). The chronic complications of diabetes include macrovascular (cardiovascular and cerebrovascular disorders), microvascular (retinopathy, neuropathy, nephropathy) and non-vascular complications. The risk of complications increases with long duration of diabetes, poor glycaemic control and hypertension. Complications are more likely to develop in the second decade of the condition, however, type 2 diabetes is often preceded by a long asymptomatic period before diagnosis and complications are often present at diagnosis (Powers 2005).

Risk factors for cardiovascular disease are similar in type 2 diabetes to people with a history of prior cardiovascular events such as heart attack or stroke and the outcomes following cardiovascular events are worse (Dushay and Abrahamson 2005). The increased risk for cardiovascular morbidity and mortality appears to be related to hyperglycaemia and other cardiovascular risk factors such as hypertension and dyslipidaemia, notably elevated trigylycerides and low HDL levels. Due to the high prevalence of atherosclerosis in diabetes, the possibility of renovascular hypertension should be considered if hypertension is difficult to control. (Powers 2005).

Retinopathy

Diabetic retinopathy and macular oedema are leading causes of adult blindness and are asymptomatic. Therefore, regular retinal screening is imperative. People with diabetes are 25 times more likely to become legally blind (Powers 2005). In addition to retinal changes, polyol accumulation causes distension of the lens and blurred vision (Balado 1999), which makes day-to-day activities such as driving and reading difficult and impacts on self-care. The risk of retinopathy increases with the increasing duration of diabetes, poor glycaemic control and hypertension.

Vigorous exercise may result in vitreous haemorrhage or retinal detachment and exercise programmes should be carefully designed (Powers 2005). A naturopath might recommend the following supplements and herbal medicines to complement conventional management strategies: lipoic acid; magnesium; *Ginkgo biloba*; *Vaccinium myrtillus*; *Vitis Vinifera*.

Neuropathy

Diabetic neuropathy affects both myelinated and unmyelinated nerves and occurs in approximately 50 per cent of people with diabetes. The incidence correlates with the duration of diabetes and hyperglycaemia (Powers 2005). Various mechanisms have been proposed including polyol accumulation (Balado 1999). Neuropathy is frequently accompanied by sensations of numbness, tingling or pain in the lower extremities. Loss of sensation in the feet significantly increases the risk of trauma and amputations. Diabetes is the leading cause of non-traumatic lower extremity amputation in the United States (Powers 2005) and loss of sensation due to neuropathy significantly increases the risk of trauma and amputations because the person does not realise their feet are damaged, which delays appropriate care. Visual problems compound the problem.

Regular foot screening, appropriate foot care and glycaemic control are imperative. Hyperglycaemia increases the risk of infection, alters blood flow and retards wound healing. Therefore, even minor injuries must be treated promptly. People with diabetes should choose footwear carefully; inspect feet daily for injury; maintain good foot hygiene, keeping the skin clean and moist, not walk around with bare feet or self-treat foot abnormalities (Powers 2005).

Autonomic neuropathy often develops in long-standing diabetes and affects multiple organs and systems including the cardiovascular, gastrointestinal and genito-urinary systems. As a result, symptoms such as gastroparesis, impaired gut motility resulting in constipation or diarrhoea, bladder-emptying abnormalities, erectile dysfunction and female sexual dysfunction may occur (Powers 2005). Improving glycaemic control, avoiding neurotoxins such as alcohol and rectifying nutritional deficiencies especially B6, B12, and folate are important (Powers 2005). Treatment strategies include: acetyl-L-carnitine; biotin; lipoic acid; omega 6 oils; vitamins B6 and B12; *Panax ginseng*.

Nephropathy

Diabetic nephropathy is the leading cause of end-stage renal disease in the United States (Powers 2005) and in Australian Aboriginals. Early nephropathy is associated with microalbuminuria, which is a marker of insulin resistance in type 2 diabetes (Dushay and Abrahamson 2005) and predicts progression to overt proteinuria and nephropathy. Hyperglycaemia contributes to the formation of glycoproteins within the kidneys, resulting in glomerulosclerosis (Balado 1999). Smoking, dyslipidaemia and hypertension are additional risk factors for nephropathy (Powers 2005). Naturopathic treatment aims to complement conventional management and may include: lipoic acid; vitamin C; vegetable protein and modest protein restriction; *Panax ginseng*.

Some herbal medicines are nephrotoxic such as aristolochic acid, which is sometimes contained in weight loss formulas, some are contaminated with toxins such as mycotoxin ochratoxin A, others are adulterated with heavy metals, yet others cause sodium retention, alter serum potassium or cause pseudoaldosteronism, often due to their oxalic acid content, others have diuretic activity and may be contraindicated in renally compromised patients (Wendell *et al.* 2005). Herbs such as *Silybum marianum* and antioxidant flavonoids demonstrate nephroprotective mechanisms in rat studies but more research is needed before these findings can be applied to humans.

Prevent long-term complications

The management of cardiovascular risk factors has already been discussed in this chapter and in Chapter 1. Hyperglycemia results in the accumulation of sorbitol, protein glycosylation and oxidative stress (Osawa and Kato 2005). In addition to controlling hyperglycaemia and lipid abnormalities, the naturopath may aim to do the following:

- Reduce sorbitol accumulation by inhibiting aldose reductase. Aldose reductase, the first rate-limiting enzyme of the polyol pathway converts glucose to fructose and appears to play a key role in the pathogenesis of microvascular complications (Chung and Chung 2005). In insulin-deficient states, more glucose enters the polyol pathway resulting in sorbitol accumulation especially in the lens and retinal blood vessels of the eye, peripheral nerves, kidney and pancreas (Pizzorno and Murray 1999). Vitamin C, flavonoids, *Glycyrrhiza glabra* and *Scuttelaria baicalensis* may reduce sorbitol accumulation. However, large doses of *Glycyrrhiza glabra* may cause hypokalaemia and pseudoaldosteronism.
- Reduce protein glycosylation using a low Glycemic Index™ high fibre diet.
- Reduce oxidative stress using antioxidant vitamins and mineral supplements and herbal medicines such as *Scuttelaria baicalensis, Vaccinium myrtillus, Vitis Vinifera.*

Acute complications

The major acute complications hypoglycaemia, ketoacidosis, hyperosmolar states and intercurrent infections are discussed in Chapter 1. These are acute emergencies and need to be assessed and managed in conventional care settings. However, naturopaths can play a preventative role and need to be able to recognise the symptoms of these emergencies in order to manage hypoglycaemia and refer the patient quickly and appropriately. They can support the person to continue self-management and to achieve appropriate glycaemic control with appropriate dietary and exercise advice. Appropriate selection of herbal medicines and supplements is also imperative.

14.4 Naturopathic Management Options

Naturopaths use a range of therapeutic options to achieve their management aims. The art of the practitioner lies in selecting suitable therapies that meet the needs of the individual patient and providing comprehensive information to assist them to implement the recommendations. The naturopath works with the patient to prioritise the aims and negotiate an attainable, sustainable and enjoyable management plan in order to achieve the best health outcomes and long-term compliance.

The naturopath should work as part of a health-care team: therefore, they have a responsibility to ensure that all health professionals caring for the patient are informed about their management recommendations. Likewise the naturopath needs to be informed of management changes implemented by other members of the team. Integration is discussed in Chapter 4. In general the naturopath uses a combination of dietary modification to promote healthy eating (see Chapter 5), exercise, stress management (see Chapter 7), energetic therapies (see Chapter 8), and herbal medicines and supplements (see Chapter 9).

Promote healthy eating

Despite advances in Western medicine, dietary and lifestyle modification remains the cornerstone of effective management of type 2 diabetes and is an important factor in the management of type 1 diabetes. Dietary modification is essential not only to the management of the diabetes itself, but also to the long-term complications, in particular the cardiovascular complications. Diets high in refined carbohydrate and low in fibre are associated with the increasing prevalence of type 2 diabetes (Gross *et al.* 2004) whereas experimental studies using low carbohydrate, high mono-unsaturated fatty acids and high fibre improve glycaemic balance (Hofman *et al.* 2004).

Naturopathic dietary advice is very similar to conventional dietary advice and considers patient's food preferences, nutritional, psychological, financial needs and practicalities, and changing requirements during life stages or illness and when complications develop. The naturopath may also consider the 'energetics' of the food, for instance whether it is warming or cooling, drying or moist, before making recommendations. Dietary compliance is a major issue and the naturopath should provide information about purchasing, storing and preparing foods as well as support and encouragement. The support of family and friends is also imperative especially in children and older people. Sometimes naturopaths recommend five small meals a day, preferably containing a combination of protein with low GI carbohydrates. This 'grazing' approach to eating can also reduce the incidence of gastroparesis, bloating and reflux in susceptible patients (Powers 2005).

Food is also considered to be a form of medicine, see Table 14.3.

Nutritional deficiencies are common in the general population, especially in older people. People with diabetes have increased requirements for certain nutrients such as antioxidants. Where possible, these should be obtained from a well-balanced diet. In some cases supplementation may be required to correct deficiency states or to provide a direct therapeutic effect. The evidence for supplementary chromium, magnesium and antioxidants is currently insufficient to suggest routine use supplementation, however, supplementary doses of these nutrients may benefit some people and should be assessed on a case-by-case basis (Guerrero-Romero and Rodriguez-Moran 2005). Self-prescribing should be discouraged because excessive doses of micronutrients may be detrimental. The prescriber should monitor patients for signs of micronutrient toxicity. Table 14.4 provides information about the most commonly prescribed supplements.

Table 14.3 Foods naturopaths commonly recommend as medicines, their beneficial effects, the issues to consider when they are prescribed and recommended doses.

Food	Beneficial effects	Considerations	Recommendations
Bitter melon *Momordica charantia*	The juice of the unripe fruit of *Momordica charantia* is used traditionally to treat diabetes. Preliminary studies suggest that constituents of bitter melon have structural similarities to insulin and exert a hypoglycaemic effect (Basch *et al.* 2003). For more detailed information, see Chapter 11.	Unpleasant taste may reduce compliance. Adverse reactions: May cause hypoglycaemic coma and convulsions in children, headaches and increased liver enzymes. Cautions/contraindications: May have additive effects with oral hypoglycaemic agents or insulin. Monitor blood glucose levels and adjust medication requirements if necessary. Monitor liver enzymes. May delay gastric emptying therefore care is required in gastroparesis.	Suggested dose: 30–60 ml fresh juice 3 times a day.
Cinnamon	A randomised controlled trial demonstrated that cinnamon 'reduces (fasting) serum glucose, triglyceride, LDL cholesterol, and total cholesterol in people with type 2 diabetes. The findings suggest the inclusion of cinnamon in the diet of people with type 2 diabetes could reduce risk factors associated with diabetes and cardiovascular diseases' (Khan *et al.* 2003).		1–6 g daily. Consider adding to porridge or stewed fruit.

Fish	Oily cold-water fish contain high levels of omega 3 essential fatty acids. Consuming fish high in omega 3 helps reduce triglyceride levels in people with type 2 diabetes and has a modest effect on hypertension (Braun and Cohen 2005). There is also a lower incidence of impaired glucose tolerance and type 2 diabetes in populations with high intakes of omega 3 containing fish (Nettleton and Katz 2005). A recent review suggests that omega 3 fatty acids are the most favourable lipid-lowering interventions with reduced risks of overall and cardiac mortality (Studer *et al.* 2005).	Fish at risk of containing high mercury levels should be minimised, these include marlin, swordfish, flake, orange roughy and catfish.	Consume oily fish 2–3 times/week.
Garlic and onions	Garlic and onions have positive benefits for the cardiovascular system modestly reducing hypertension and cholesterol levels (Braun and Cohen 2005) and may also reduce blood glucose levels.	Sensitivity occurs in some people.	These foods can be consumed regularly as part of a healthy diet.
Honey	Honey has traditionally been used to promote wound healing and a series of case reports suggest that honey impregnated dressings may improve neuropathic foot ulcers (Eddy and Gideonsen, 2005, Dunford 2005; van der Weyden 2005).	A theoretical concern exists that the honey may feed bacteria in the ulcer.	Impregnate dressings with manuka or Medihoney™.
Oats	Oats delays glucose absorption and reduces post-prandial hyperglycaemia. It may also reduce total and LDL cholesterol and hypertension reducing requirements for medications (Braun and Cohen 2005).	Despite concerns for people with Coeliac disease due to gluten content, long-term studies suggest that it is generally well tolerated (Braun and Cohen 2005).	Consume wholegrain oat-based cereals regularly as part of a healthy diet.

Table 14.4 Commonly prescribed supplemental nutrients and antioxidants their beneficial effects, the issues to consider when they are prescribed and recommended doses.

Nutrient	Beneficial effects	Cautions/contraindications	Suggested dose
Biotin	Enhances insulin sensitivity, lowers fasting and postprandial blood glucose levels and improves diabetic neuropathy (Mitchell and Mitchell 2003; Pizzorno and Murray 1999).	May require reassessment of insulin requirements.	Type 1 diabetes 16 mg/day; Type 2 diabetes 9 mg/day. Food sources: egg yolk, diary products, legumes, brewer's yeast, sardines (Note: eating raw eggs can cause a biotin deficiency).
Carnitine	Studies have demonstrated that acetyl-L-carnitine is efficacious in alleviating symptoms, particularly pain, and improves nerve fibre regeneration and vibration perception in patients with established diabetic neuropathy (Sima et al. 2005).		Suggested dose: 1,000 mg/day acetyl-L-carnitine

Chromium	Chromium is a component of the glucose tolerance factor (GTF) and works closely with insulin to facilitate the uptake of glucose into cells. Chromium is essential for insulin sensitivity and deficiency may result in insulin resistance (Braun and Cohen 2005). Chromium supplementation improves insulin sensitivity, reduces post-prandial and fasting hyperglycaemia, reduces total and LDL cholesterol and triglycerides and modestly increases protective HDL cholesterol (Braun and Cohen, 2005) A recent meta-analysis reported no effects on glycaemic control in people without diabetes (Althuis et al. 2002) and chromium appears to be more effective in people with Type 2 diabetes who are chromium depleted (Braun and Cohen 2005).	Chromium supplementation may reduce exogenous insulin requirements in Type 1 diabetes (Braun and Cohen 2005). Monitor blood glucose and lipid levels and adjust medication doses if necessary.	200–1000 mcg/day as chromium picolinate Food sources: wholegrains, meat, cheese, brewer's yeast, eggs, bananas, spinach, mushroom, broccoli.
Coenzyme Q10	CoQ10 is an important antioxidant, which is essential for normal myocardial function. It improves insulin secretion and sensitivity (Mitchell and Mitchell, 2003) and reduces hypertension (Braun and Cohen 2005). As CoQ10 can be inhibited by HMG CoA reductase inhibitors, concurrent supplementation of CoQ10 may be prudent		100–150 mg/day. Food sources: meat, seafood, wholegrains, green leafy vegetables, fruit, dairy products.

Table 14.4 (Continued)

Nutrient	Beneficial effects	Cautions/contraindications	Suggested dose
	when taking these medications (Braun and Cohen 2005). CoQ10 also reconstitutes vitamin E back into its unoxidised state allowing it to continue neutralising free radicals (Braun and Cohen 2005).		
Flavonoids	Flavonoids such as quercetin prevent the accumulation of sorbitol, promote insulin secretion (Pizzorno and Murray 1999) and strengthen vascular walls, which prevents damage from hyperglycaemia.		1–2 g mixed flavonoids/day. Food sources: onions, buckwheat, grapefruit pith.
Lipoic acid	Lipoic acid (thioctic acid) is an important antioxidant and may play a preventative role and reduce the progression of diabetic nephropathy, retinopathy and neuropathy and insulin sensitivity (Mitchell and Mitchell 2003; Bonnefont-Rousselot 2004; Packer et al. 2001).		250–800 mg/ day. Food sources: potato, red meat, spinach, brewer's yeast.
Magnesium	Magnesium is involved in glucose metabolism, moderately reduces hypertension has a preventative role in reducing complications such as diabetic retinopathy and cardiovascular disease and may maintain beta cell functional and improve insulin sensitivity. Magnesium deficiency is common in diabetes and may increase insulin secretion and insulin resistance (Mitchell and Mitchell 2003; Yokota 2005).		300–500 mg/day; should be taken with 50 mg B6 to assist absorption into the cell. Food sources: green leafy vegetables, wholegrains, legumes, tofu, nuts, seeds, mineral water.

| Niacin | Niacin also affects glucose tolerance and assists in regulating carbohydrate, fat and cholesterol metabolism. Niacinamide (nicotinamide) may have a role in preventing the development of Type 1 diabetes preventing damage to beta cells and improving the function of residual beta cells. It is also an antioxidant and high dose supplementation improves lipid profiles by reducing triglycerides, total and LDL cholesterol and increasing HDL cholesterol (Braun and Cohen 2005). | Niacin may cause relatively severe flushing in some individuals. The sustained release form is associated with fewer side effects and has less effect on glucose metabolism resulting in less frequent dosing and improved compliance (Dushay and Abrahamson 2005). High doses of niacin must be used cautiously in people with impaired glucose tolerance because it may cause insulin resistance and increase fasting hyperglycaemia (Braun and Cohen 2005; Powers, 2005), therefore, blood glucose should be monitored carefully and medications adjusted as necessary. | 25 mg/kg body weight; children 100–200 mg/day. Food sources: fruit, legumes, meat, wheat bran and organ meats. |
| Omega 3 oils | A recent review suggests that omega 3 fatty acids are the most favourable lipid-lowering interventions with reduced risks of overall and cardiac mortality (Studer *et al.* 2005). Epidemiological studies report a lower incidence of impaired glucose tolerance and Type 2 | | 1–2 g/day. |

Table 14.4 (Continued)

Nutrient	Beneficial effects	Cautions/contraindications	Suggested dose
	diabetes in populations with high intakes of omega 3 containing fish. Clinical trials show that omega 3 consumption has a cardioprotective role in Type 2 diabetes reducing cardiovascular mortality rates. Omega 3 oils reduce triglyceride levels, increase protective HDL, improve endothelial function, reduce platelet aggregation and have a modest effect on hypertension (Braun and Cohen 2005; Nettleton and Katz 2005). Preliminary reports suggest that consuming omega 3 oils in conjunction with a low saturated fat diet may reduce the progression of impaired glucose tolerance to Type 2 diabetes in overweight people (Nettleton and Katz 2005).		
Omega 6 oils	Omega 6 oils such as Evening Primrose and Borage oil reduce CRP and may help to protect against diabetic neuropathy (Mitchell and Mitchell 2003).	EPO may lower seizure threshold in people with epilepsy.	Evening primrose oil equiv. 500–2800mg GLA/day in conjunction with omega 3 oils

Vanadium	May increase insulin sensitivity by acting as an insulin mimetic (Mitchell and Mitchell, 2003) and reduce fasting glucose levels.	Doses required to exert an insulin-mimetic effect are potentially toxic therefore vanadium should be limited to dietary intake or in formulations with other nutrients.	Cereal grains, sunflower seeds, black pepper, mushrooms, shellfish, parsley, dill seed.
Vitamin B6, B12 and Folic acid	Deficiency of B6 is associated with diabetic neuropathy and may reduce the severity of gestational diabetes. Vitamin B12 may reduce the symptoms associated with diabetic neuropathy (Braun and Cohen 2005; Pizzorno and Murray 1999; Powers 2005). Vitamins B6, B12 and folate are required to maintain nerve function and for the metabolism of homocystine. Elevated homocystine has been associated with increased risk of cardiovascular disorders. While it is currently unclear whether homocystine is a cause or consequence of cardiovascular disease the supplementation of B6, B12 and folate may be beneficial (Braun and Cohen 2005).	B6:100–150 mg/day (Braun and Cohen 2005; Pizzorno and Murray 1999). B12: 250–3,000 µg/day (Braun and Cohen, 2005; Pizzorno and Murray 1999). Folate: 500–5000 µg/day (Braun and Cohen 2005)	Food sources: B6: fish, legumes, organ meats, eggs, nuts, potatoes, bananas. B12: meat, fish, oysters, dairy. Folate: green leafy vegetables, sprouts, legumes, nuts.

Table 14.4 (Continued)

| Vitamin C | Vitamin C is a useful antioxidant that also reconstitutes vitamin E back into its unoxidised state allowing it to continue neutralising free radicals. It also helps prevent accumulation of sorbitol in cells and assists in insulin modulation and hypertension (Braun and Cohen 2005) and reduces CRP (Mitchell and Mitchell 2003). Vitamin C deficiency increases the risk of developing gestational diabetes mellitus (Zhang *et al.* 2004). Vitamin C requires insulin for transport into cells, consequently some people with diabetes may have low intracellular vitamin C levels (Mitchell and Mitchell 2003). People with diabetic nephropathy have increased ascorbic acid clearance resulting in a reduction in antioxidant defence and an increased risk of cardiovascular morbidity and mortality (Hirsch *et al.* 1998). | Doses500–3,000 mg/day; 2,000 mg/ day to reduce sorbitol accumulation (Pizzorno and Murray 1999). Food sources: fruit, vegetables and sprouts including; blackcurrants, strawberries, broccoli, capsicum, potato, Brussel sprouts, citrus fruit. |

Vitamin E	Diabetes is associated with increased free radical production and a reduction in antioxidant defences, as a result people with diabetes may have an increased requirement for vitamin E (Osawa and Kato 2005) and a vitamin E deficiency may correlate with an increased risk of developing diabetes (Salonen et al. 1995). Vitamin E is an important antioxidant, reduces hypertension, CRP and LDL oxidation and may improve insulin sensitivity (Mitchell and Mitchell 2003). In the process of neutralising free radicals vitamin E becomes oxidised. Other antioxidants such as vitamin C, CoQ10 and Vitis Vinifera recycle vitamin E back into its unoxidised state allowing it to continue neutralising free radicals (Braun and Cohen 2005).	Recently some of the reported cardiovascular benefits of vitamin E have been refuted and suggestions made that vitamin E may actually increase the risk of heart failure (Lonn et al. 2005). Obtaining vitamin E from dietary sources is the preferred option.	900 iu/day. Food sources: nuts, seeds, green leafy vegetables, cold-pressed vegetable oils, sweet potatoes, soy beans, dairy.
Zinc	Zinc is an important antioxidant and may improve insulin resistance and protect the beta cells (Pizzorno and Murray 1999, Braun and Cohen, 2005). Deficiency is common in diabetes and may arise as a result of excessive excretion (Pizzorno and Murray 1999). Zinc deficiency is a risk factor for cardiac oxidative damage and supplementation with Zn provides significant prevention of oxidative damage to the heart (Song et al. 2005).	High dose, long-term use is not advisable as it may result in immunosuppression.	30 mg/day. Food sources: oysters, wholegrains, nuts, seeds, legumes, meat, seafood, eggs.

Exercise

Naturopaths promote regular exercise to reduce the risk of developing type 2 diabetes and prevent cardiovascular disease (Steyn *et al.* 2004; Dushay and Abrahamson 2005). Exercise helps weight management, improves insulin sensitivity, up regulates insulin receptors, lowers plasma glucose, reduces blood pressure, increases HDL and reduces triglycerides, increases chromium levels and maintains muscle mass (Pizzorno and Murray 1999; LaMonte and Yanowitz 2002; Gilliam 2004; Steyn *et al.* 2004; Dushay and Abrahamson 2005; Powers 2005).

As a result of the positive benefits of exercise, the requirements for oral glucose-lowering agents insulin, antihypertensives or lipid lowering and herbal medications may need to be reviewed (Gilliam 2004). Special care also needs to be taken in the presence of injury, foot problems, retinopathy, arrhythmias, cardiac disease or microvascular complications. People taking insulin or glucose-lowering agents need to be given advice about preventing hypoglycaemia (Gilliam 2004; Powers 2005). For best outcomes exercise should be combined with a sensiblediet.

The person's current fitness levels, and their likes and dislikes, time and financial constraints need to be considered when recommending an exercise programme. Specific, measurable recommendations should be made in order to monitor the person's progress and compliance, and blood glucose levels should be monitored. Kilojoule requirements may also need to be reassessed. Cardiovascular function tests may be required before people who are not exercising commence an exercise programme. The naturopath should refer these people to their doctor.

Naturopaths usually recommend people begin exercising slowly in small blocks, for example, 10 minutes at a time and progressively increase the duration and intensity to 30–60 minutes each time, four to six times per week. Likewise, weight training should commence with light weights and increase progressively over time. Exercises that improve core strength and stability such as tai chi, yoga or Pilates are useful to improve balance and reduce the risk of falls especially in older people. However, apart from the most basic exercise advice, few naturopaths are adequately trained in this area and referral to an exercise physiologist may be beneficial.

Stress management

As already indicated, elevated prolonged stress is multifactorial and may include the day-to-day diabetes self-management tasks. Stress management reduces stress hormones (Wolkowitz *et al.* 2001) and improves depression and hypertension. A recent study of a stress management programme based on yoga indicated a potential role in reducing lipid and glucose profiles (Bijlani *et al*. 2005).

Naturopaths recommend a range of stress management techniques such as meditation, visualisation, yoga, tai chi, qi gong, exercise, listening to music, massage, prayer, social activities with friends or family, walking in nature and journal writing. The naturopath may provide information about these various techniques or refer to an appropriate practitioner depending on their level training in the relevant technique. It is important that stress management activities suit the individual. In some cases counselling may be necessary.

Energetic remedies

Energetic therapies are discussed in Chapter 8. Many naturopaths employ energetic remedies to assist emotional well-being particularly flower essences such as Bach Flower, Californian or Australian Bush Flower remedies. Flower essences have a long history of traditional use. Initially it is likely that the dew that formed on certain flowers was consumed often with the flower itself, to treat emotional imbalances. In modern times flower essences are generally prescribed in drop doses using commercially prepared stock remedies. The naturopath undertakes an individual assessment to determine which flower essences are required and may prepare a flower essence remedy that contains a combination of a number of different essences.

Arthritis is a very common disease and many people with diabetes present with this condition. Naturopaths often prescribe glucosamine for osteoarthritis and many people self-prescribe it. Some experts suggest glucosamine may contribute to hyperglycaemia, however, no effects on HbA_{1c} were found in a randomised double-blind placebo-controlled trial (Scroggie *et al*. 2003). Nevertheless, as with other supplements and herbal medicines, practitioners and patients need to be aware of possible reactions and interactions that can occur as a result of using concomitant therapies for coexisting conditions.

Herbal medicines

Table 14.5 provides details of herbal medicines commonly prescribed by naturopaths. Interactions can and do occur between conventional and herbal medicines and these must be considered thoroughly before prescribing. Cautions and contraindications, including those for pregnancy, should also be observed. See also Chapters 9, 10 and 11 where herbal medicines are discussed in more detail, including Ayurvedic and Chinese herbal medicines.

Table 14.5 Commonly prescribed herbal medicines their beneficial effects, the issues to consider when they are prescribed and recommended doses.

Herb	Beneficial effects	Cautions/contraindications	Suggested dose
Codonopsis pilosula (codonopsis)	Traditionally used in naturopathic medicine to regulate blood glucose levels and to assist the body in coping with the effects of stress.		30–60 ml/week; usually taken as part of a combination formula in divided doses 2–3 times/day.
Galega officinalis (goat's rue)	Traditionally used in diabetes to regulate blood glucose levels, *G. officinalis* is the herbal source from which Metformin was developed (Vuksan and Sievenpiper 2005).	Monitor requirements for diabetes medications.	30–60 ml/week; usually taken as part of a combination formula in divided doses 2–3 times/day.
Ginkgo biloba (ginkgo)	Improves blood flow to peripheral tissues and may assist in peripheral vascular diseases, common in diabetes. It has also been shown to improve diabetic retinopathy in animal studies (Pizzorno and Murray, 1999, Braun and Cohen 2005).	Check possible drug interactions before prescribing.	21–28 ml/week (standardised to 24 per cent ginkgo flavoglycosides); usually taken as part of a combination formula in divided doses 2–3 times/day.
Glycyrrhiza glabra (licorice)	*Glycyrrhiza glabra* has demonstrated an ability to inhibit aldose reductase in vitro and thus suppress sorbitol accumulation (Braun and Cohen 2005).	*G. glabra* has the capacity to increase blood pressure and reduce cortisol breakdown resulting in increased levels of circulating cortisol. As these factors are often not desirable in people with diabetes its use is limited. Various contraindications also exist with a number of medications and these should be checked prior to prescribing.	15–40 ml/week; usually taken as part of a combination formula in divided doses 2–3 times/day.

Gymnema sylvestre (gymnema)	When applied to the tongue *Gymnema sylvestre* numbs the sweet taste receptors, which can reduce the consumption of sweet foods. It increases beta cell permeability in vitro resulting in increased insulin release (Mitchell and Mitchell 2003) and may improve fasting blood glucose levels and enhance insulin action, therefore reducing insulin requirements in Type 1 diabetes and the use of oral hypoglycaemics in Type 2 diabetes. It does not appear to affect insulin levels in people without diabetes (Pizzorno and Murray, 1999).	Medication doses may need to be adjusted if *G. sylvestre* is taken concurrently. In people with insulin resistance and hyperinsulinaemia, *G. sylvestre's* insulin-promoting effects may not be desirable.	Liquid forms should be used if the aim is to numb the sweet taste buds; 5–10 drops in a mouthful of water is sufficient. 25–75 ml/week; usually taken as part of a combination formula in divided doses 2–3 times/day after meals.
Panax ginseng (Korean ginseng)	*Panax ginseng* may assist in improving fasting blood glucose levels; reduce triglycerides and increase HDL cholesterol and prevent complications associated with diabetic neuropathy (Braun and Cohen 2005).	Conflicting evidence exists as to whether *P. ginseng* increases blood pressure (Braun and Cohen 2005). People with hypertension or taking antihypertensive medications should only take *P. ginseng* under medical supervision.	7–40 ml/week; usually taken as part of a combination formula in divided doses 2–3 times/day.
Panax quinquefolius (American ginseng)	*Panax quinquefolius* appears to reduce postprandial glycemia in people with Type 2 diabetes by enhancing insulin secretion (Vuksan *et al.* 2001).	The lack of standardisation of herbs such as *P. quinquefolius*, provides a challenge for demonstrating reproducible efficacy in clinical settings (Vuksan and Sievenpiper 2005). Monitor requirements for diabetes medications.	1,000–3,000 mg *P. quinquefolius* up to 40 minutes prior to or with a meal.

Table 14.5 (Continued)

Herb	Beneficial effects	Cautions/contraindications	Suggested dose
Scuttelaria baicalensis (baical skullcap)	Preliminary evidence suggests that *Scuttelaria baicalensis* possesses antioxidant and neuroprotective properties; reduces blood pressure, cholesterol and triglycerides; protects against vascular disorders; slows the absorption of glucose by inhibiting intestinal sucrase and inhibits 5-alpha-aldose resulting in reduced sorbitol levels (Braun and Cohen 2005).		30–60 ml/week; usually taken as part of a combination formula in divided doses 2–3 times/day.
Trigonella foenum graecum (fenugreek)	May delay glucose absorption, reduce fasting glucose levels, enhance insulin sensitivity and reduce cholesterol levels in people with diabetes (Mitchell and Mitchell, 2003, Braun and Cohen 2005).	Monitor requirements for diabetes medications.	As fibre and steroidal saponins appear to be the active constituents in fenugreek the de-fatted seed extract is considered to be the most effective dose form. 25–100 g/day de-fatted fenugreek seed powder.

Vaccinium myrtillus (bilberry)	*Vaccinium myrtillus* may assist in protecting small blood vessels from damage due to its flavonoid content. The anthocyanadins in *V. myrtillus* are antioxidants and have a particular affinity for the blood vessels of the eye, which may assist in preventing diabetic retinopathy, cataracts, glaucoma and blindness. It may also reduce blood glucose levels and triglycerides (Braun and Cohen 2005).	*V. myrtillus* contains tannins, which may affect the absorption of some medicines and nutrients. *V. myrtillus* doses should, therefore, be given separately from food and medicines by at least 2–3 hours. Monitor requirements for diabetes medications. *V. myrtillus* may also cause constipation in some people.	Fluid extract 1:2–20–40 ml/week; usually taken as part of a combination formula in divided doses 2–3 times/day.
Vitis vinifera (grape seed extract)	A powerful antioxidant that helps to reconstitute vitamin E back into its unoxidised state allowing it to continue neutralising free radicals. It may also be of assistance in stabilising diabetic retinopathy (Braun and Cohen 2005).	Cautions/contraindications: Suspend use one week prior to surgery due to antiplatelet effects.	Suggested dose: Due to the unpleasant taste, tablet/capsule forms are most applicable in practice.

References

AANP The American Association of Naturopathic Physicians. Available from: http://www. naturopathic.org/naturopathic_medicine/definitions.aspx.

Althuis M, Jordan N, Ludington E, Wittes J. Glucose and insulin responses to dietary chromium supplements: a meta-analysis. *American Journal Clinical Nutrition* 2002; **76**(1): 148–155.

Balado D. (ed.) *Nutritional Management of Diabetes Mellitus*. 9th edn. Baltimore, MD: Williams & Wilkins. 1999, pp. 1370–1393.

Basch E, Gabardi S, Ulbricht C. Bitter melon (*Momordica charantia*): a review of efficacy and safety. *American Journal of Health System Pharmacology* 2003; **60**(4): 356–359.

Bijlani R, Vempati R, Yadav R, Ray R, Gupta V *et al*. A brief but comprehensive lifestyle education program based on yoga reduces risk factors for cardiovascular disease and diabetes mellitus. *Journal of Alternative and Complementary Medicine* 2005; **11**(2): 267–274.

Bonnefont-Rousselot D. The role of antioxidant micronutrients in the prevention of diabetic complications. *Treat Endocrinology* 2004; **3**(1): 41–52.

Braun L, Cohen M. *Herbs and Natural Supplements: An Evidence Based Guide*. Australia: Elsevier, 2005.

Chung S, Chung S. Aldose reductase in diabetic microvascular complications. *Current Drug Targets* 2005; **6**(4): 475–486.

Dunford C. The use of honey-derived dressings to promote effective wound management. *Professional Nurse* 2005; **20**(8): 35–38.

Dushay J, Abrahamson M. Insulin resistance and type 2 diabetes: a comprehensive review. *Medscape* [Online]. 2005.

Eddy J, Gideonsen M. Topical honey for diabetic foot ulcers. *Journal of Family Practice* 2005; **54**(6): 533–535.

Frishman W, Sinatra S, Kruger N. Nutriceuticals and cardiovascular health. In: Frishman W, Weintraub M, Micozzi M (eds), *Complementary and Integrative Therapies in Cardiovascular Disease*. Mosby, MO: Elsevier 2005; pp. 58–85.

Gilliam I. An exercise prescription for diabetes. *Journal of Complementary Medicine* 2004; **3**(4): 35–38.

Gonzalez-Bono E, Rohleder N, Hellhammer D, Salvador A, Kirschbaum C. Glucose but not protein or fat load amplifies the cortisol response to psychosocial stress. *Hormones and Behavior* 2002; **41**(3): 328–333.

Gross L, Li L, Ford E, Liu S. Increased consumption of refined carbohydrates and the epidemic of type 2 diabetes in the United States: an ecologic assessment. *American Journal Clinical Nutrition* 2004; **79**(5): 774–779.

Guerrero-Romero F, Rodriguez-Moran M. Complementary therapies for diabetes: the case for chromium, magnesium, and antioxidants. *Archives Medical Research* 2005; **36**(3): 250–257.

Hirsch I, Atchley D, Tsai E, Labbe R, Chait A. Ascorbic acid clearance in diabetic nephropathy. *Journal of Diabetes Complications* 1998; **12**(5): 259–263.

Hofman Z, van Drunen J, de Later C, Kuipers H. The effect of different nutritional feeds on the postprandial glucose response in healthy volunteers and patients with type II diabetes. *European Journal Clinical Nutrition* 2004; **58**(11): 1553–1556.

Huerta M, Roemmich J, Kington M, Bovbjerg V, Weltman A *et al*. Magnesium deficiency is associated with insulin resistance in obese children. *Diabetes Care* 2005; **28**(5): 1175–1181.

Khan A, Safdar M, Ali Khan M, Khattak K, Anderson R. Cinnamon improves glucose and lipids of people with type 2 diabetes. *Diabetes Care* 2003; **26**(12): 3215–3218.

LaMonte M, Yanowitz F. Aerobic exercise for lowering blood pressure: a meta-analysis. *Clinical Journal Sports Medicine* 2002; **12**(6): 407.

Lonn E, Bosch J, Yusuf S, Sheridan P, Pogue J *et al*. Effects of long-term vitamin E supplementation on cardiovascular events and cancer: a randomized controlled trial. *Journal American Medical Association* 2005; **293**(11): 1338–1347.

Mitchell D, Mitchell P. Diabetes. *Journal of Complementary Medicine* 2003; **2**(5): 14–19.

Nettleton JA, Katz R. n-3 long-chain polyunsaturated fatty acids in type 2 diabetes: a review. *Journal American Dietetics Association* 2005; **105**(3): 428–440.

Osawa T, Kato Y. Protective role of antioxidative food factors in oxidative stress caused by hyperglycemia. *Annals of the New York Academy of Sciences* 2005; **1043**: 440–451.

Packer L, Kraemer K, Rimbach G. Molecular aspects of lipoic acid in the prevention of diabetes complications. *Nutrition* 2001; **17**(10): 888–895.

Pham P, Pham P, Pham P, Pham S, Pham H, *et al*. Lower serum magnesium levels are associated with more rapid decline of renal function in patients with diabetes mellitus type 2. *Clinical Nephrology* 2005; **63**(6): 429–436.

Pizzorno J, Murray M. *Diabetes Mellitus: Textbook of Natural Medicine*. Edinburgh: Churchill Livingstone. 1999; pp. 1193–1218.

Powers A. Diabetes mellitus. In: Kasper, D. (ed.), *Harrison's Principles of Internal Medicine*. vol. 2: New York: McGraw-Hill, 2005; pp. 2152–2179.

Robertson R, Tanaka Y, Takahashi H, Tran P, Harmon J. Prevention of oxidative stress by adenoviral overexpression of glutathione-related enzymes in pancreatic islets. *Annals of the New York Academy of Sciences* 2005; **1043**: 513–520.

Salonen J, Nyyssonen K, Tuomainen T, Maenpaa P, Korpela H *et al*. Increased risk of non-insulin dependent diabetes mellitus at low plasma vitamin E concentrations: a four year follow-up study in men. *British Medical Journal* 1995; **311**(7013): 1124–1127.

Schulze M, Liu S, Rimm E, Manson J, Willett W, Hu F. Glycemic index, glycemic load, and dietary fiber intake and incidence of type 2 diabetes in younger and middle-aged women. *American Journal Clinical Nutrition* 2004; **80**(2): 348–356.

Scroggie D, Albright A, Harris M. The effect of glucosamine-chondroitin supplementation on glycosylated haemoglobin levels in patients with type 2 diabetes mellitus: a placebo-controlled, double-blinded, randomised controlled trial. *Archives of Internal Medicine* 2003; **163**(13): 1587–1590.

Sima A, Calvani M, Mehra M, Amato A. Acetyl-L-carnitine improves pain, nerve regeneration, and vibratory perception in patients with chronic diabetic neuropathy: an analysis of two randomized placebo-controlled trials. *Diabetes Care* 2005; **28**(1): 89–94.

Song Y, Wang J, Li X, Cai L. Zinc and the diabetic heart. *Biometals* 2005; **18**(4): 325–332.

Steyn N, Mann J, Bennett P, Temple N, Zimmet P *et al*. Diet, nutrition and the prevention of type 2 diabetes. *Public Health Nutrition* 2004; **7**(1A): 147–165.

Studer M, Briel M, Leimenstoll B, Glass T, Bucher H. Effect of different antilipidemic agents and diets on mortality: a systematic review. *Archives of Internal Medicine* 2005; **165**(7): 725–730.

van der Weyden E. Treatment of a venous leg ulcer with a honey alginate dressing. *British Journal of Community Nursing* 2005; Supplement: S21, S24, S26–27.

Venn B, Mann J. Cereal grains, legumes and diabetes. *European Journal Clinical Nutrition* 2004; **58**(11): 1443–1461.

Vuksan V, Sievenpiper J. Herbal remedies in the management of diabetes: lessons learned from the study of ginseng. *Nutrition Metabolism Cardiovascular Disease* 2005; **15**(3): 149–160.

Vuksan V, Sievenpiper J, Xu Z, Wong E, Jenkins A *et al*. Konjac-Mannan and American ginsing: emerging alternative therapies for type 2 diabetes mellitus. *Journal of American College Nutrition* 2001; **20**(5 Suppl): 370S–380S; discussion 381S–383S.

Wilson B, Gondy A. Effects of chromium supplementation on fasting insulin levels and lipid parameters in healthy, non-obese young subjects. *Diabetes Research Clinical Practice* 1995; **28**(3): 179–184.

Wolkowitz O, Epel E, Reus V. Stress hormone-related psychopathology: pathophysiological and treatment implications. *World Journal of Biological Psychiatry* 2001; **2**(3): 115–143.

Yokota K. Diabetes mellitus and magnesium. *Clinical Calcium* 2005; **15**(2): 203–212.

Zhang C, Williams M, Frederick I, King I, Sorensen T *et al*. Vitamin C and the risk of gestational diabetes mellitus: a case-control study. *Journal Reproductive Medicine* 2004; **49**(4): 257–266.

15 Complementary Approaches to Managing Pain

Trish Dunning and Leon Chaitow

15.1 Introduction

Almost everybody experiences pain at some stage in their lives and pain is the most common reason people seek health care. Persistent pain occurs in up to half the world's population and more than 50 per cent of chronic pain sufferers describe their pain as severe (Breen 2002). Chronic pain has significant negative physical, psychological and social consequences and affects quality of life, self-esteem and motivation, and health service utilisation (Breen 2002; MacDonald 2003; Murphy-Ende 2003; Haetzman et al. 2003). Haetzman et al. (2003) found 18.2 per cent of n = 840 consulted a complementary therapist for chronic pain and 15.7 per cent were taking complementary medicines and usually used these therapies in combination with conventional medicines. Adolescents use complementary pain management strategies and family members often influence their choice (Braun et al. 2005). Most indicate they were not asked about complementary therapy use but ∼ 15 per cent choose not to disclose. Many physical and psychological disorders, and their diagnostic investigations and treatments, cause pain. Pain has such an impact on health care that it has been described as the '5th vital sign' (Campbell 1995).

The prevalence of acute pain among hospitalised patients is also high, occurring in 58–75 per cent of admissions, and may result from disease, injury or surgical procedures (Acute Pain Management Guideline Panel 1992). Acute pain triggers a metabolic stress response that can cause hyperglycaemia. Post-operative pain can delay the return to normal bowel function that may exacerbate diabetic gastroparesis. The Acute Pain Management Panel (1992) recommended an aggressive and flexible approach to managing acute pain, using strategies that incorporate stress management and non-pharmacologic and pharmacologic therapies. There is good evidence for the effectiveness of behavioural therapies, electrical nerve stimulation, acupuncture, and relaxation therapies in managing post-operative pain

Table 15.1 Some common conditions that cause pain in people with diabetes.

Acute	Chronic
Minor cuts, burns, insect bites	Concomitant diseases such as arthritis.
Acute conditions such as:	Nerve entrapment such as carpel tunnel syndrome.
fractures and other trauma	Diabetes complications especially:
surgical emergencies	peripheral neuropathy
ketoacidosis (abdominal pain)	autonomic neuropathy
Myocardial infarction (MI)	cardiac disease.
(although MI may be 'silent')	Vascular and arterial leg ulcers.
	Amputation.
	Frequent blood glucose monitoring, especially
	when the fingers are sensitive and is a cause
	of infrequent monitoring

(Spencer and Jacobs 1999: 217). Therefore, in a Quality Use of Medicine approach, these therapies could complement or replace conventional analgesia.

Pain may affect self-care and compromise metabolic control. The prevalence of pain among people with diabetes is unknown. They experience pain for the same reasons as non-diabetics, in addition to pain related to diabetes and its complications, see Table 15.1. Therefore, the prevalence of pain is likely to be similar to, or even higher, in people with diabetes than in non-diabetics. Pain management in people with diabetes is often overshadowed by the focus on metabolic control and achieving metabolic targets. For example, most studies of pain management of neuropathic pain use blood glucose as a major outcome indicator. In addition, pain is poorly assessed and managed in the elderly, especially those over 65, who have a high prevalence of diabetes, and often in palliative care situations (McCaffrey and Rolling Ferrell 1991). Some of the reasons for inadequate pain management are shown in Table 15.2.

Table 15.2 Some reasons for inadequate pain management. Pain is more likely to be under treated in people over 65 years (McCaffery and Rolling Ferrel 1991). The reasons may be fear of causing respiratory distress, mistaken belief that the elderly do not experience the same pain intensity and the individual under-reporting pain.

Clients with pain	Health professionals
Reluctance to take medicines.	Belief that the pain will 'go away by itself'.
Not taking medicines is an effective way to	Not appreciating the severity of the pain.
minimise pain for example using low doses	Fear that analgesia will mask important
or prolonged dose intervals.	signs and symptoms and obscure or
Not asking for analgesia because they do not	delay the diagnosis.
want to appear to be 'demanding' or 'addicts'.	Fear of causing addiction.
Fear of becoming addicted.	Concerns about causing side effects such
Unpleasant side effects of some analgesic agents.	as respiratory depression and nausea and
	vomiting.
	Inadequate education about pain
	assessment and management strategies.

15.2   What Is Pain?

Physical pain cannot be separated from its psychological effects. As Sinclair (2002) stated, 'The most universal form of stress is pain.' People vary in their experiences and reported severity of pain, which may be unrelated to the underlying pathology or the extent of tissue damage (The International Association for the Study of Pain 1986). Merskey and Bogdus (1994) defined pain as: 'An unpleasant sensory and emotional experience associated with actual or potential tissue damage or described in terms of such damage.' This definition clearly links physical and emotional factors, and highlights the fact that the degree of pain experienced is not necessarily correlated with the degree of injury. In addition, the definition suggests that pain perception is a complex phenomenon involving sensory, emotional and cognitive processes that can be modified by circumstances. Pain is also defined as 'whatever the person says it is, existing wherever the experiencing person says it does' (McCaffery and Beebe 1989: 7). McCaffrey and Beebe's (1989) definition, although old, highlights the individual, subjective nature of pain. Further, it suggests health professionals must accept the person's assessment of their pain severity.

Pain can be categorised as: acute, chronic, and cancer-related pain. Acute pain is usually short-lived and resolves when the precipitating event resolves. Chronic pain can be persistent or occur intermittently (flare-ups), and may become the primary health condition requiring management. Cancer-related pain can be either acute or become chronic with associated flare-ups. Unrelieved pain can affect all the body systems, as indicated, and produces its own physical and emotional symptoms. These effects compromise important diabetes management strategies, such as exercise and self-care and may engender depression, which in turn affects motivation and the ability to achieve metabolic targets. Pain interferes with REM sleep and contributes to sleep deprivation. It is also becoming clear that these factors increase sensitivity to pain (Roth 2005). Therefore managing sleep is part of pain management.

15.3   Pathophysiology of Pain

Pain consists of four nerve-related aspects: sensory, feeling pain; arousal, being aware or alert to pain; emotional, being distressed by pain; cognitive, the context in which the pain occurs and its meaning to the individual (Spinella 2005).

Several theories have been developed to explain pain, the best known being the gate control theory (Melzack and Wall 1965). The gate control theory is outdated because recent research demonstrates that pain perception is a dynamic, rapidly changing, phenomenon involving a more complex interplay between the peripheral nerves, the central nervous system and the ascending and descending pathways, than the gate control theory suggests (Power and Colvin 2001).

Ascending system

Once tissue injury occurs, the damaged cells and surrounding capillaries produce algesic substances (bradykinin, serotonin, substance P, potassium and prostaglandins), which activate nerve endings and sensitise them to other chemical, thermal, or mechanical stimuli and induce a state of hyperalgesia. Prostaglandin plays a central role in sensitisation. In hyperalgesic states the nerve pain threshold is significantly lowered so that even mild stimuli cause pain. Once nocioceptors are stimulated they generate an electrical impulse, which carries the pain signal along the peripheral nerves, to the central nervous system via alpha delta C fibres (Hawthorn and Redmond 1998). Primary afferent fibres enter the spinal cord through the dorsal horn, or dorsal root, where they are modulated by the descending influences of the brain and/or excitatory or inhibitory peptides.

Neurotransmitters, such as substance P, facilitate the transmission of pain stimuli from first-order neurones to second-order neurones across nerve synapses. The second-order neurones cross the spinal cord at the anterior commissur and reach the brain via the spinothalamic tract where they are relayed to the reticular formation, which controls the initial response to the injury: the hypothalamus, which triggers neuroendocrine responses such as tachycardia and sweating; and the thalamus where the intensity and site of the pain are interpreted. Third-order neurones project from these areas of the brain to the limbic system, which triggers psychological responses to the pain, and to the somosensory cortex, where memories and experiences are integrated.

Descending system

Endogenous opioids are activated when the pain stimuli reach the brain. These arise from the hypothalamus, periductal grey matter and nucleus raphe magnus in the brain stem, and interrupt pain transmission. Endogenous and exogenous opoids bind to opoid receptors and inhibit the release of neurotransmitters. Thus, several types of nerve fibres are involved in pain processing: Alpha, alpha beta and alpha delta fibres, which are large, myelinated fibres that usually transmit localised intense pain rapidly. Alpha beta fibres transmit low intensity mechanical messages and respond to touch and pressure, for example, they can be stimulated by massage (Hawthorn and Redmond 1998) and chronic pain. Massage, heat and cold, and TENS all activate alpha beta fibres, and override ascending pain stimuli being transmitted via the alpha delta and C fibres. C fibres, which are unmyelinated, transmit signals slowly. They respond to pain and temperature and often cause dull, aching, or burning pain, for example, diabetic neuropathic pain.

Effects of pain

The effects of pain may be short term or chronic or long term. Short-term or immediate effects include tachycardia, a rise in blood pressure, increased respiratory rate, pupil dilatation, increased perspiration and muscle tension, and psychic arousal. Specific types and locations of pain may produce other symptoms such as hypotension, nausea and vomiting, with abdominal pain (Merskey and Bogdus 1994; Hawthorn and Redmond 1998). Acute pain is a warning that something is wrong and usually dissipates when the triggering factor resolves. Greuner (2004) suggested inadequate treatment of acute pain could 'facilitate the development of chronic pain'.

Chronic or long-term pain can result in various debilitating disorders that reduce mobility and affect quality of life and psychological well-being. Stress and anxiety, fear of losing control, and, in the long term, depression, are common (Breen 2002). These consequences affect concentration and cognitive ability (Hallberg and Carlsson 2000). For people with diabetes this might mean they have difficulty concentrating during diabetes education sessions, and taking in medical advice during consultations, if pain is not adequately managed.

Assessing pain

A careful appropriate assessment is essential to managing pain. However, it is difficult to assess pain, especially when comorbidities and impaired cognition are present, and in the elderly, children, and people from culturally different backgrounds such as Aboriginal peoples (Fenwick and Stevens 1998). Asking the patient to describe their pain can provide clues to the type of fibres involved and indicate possible management strategies. Using a variety of descriptive terms when asking patients to describe their pain is important, because people do not always know how to describe their pain. Several assessment procedures are used: observation, taking a verbal history of the physical and psychological symptoms, physical examination, determining methods the patient uses to manage pain, including the current episode, and their relative effectiveness.

Assessment involves:

- Careful observation of non-verbal cues and checking assumptions and interpretation. For example, a quiet and withdrawn child may be in pain or may be fearful of strangers. The behaviour should be observed over time and changes noted.
- Using pain-rating scales, which may be pictorial such as a series of faces ranging from a happy smile to downturned mouth and frown.
- Physical signs such as tachycardia, or guarding.

Issues to note when conducting a pain history:

- onset, duration and pattern of the pain;
- site of the pain and where it radiates. If the pain is chronic, the frequency and duration of flare-ups and their association with any specific activity.
- type or character of the pain including the intensity at rest and during movement, for example, allodynia, hyperalgesia, dysesthesia;
- limitations to mobility and manual dexterity;

- factors that aggravate or relieve the pain;
- symptoms that accompany the pain such as sleep deprivation or lowered mood;
- emotional responses to pain and the client's beliefs about the pain;
- expectations of treatment;
- the treatments that have improved the pain in the past;
- possible secondary gain from the pain process.

Investigations such as blood tests (ESR, C-reactive protein, white cell count), electrical nerve conduction studies and radiological imaging may be indicated to determine the underlying cause of the pain. In some cases, especially chronic pain, referral to an appropriate specialist or pain management clinic (conventional or complementary) can be beneficial.

15.4 Measuring Pain Severity

A range of pain assessment tools is used to measure pain. It is particularly helpful to use several tools over a period of time. Some, such as the McGill Pain Questionnaire, are useful initially to assess acute pain. However, the McGill Questionnaire does not take into account past experiences, cultural and psychological factors or associated fears that influence an individual's pain perception – the personal meaning of pain. Although most pain measurement tools are subjective, they enable repeat measures to be made that assist with identifying pain patterns.

Visual analogue, Likert, and descriptive pain intensity scales are widely used to rate pain severity before and after treatment to assess treatment effectiveness, see Figure 15.1. Some people have difficulty understanding visual analogue scales and a range of pictorial and binary scales have been developed, for example, the pictorial face pain scale (The Association for the Study of Pain at the Sydney

Example word category rating scales	Example visual analogue scales.
People place a tick ☑ next to the word that best describes their pain.	The lines are usually 10 cm and people place a mark on the line to indicate their response.
A) Pain intensity. none 0 slight 1 moderate 2 severe 3	Please place a mark on the line that best describes your pain ├─────────────────────────────┤ Least possible pain Worst possible pain
B) Pain relief. none 0 slight 1 moderate 2 good 3 complete 4 Please circle the response that best describes your pain/pain relief.	Please place a mark on the line that best describes your pain relief. ├─────────────────────────────┤ No pain relief Complete pain relief

Figure 15.1 Word category rating scales and visual analogue scales that can be used to rate pain a), and the effects of pain management techniques. b) Visual analogue scales are well validated for clinical use and are widely used to assess both acute and chronic pain.

Children's Hospital). Although this scale was developed for children, people who cannot communicate verbally or speak English can use it. However, other indicators of pain need to be considered when patients are comatose or cognitively impaired. These include non-verbal body clues such as guarding, grimacing, moaning, and thrashing about, or changed behaviour patterns.

Multidimensional tools that assess pain perception, functional effects and mood are particularly useful to measure chronic pain and include:

- McGill Pain Questionnaire
- Pain Disability Index
- SF36 Short Form 36 Health Survey and a range of specialised scales such as the Oswestry low back pain scale.
- Nijmegen questionnaire, which is a validated tool that can rapidly quantify the degree to which altered breathing patterns may be a feature. (van Dixhoorn 1985, Vansteenkiste *et al.* 1991). Breathing patterns are particularly important because hyperventilation modifies pain perception (lowered threshold) and influences circulatory efficiency, which is of particular relevance to people with diabetes (Pryor and Prasad 2002).

Anxiety exacerbates pain; therefore, anxiety scales such as the State Trait Anxiety Inventory are sometimes used together with pain rating scales. Figure 15.2 provides an overview of important factors to consider when assessing pain.

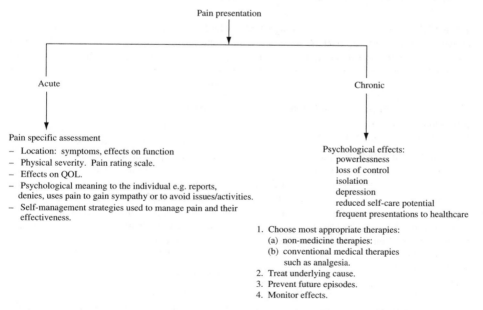

Figure 15.2 Outline of important factors to consider when assessing pain. The aim of pain management is to achieve balanced analgesia using an appropriate therapy or therapies with the fewest side effects at the lowest doses. Totally suppressing the pain may not be the best option. QOL = quality of life.

15.5   Managing Pain

Pain management strategies must be individualised especially if the pain is chronic, which usually requires self-care (Edworthy 2000). Managing negative cognitive and behavioural patterns that often accompany chronic pain may be necessary to help the individual develop effective pain coping strategies. Therefore, the individual is a pivotal member of the pain management team and this philosophy is consistent with complementary therapy philosophy and diabetes management strategies that aim for patient empowerment, patient-centred care and team care in a therapeutic relationship are important aspects of pain management.

Early treatment often enables non-pharmacological methods or lower doses and less potent pharmacological substances to be used. Diet and mental health are key considerations. Table 15.3 outlines the commonly used conventional and complementary pain management techniques. Pain management strategies relieve pain by removing the cause, neutralising the effect of the stimulus, relieving associated discomfort, suppressing the disease process or the pain, and altering the individual's perception of their pain. Pain management techniques may include: masking pain messages or reducing their intensity; reducing pain transmission; changing the way the patient interprets the pain; reducing the inflammatory response; educating the person to understand their pain and pain self-management techniques. Although the gate control theory is outdated, it is a useful way to explain pain and its management to patients.

Table 15.3   Commonly used pain management methods. Often combinations of complementary, conventional or both approaches can be used and sometimes combined therapies enable lower doses of pharmacological agents to be used, which is in keeping with Quality Use of Medicines.

Conventional	Complementary
Non-pharmacological: Rehabilitation programmes, structured exercise programs, rest and immobilisation. Pharmacological: • Opioids, which bind to opioid receptors in the central nervous system, e.g. morphine, codeine, pethidine, oxycodeine, methadone, fentanyl and tramadol that also has spinal non-opioid spinal and central nervous system effects • Non-steroidal anti-inflammatory agents (NSAIDS) • Paracetamol • Local anaesthetics, regional anaesthesia, nerve blocks • Anticonvulsants and antidepressants for neuropathic pain • Counter Erritants	Non-pharmacological: • Psychological approaches including education, cognitive therapies, hydrotherapy, relaxation training, breathing retraining, distraction, meditation and guided imagery, humour, hypnosis, biofeedback and music • Physical approaches including massage, acupuncture, shiatsu, Therapeutic Touch, TENS, manipulative therapies such as chiropractic Pharmacological: • Analgesic and anti-inflammatory herbs • Analgesic and anti-inflammatory essential oils • Homeopathy • Antioxidants and dietary supplements

Complementary and conventional therapies both include pharmacological and non-pharmacological methods. Where pharmacological methods are used, they should be applied within the Quality Use of Medicines Framework (Australian Department for Health and Ageing 2002; Dunning 2005). This chapter focuses on complementary pain management approaches. Complementary therapies can be used alone, in combination, or combined with conventional approaches. Non-pharmacological complementary therapies may avoid adverse medicine-related events especially where multiple medicines are used, which is often the case in diabetes.

Many complementary approaches address the physical, psychological and spiritual aspects of pain and recognise that the responsibility for pain management is shared between the health professional and the patient, which helps people feel more in control of the outcomes (Stevenson 1995).

Non-pharmacological complementary pain management approaches

Non-pharmacological complementary methods can be loosely divided into physical and psychological techniques, which can be used alone, combined with other complementary therapies or pharmacological methods to enhance their analgesic effects (Jakobsson 2005).

Nutrition

Eating a well-balanced diet to promote normal growth and repair and control blood glucose and lipids. If inflammation is contributing to pain, anything that reduces or modifies the inflammation is likely to reduce the level of perceived pain. Ideally, anti-inflammatory strategies limit, rather than eliminate the inflammatory process, which is an integral aspect of tissue healing. A major feature of inflammation involves prostaglandins and leukotrienes that are largely dependent on the presence of arachidonic acid, found abundantly in animal fats. Useful anti-inflammatory strategies include:

- reducing or eliminating arachidonic acid, one of the main precursors of inflammatory leukotrienes and prostaglandins by reducing or eliminating dietary animal fats (Donowitz 1985, Ghosh and Myers 1998);
- increasing the intake of cold water fish, or fish oil in capsule form, which provides anti-inflammatory eicosapentenoic acid (EPA) (Moncada 1986);
- vitamin B supplements may prevent moderate nerve damage.

Physical therapies

Manipulative therapies

Manipulative therapies include acupuncture, osteopathy, chiropractic, massage, kinesiology, and trigger point therapy. Once serious spinal pathology is ruled out, manipulative therapies can provide symptomatic relief and restore function

(Shekelle 2002). Serious complications from manipulation have been reported. The safety of acupuncture is well documented (Rampes and James 1995) but some adverse events have been recorded and include bleeding, needle pain, tiredness and very rarely syncope and hepatitis from unsterile needles.

Chiropractic and osteopathic manipulation are frequently used methods of relieving musculoskeletal pain and are often used to treat chronic headache, back and neck pain and sciatica. Soft tissue manipulation methods that focus on deactivation of pain-inducing myofascial trigger points can also improve function where muscles have become excessively tense, see Chapter 16 (Chen *et al.* 1993; Hong *et al.* 1996; Simons *et al.* 1999).

Acupuncture

Acupuncture can be applied using needles, pressure to specific points on the body or laser and is often combined with moxibustion, which involves burning a small piece of a herb called moxa (*Artemisia vulgaris*) that is attached to the needle handle, in order to generate heating of the needle. Other substances, such as a salt, may also be placed over the appropriate acupoint, theoretically to stimulate *chi*, see Chapter 11. The World Health Organization (WHO) lists over 40 conditions for which acupuncture can be used that covers most body systems as well as emotional problems such as anxiety and depression. Many medical doctors qualify as acupuncturists or refer to acupuncturists. Appropriate infection control procedures for acupuncture needles must be followed.

Acupuncture analgesia is one of the most frequently researched complementary therapies. It most probably works through stimulating the release of neurotransmitters such as endorphins, monoamines and serotonin, which block pain signals (Kiser 1983; Baldry 1993; Yoon-Hang Kim 2004a).

Significant improvement in neuropathic pain has been demonstrated using acupuncture (Abuaisha *et al.* 1998). Abuaisha *et al.* provided acupuncture for 46 patients with chronic painful neuropathy to determine long-term effectiveness. Initial treatment consisted of six courses of acupuncture over ten weeks. Forty-four completed the course: 63 per cent were already receiving standard conventional neuropathy medications. Some 77 per cent showed significant pain reduction. These were followed up for 18–72 weeks and 67 per cent were able to stop or reduce their conventional analgesia and only 24 per cent required further acupuncture during the follow-up period but neurological parameters and HbA_{1c} did not change. No side effects were observed. The authors concluded acupuncture is a safe, effective treatment for painful peripheral neuropathy but the mechanism of action remains unclear.

PAIN® GONE, is a form of acupuncture where a 'self-activated crystal stimulator,' appears to effectively control acute and chronic pain (www.paingone.com.au 2002). A small electrical current (1–2 Hz) is delivered to acupuncture points through a small pen-like device. It is available from pharmacies and surgical supply outlets in Australia and has TGA approval, however, more quality research is needed.

Applied Kinesiology (AK)

AK involves testing muscle strength after the muscles are challenged to gather information as part of a normal diagnostic assessment and aims to restore neuromuscular function. A basic concept of AK, held in common with other complementary therapies, is that the body is self-correcting and self-regulating. Chiropractor George Goodheart (1980) who developed AK, stated:

> Applied Kinesiology is based upon the fact that body language never lies. The opportunity of understanding body language is enhanced by the ability to use muscles as indicators of body function . . . Once muscle weakness has been ascertained, a variety of therapeutic actions become available.

AK practitioners believe that many standard diagnostic procedures fail to detect significant changes of function until they are two standard deviations from the norm. That is, when the normal negative feedback control mechanisms of homeostasis have failed. AK aims to detect what could be termed 'noise in the system', which detracts from system performance to arrive at a functional diagnosis (Walther 1988). AK may be relevant to assessing the early stages of peripheral neuropathy but no definitive information is available. Widely used approaches within AK include: adjusting spinal and extremity joints; observing actions to normalise, posture and gait; soft tissue techniques; neural receptor treatment; balancing meridian; balancing the craniosacral system; nutritional therapy.

Exercise

Exercise is one of the preventative health strategies Hippocrates recommended to achieve a healthy lifestyle and is central to diabetes management. A number of exercise techniques are used as part of pain management strategies to improve mobility, fitness and strength. Exercise also has positive benefits for blood glucose and lipid levels by improving insulin sensitivity and blood flow, cardiovascular fitness, weight control, and reduces blood pressure and minimises falls risk.

Common exercises include resistance training, yoga, Qi gong and tai chi, which are integral aspects of some complementary medicine systems such as Chinese medicine, see Chapter 11, and Ayurveda, Chapter 10. People commencing an exercise regime should have a thorough physical assessment before they commence and be educated about foot care and managing hypoglycaemia if they are taking insulin or oral hypoglycaemic agents.

Hydrotherapy

Hydrotherapy has been used for centuries (Coccheri 2002). In order to be considered holistic, hydrotherapy should meet several basic criteria:

- Treatment should aim to assist homeostatic mechanisms and not suppress symptoms (Standish 1992).

- Treatment should not create new problems or overload adaptive capacity.
- Treatment should take account of the individual's unique requirements, current state of vulnerability and ability to respond to stimuli. The levels of heat/cold used and the duration of exposure should be tailored to match these requirements especially when the person has peripheral neuropathy, which puts their feet at risk of burns when hot water is used. Therefore, hot applications to the feet or legs and full body heating treatments such as saunas and hot immersion baths should be avoided. The latter may also precipitate hypotension and lead to other adverse events such as falls.
- Where hydrotherapy is used repetitively over long periods of time, the degree and length of exposure to the treatment are usually gradually increased.

Hydrotherapy variables are as follows:

- Hot, warm, neutral cool or cold water can be used for seconds, minutes or hours; alternately (hot followed by cold etc.) or constantly; applied directly to the body, or 'held' in saturated material such as cotton or linen, sometimes insulated by a woollen (or other) covering, after application.
- Part, or all, the body can be placed into water to achieve a variety of effects, including exercising in a reduced gravitational environment.
- Jets can be sprayed at the body, or parts of it, involving both thermal and mechanical effects and/or to effect circulation.
- Douching can be used to apply water to orifices.
- Ice may be applied to inflamed areas or for profound reflex effects (Kuznetsov 2000).
- Steam can be inhaled.
- Water may used in a pure form, or with substances suspended in it such as Epsom salts, sea salt, oatmeal 'milk', essential oils (Mancini 2003). Alternatively Sea water may be used (thallasotherapy).
- Mud, clay and/or peat and other colloidal suspensions may be used for specific effects.

Two main types of hydrotherapy are used: external and internal. External hydrotherapy includes:

- Hot and cold contrast which is believed to stimulate endocrine function and reduce congestion. Heat and cold packs have counter-irritant effects.
- Hot water including saunas, sweat baths and hot compresses, which increase local blood flow induce relaxation and reduce pain. Gel packs and wheat bags are other ways of using heat. Hot water or hot packs may be contraindicated for people with neuropathic feet because of the risk of burns, which puts the person at risk of ulcers and amputation.
- Cold water, ice or cold packs, which causes an initial vasoconstriction followed by vasodilation. Therefore, cold applications may actually improve circulation, unlike hot applications which produce venous stasis and retard circulation. Improving the circulation may reduce swelling and inflammation, thereby relieving local pressure and improve tissue oxygenation.

- Baths.
- Poultices, which can be hot or cold, may use clay, comfrey or charcoal depending on the indication for the compress. For example, comfrey reduces local oedema and reduces pain by relieving pressure from oedema. Poultices can also be warming and help relieve arthritic pain.

Internal hydrotherapy includes:

- Steam inhalation, often using essential oils, can reduce upper airway congestion but may be contraindicated if the person has asthma, heart disease, is frail, or at risk of burns.
- Fluid replacement in dehydrated states, which is standard conventional management.
- Colonic irrigations to flush out toxins. These can precipitate dehydration and ketoacidosis or hyperosmolar states.

Transcutaneous electrical nerve stimulation (TENS)

TENS involves placing gel-covered pads to the area over or beside the pain and delivering a mild electric current to mask the pain by stimulating local nerves. TENS is effective for acute pain but is particularly useful for chronic pain low back pain (Siddall 1991). One advantage is that TENS can be self-applied, which enhances the patient's independence and self-efficacy.

Blood flow is an important factor in wound healing and is often compromised in the lower extremities of people with diabetes. Ghen (1998) examined the effect of high voltage pulsed current on blood flow to the feet in people at risk of diabetic foot ulcers using a repeat measure study design. Transcutaneous oxygen levels were measured at baseline, 30 and 60 minutes (n = 132). Transcutaneous oxygen levels decreased from baseline following electrical stimulation in 73 per cent of people. Ghen concluded that electrostimulation was only effective at increasing blood flow in a small subset by an unknown mechanism.

Magnet therapy

Magnets are used in conventional medicine as diagnostic tools, for example, nuclear magnetic resonance imaging and pulsed electromagnetic field used to stimulate fracture healing. In complementary care, they are often used to manage musculoskeletal pain. They may exert their effect by moving ions associated with blood flow to induce an electrical current in soft tissue and joints (Kolasinski 2005). Magnets may modify cell membrane potential and desensitise sensory neurons, thus they may have a role in peripheral neuropathy as well as musculoskeletal pain. Apart from medical equipment, magnets are placed in mattresses, innersoles and bracelets. There is no evidence of any serious adverse events provide the product specifications are followed.

Massage and touch therapies

Massage is an instinctive response to pain and may reduce pain by stimulating alpha beta fibres and limit the number of pain impulses reaching the brain. Alternatively it may stimulate the endorphin release (Kaada and Torsteinino 1989), however, good quality evidence of pain relief is lacking and many available studies have methodological flaws (Vickers 1996: 86). Massage has been shown to improve mood and sleep patterns (Field *et al.* 2002), joint mobility, induce relaxation, reduce stress and reduce spinal cord excitability in a small sample (Morelli *et al.* 1991), see Chapter 7.

Cherkin (2001) demonstrated that massage is an effective short-term treatment for low back pain compared to acupuncture in a randomised control trial (n = 262). The massage group used fewer medicines and reported improved symptoms and lower disability. Appropriate diet, mobilisation, exercise and, if necessary, analgesia are effective and preferred by patients, see Chapter 13. The postulated mechanisms of pain relief using massage may not account for its actual analgesic effects. Other potential mechanisms of pain modulation include altering the individual's perception of pain, the analgesic properties of some essential oils (when they are combined with massage), and skin stimulation and increase temperature (Naliboff and Tachiki 1991). Many health professionals have regular massages and health insurance companies in Australia cover massage when it is a prescribed treatment.

Touch is a key aspect of massage. Physical contact is vital to human development and conveys caring and understanding in a health professional context. Two other major types of touch include Healing Touch (HT) and Therapeutic Touch (TT). HT and TT are energy-based therapies. TT does not involve actual physical contact; the practitioner's hands are moved through the patient's energy field. Significant reductions in headache and post-operative pain over placebo have been demonstrated (Dossey 1995; Stevenson 1994).

Reflexology

Pain relief is one of the earliest recorded indications for reflexology (Wright no date), see Chapter 13. Reflexologists view pain as an emotional as well as physical condition and often concentrate on stimulating the solar plexus point on the feet or hands or endocrine and circulatory systems, and lymphatic points to remove toxins. One postulated mechanism is that reflexology pressure causes numbness by exerting pressure and releasing tension and inducing relaxation that assists the person to remain calm when acute pain is present. Specific points may be activated in acute pain but usually the whole foot or hand is worked to manage chronic pain. For example, Li 4 (the great eliminator) may be worked to relieve pain in the upper body. SP 21 may be activated to help boost the immune system. Stress reduction aid in blood glucose control and pain perception. However, reflexology is under-researched and many studies are methodologically flawed.

Psychological approaches

Psychological approaches involve stress management and enhancing coping. Psychological factors (depression) can affect the outcome of cardiovascular disease (National Heart Foundation 2003). Thus appropriate pain management may contribute to improved outcomes. Psychological approaches are discussed in Chapter 7.

Biofeedback

Types of biofeedback include electromyography and thermal. Biofeedback is often combined with other non-pharmacological therapies such as relaxation techniques. Education from a suitably qualified practitioner is required for individuals to learn biofeedback techniques (Alternative Medicine Alert 2005). Biofeedback is often used with relaxation and other pain management strategies. People learn to control body functions such as blood pressure, heart rate and muscle tension. Studies in both type 1 and type 2 diabetes indicate biofeedback does not reduce pain but has positive benefits for depression (McGrady et al. 1991; Jablon et al. 1997).

McGrady et al. (1991) undertook a randomised controlled study to test the effect of a ten-week course of biofeedback-assisted relaxation in 18 adults with type 1 diabetes comparing pre- and post-treatment insulin doses. Significant lower blood glucose was observed in the biofeedback group that could not be explained by increased insulin doses. McGrady et al. recommended stress management is considered as a complementary management strategy in type 1 diabetes. While this study does not directly concern pain management, improved control has been shown to delay or prevent the onset of diabetes complications, which are a major cause of pain in people with diabetes.

Likewise, Jablon et al. (1997) used EMG biofeedback combined with progressive relaxation in 20 people with type 2 diabetes using a pre- and post-test design. Outcomes measures were glucose tolerance, fasting and two-hour post-prandial blood glucose levels, fructosamine and stress reduction using physiological measures and self-complete questionnaires. Significant stress reduction was noted using the State Trait Anxiety Scale and reduced muscle activity and skin conductance, but no changes were found in metabolic parameters.

Distraction

Distraction therapies aim to help people focus on something other than their pain. People often use distraction unconsciously, for example, watching television. Distraction alone may help people manage mild pain but additional or other strategies are usually required to manage moderate to severe pain. However, some people report feeling irritable, tired and have more pain after using the distraction techniques suggested so patient selection is important (Alternative Medicine Alert 2005). Many of the psychosocial pain management strategies such as relaxation, meditation and guided imagery involve distraction.

Humour may be a form of distraction and may help people relax and put their problems into perspective and promote hope. These factors have positive benefits physically and enable people to cope with their pain – and their diabetes. Likewise, creative arts such as painting and writing can be relaxing and cathartic and could be incorporated into holistic education and management. The arts may affect health professionals' performance. For example, music is often played in operating theatres and a recent study showed classical music led to marginally more accurate monitoring than rock music (Rouse 2005). People who listened to music intraoperatively or post-operatively reported significantly lower pain one and two hours post-operatively than a control group.

Relaxation

Relaxation therapies aim to reduce stress. Reducing stress has positive benefits not only for pain relief but also in improving immune system function, coping ability and general well-being. Early studies showed stress is an important component of pain (Morgan 1984). Stress can be acute and of short duration or become chronic, as may be the case with diabetes. Metabolic effects include increased fat metabolism and hyperglycaemia.

Relaxation therapies prevent some types of pain from exacerbating by reducing muscle tension. They also promote sleep and reduce stress and anxiety, which enhances people's coping abilities and positively affects other concomitant pain management therapies (Alternative Medicine Alert 2005). Generalised relaxation appears to be more effective than relaxing specific body areas. It can be difficult for people with severe pain to relax. Potential adverse events include shortness of breath with deep breathing and sleeping in inappropriate positions that can cause discomfort such as neck and back pain (National Institute Health Technology Statement 1999).

Although relaxation reduces pain, Lane *et al.* 1993 did not find any significant improvement in glycosylated haemoglobin after intensive conventional treatment followed by biofeedback-assisted relaxation training for eight weeks over conventional treatment alone. However, blood glucose was lower and improvements in anxiety occurred in a subgroup of the relaxation group ($n = 38$). Lane *et al.* recommended further research to determine whether relaxation training in addition to conventional treatment could provide added benefits by reducing stress. It should be noted that pain management was not the prime focus of Lane *et al.*'s study.

Breathing rehabilitation

Anxiety resulting from illness and pain encourages rapid, upper-chest breathing. Breathing rehabilitation reduces or eliminates many of the negative effects of breathing pattern disorders (Han *et al.* 1996), which includes increased excitability of both cutaneous and motor axons (Seyal 1998) and increased pain perception, by lowering pain thresholds and decreasing excitability of hippocampal neurons (Lum 1994).

Meditation and guided imagery

Meditation is the intentional self-regulation of awareness of the present, see Chapter 7. Two major techniques are used: Concentration meditation, the best-known types being transcendental meditation and mindfulness meditation. In these meditation types attention is focused on a single aspect such as breathing or a visual object or sound and the attention span progressively increases as the individual becomes more skilled. Meditation is one aspect of Chinese medicine and Ayuverda and can help distract people from their pain due to 'uncoupling of the sensory dimension of the pain experience' (Yoon-Hang Kim 2004b). Enhanced immune modulation has also been reported. Guided imagery refers to helping people create mental pictures that try to evoke all the senses. It may be used with relaxation and meditation.

Pharmacological approaches

Herbal therapies

Many herbal preparations are used to manage pain. Most have a long history of safe traditional use and some have demonstrated effectiveness in randomised control trials, see Chapter 9. Some herbs are toxic if they are overused, inappropriately combined including with conventional medicines, or used in situations such as renal disease. If used inappropriately, herbs may mask pain and/or delay the diagnosis of the cause of the pain in the same way as conventional analgesic medicines. Table 15.4 lists some commonly used analgesic herbs. Complementary pharmacological preparations need to be considered in the light of the overall management plan and pain management strategies and within the principles of Quality Use of Medicines, and outcomes need to be monitored.

Counter-irritants

Counter-irritants, including herbs such as chilli peppers (capsaicin) and ginger (gingerols), act on pain receptors to deplete substance P and are used by conventional practitioners to manage painful peripheral neuropathy. They produce an initial burning sensation before inhibition occurs and people often stop using them for this reason. Gingerols do not appear to cause initial discomfort. Tiger Balm™, which is often used for joint pain has counter-irritant as well as other analgesic effects. It contains essential oils of clove, menthol, cassia, camphor, cajuput and sometimes peppermint. Cupping is a non-pharmacological counter-irritant method used in Chinese medicine where hot glass or bamboo cups are placed on the skin to create a vacuum suction to draw out toxic substances, see Chapter 11.

The ability of capsaicin to reduce pain by 'desensitising' nocioreceptros with repeat applications was first described in 1961. Capsaicin receptors are found on the afferent neuronal membranes of C fibres, which are sensitive to all three pain

Table 15.4 Some commonly used herbs, supplements and homeopathic remedies with analgesic properties and the main types of pain they are traditionally used to treat. The number after the name of the homeopathic remedy indicates the correct dilution for specific types of pain. Appropriately qualified practitioners using Quality Use of Medicines should prescribe these medicines.

Herb	Pain
Cayenne/capsiain – releases substance P. Causes initial reddening then reduction in pain.	Peripheral neuropathy, used as a cream
Aloe vera – extract or gel squeezed from the fresh plant, formulation.	Sunburn, wounds, and gastrointestinal inflammation. May cause hypoglycaemia – laxative effect
Chamomile – anti-inflammatory, antispasmolytic.	Used in compresses, tea or essential oils. Neuralgia, digestive disturbances, sedative
Bromelain	
Clove	Dental pain applied locally
Ginger	Travel sickness, digestive discomfort, nausea grated as a compress for joint pain May reduce prostaglandins
Willow, Wintergreen, meadowsweet, which contain salicin, which is converted to salicylic acid (salicylate).	External use for joint pain often as an essential oil May also reduce fever
Arnica	External use on unbroken skin to reduce bruising, in compresses or ointment
Calendula	Skin conditions and sunburn. Can be used on broken skin. Gastrointestinal discomfort
Echinacea	Pain associated with infection, indigestion, boost immunity
Passionflower	Antispasmolytic and to reduce insomnia associated with pain
Peppermint	Carminative. Digestive upsets
Raspberry leaf	Menstrual pain
Red sage	Painful throat and mouth
Slippery elm	Demulcent. Acute digestive upset. It 'coats' the intestine so may reduce glucose uptake and predispose to hypoglycaemia
Viburnum opulus	Spasmodic cramps
Feverfew	Antiinflammatory and antispasmolytic, headache
Lavender	Antiinflammatory, sedative, carminative, skin
New Zealand green mussel	Osteoarthritis
Shark cartilage	Osteoarthritis
Proprietary herbal anti-inflammatory blends	
Rosemary, hops and olive leaf	Osteoarthritis. Reduce cardiovascular risk
Boswellia, ginger and turmeric	Reduces prostaglandin E2, COX and lipooxygenase. Antioxidant. Arthritis. Also has antiplatelet activities

Quercetin	Inhibits leucotrine, prostaglandin and histamine. antioxidant. Gout, skin sensitivities
Crampeze (Rutin, Vitamin B6, magnesium salts)	Reduce cramps
GenFlex osteoarthritis solutions	Glucosamine hydrochloride and chondroitin sulphate, manufacturers recommendusing with exercise and analgesis as needed

Supplements

Calcium	Leg cramps
Chondroitin	Osteoarthritis ± glucosamine
Glucosamine	Antiinflammatory arthritis ± chondroitin
B group vitamins	Neuropathic pain
Zinc	Neuropathic pain
Omega 3 fish oils	Inhibit COX Increase anti-inflammatory prostaglandins Reduce cardiovascular risk

Homeopathic preparations

Aconitum 12x	Severe pain
Apis 12x	Bites and stings
Arnica 6x	
Arnica 3x	Bruising
Chamomile 3x	General anxiety associated with pain
Hypericum 6x	Open wounds and cuts
Rhus tox 6x	Muscular aches and pain

modalities (chemical, thermal, mechanical). Capsaicin is usually formulated as a topically applied cream used 3–4 times per day for 4–6 weeks. A similar product, Aloe MSM Gel, applied as a massage, causes a similar initial burning sensation but does not contain either ginger or capsaicin. It contains other essential oils/herbs with analgesic properties such as rosemary and willow bark although these herbs are not necessarily counter-irritants. The effect of MSM gel effect on neuropathic pain has not been tested but anecdotally it reduces joint pain. Counter-irritants may be most effect as an adjuvant therapy.

Analgesic herbal formulations

Analgesic herbs are available in a variety of formulations such as tinctures or extracts, capsules, lozenges, teas, poultices, oils, ointments or salves, and bath products, see Chapter 9. Analgesia may be specifically formulated for the individual or a manufactured product purchased from reputable suppliers and used according to directions. The botanical names of the herb and parts of the plant used should be included on the label. Pain reduction may be secondary to other effects such as reducing oedema. For example, Koll *et al.* (2004) demonstrated significant reduction in pain and oedema and increased mobility in unilateral uncomplicated ankle sprains using a cream prepared from comfrey (*Symphytum officinale*) root 2gm applied four times a day in a multicentre randomised control trial (n = 148). Anecdotally moistened chopped comfrey leaves wrapped in a cloth and applied as a poultice has the same effect.

Homeopathic medicines

Homeopathy was discussed in detail in Chapter 8. Generally, the individual's personality as well as their pain is considered when selecting homeopathic remedies except in emergency situations. Repeat doses of homeopathic remedies are not usually recommended unless the pain is not reduced or returns. Homeopathic remedies are generally taken sublingually between meals. The correct dilution is important when using homeopathic remedies (Chaitow 1993), see Table 15.4.

Flower remedies

Flower essences are a form of vibrational remedy. A range of flower remedies is available such as Back Flower and Australian Bush Flowers. Essentially, the remedies consist of the imprint of the flowers in a water or alcohol base and no part of the flower remains in the preparation. 'Rescue Remedy' is used to reduce anxiety and fear and can be used before undertaking a procedure such as changing a dressing or with psychotherapies. There is limited research to support using Flower Remedies but they appear to be safe.

Essential oils (aromatherapy)

Essential oils can be used to manage the multidimensional, individual nature of pain from a variety of causes. The application method such as massage also plays a part in pain management as noted earlier in this chapter and in Chapter 6. A range of factors needs to be considered before using essential oils, see Chapter 6.

Table 15.5 lists a range of essential oils traditionally used as analgesic agents and the type of pain they are commonly used for. Peppermint oil has been shown to reduce gastric motility by direct action on the gut caleum channels to relax gastrointestinal smooth muscle (Koch 1998) but it may be contraindicated in autonomic neuropathy with gastroparesis. Inhaling odorants reduces autonomic functions, thus essential oils may be more useful in chronic pain management than sharp acute pain and may increase arousal (Saeki and Tanaka 2005).

Table 15.5 Essential oils reputed to have analgesic properties. Analgesia may be due to an effect on nerves, antispasmodic or anti-inflammatory properties and other mechanisms. Not all indications are evidence based.

Essential oil	Type of pain the essential oil is traditionally used to treat
Callitris intratropica	local bites and stings, small cuts joint pain and swelling
Eucalyptus citriodora, E dives, E globulus	muscular pain respiratory tract pain
Kunzea ambigua	arthritic
Ocimum basilium	headache
White birch	joint pain
Piper nigrum	muscular
Gaultheria procumbens	muscular
Carum cavi Elettaria cardamonum Corandrum sativum Anthum gravedens Foeniculum vulgare Zingiber officinale Mentha piperita	indigestion, flatulence, bloating
Anthemis nobilis	dull muscular pain
Eugenia caryophyllata	tooth ache tension headache rheumatism arthritis
Zingiber officinalis	arthritis and rheumatism digestive upsets
Lavandin	muscle stiffness and aches
Cymbopogon citratus	headache
Origanum marjoranum	migraine muscle pain and stiffness indigestion
Myristica fragrans	muscular aches neuralgic pain
Mentha piperita	headaches toothache aching feet and legs muscular aches
Pimenta officinalis	neuralgia and muscle spasm depletes substance p.

15.6 Common Types of Pain Associated with Diabetes

As already indicated, people with diabetes experience the same types of pain from the same causes as non-diabetics. Commonly encountered types of pain associated with diabetes are angina, claudication, peripheral neuropathy, gastroparesis associated with autonomic neuropathy, neuropathic vascular ulcers, and hypoglycaemic headache.

Angina

Angina symptoms may be mild or not recognised (silent) in people with diabetes due to autonomic neuropathy, which increases their risk of an adverse outcome. Angina is a serious condition and conventional medicines such as aspirin, beta blockers, calcium channel blockers and nitrates are usually required. Complementary therapies may have a role in reducing the associated anxiety and controlling breathing. Some therapies include dietary management to reduce animal fats, salt intake, sugar and alcohol; and dietary supplements such as:

- carnitine, which reduces free fatty acids in cardiac muscle and oxidative cellular damage;
- co-enzyme Q_{10} reduces LDL and cholesterol as well as systolic and diastolic blood pressure and HbA_{1c}. Fewer cardiac events and deaths were reported compared to a control group but fatigue was greater in the CQ_{10} group (Alternative Medicine Alert 2003).
- magnesium to reduce pump stress by relaxing blood vessels.

Chest pain is a very important warning sign and warrants immediate investigation especially in people with diabetes. The patient's perception of the pain significantly affects the severity of the pain as well as their confidence, self-esteem and activity levels. The Lifestyle Heart Trial found a combination of lifestyle, gentle exercise, meditation and progressive relaxation reduced fear and the psychological impact of chest pain (Ornish 1991). Deep breathing reduced blood pressure and other autonomic effects after coronary artery bypass grafts (Miller and Perry 1990).

Herbal therapies include hawthorn (*Crataegus laevigata*), which has inotropic effects mainly due to its flavonoid and procyanidin content. It increases the force of myocardial contraction, increases coronary blood flow and reduces oxygen demand, reduces the blood pressure and may reduce the incidence of arrhythmias. Hawthorn also has antioxidant and lipid-lowering effects. Interactions may occur with conventional anti-hypertensives and anti-anginal conventional medicines. Sometimes *Ammi visnaga* or *Khella* are used alone or combined with hawthorn and act in a similar way to calcium channel blockers.

Peripheral neuropathy

Chronic neuropathic pain is common in people with diabetes and is under-diagnosed in people suffering acute pain. Neuropathic pain frequently involves central and peripheral sensation (NHMRC 1999) and affects work, sleep, leisure time and quality of life (Schmaden 2002). Medicine-related adverse events are common in the treatment of neuropathic pain where people are often old and on multiple medicines (Dwokin 2003). Therefore, non-pharmacological treatments or combined pharmacological methods at lower doses may reduce some of these adverse events. Conventional medicines used to manage peripheral neuropathy include amitriptyline, gabapentin, lignocaine, tramadol. An important consideration

Table 15.6 Factors that indicate neuropathic pain may be present.

Continuing pain where there is no tissue damage present especially in the presence of neurological deficits.

Presence of pain despite sensory loss.

Allodynia.

Hyperalgesia

Dysaesthesia

Non-nocioception pain such as burning, pulsing, stabbing pain.

Continued and increasing pain after repeat stimulation (hyperpathia), which may radiate into surrounding areas.

Poor response to opoids.

---

is that many people with neuropathic pain also experience pain from other causes and these may need to be treated as well. Table 15.6 outlines some of the factors that indicate neuropathic pain is present. These factors should be assessed in conjunction with a pain rating scale, pain history and pain diagram. Consideration needs to be given to people with special needs, such as children, those with hearing and cognitive deficits, and people who do not speak English.

Abuaisha *et al.* (1998) showed significant improvement in 77 per cent of 46 patients treated for peripheral neuropathy with up to six courses of classical acupuncture. Patients were followed up for 18–52 weeks and 67 per cent were able to reduce or stop their conventional treatment. However, their peripheral neuropathic status remained unchanged. In another study by Alvara *et al.* (1998), 23 patients with type 2 diabetes with peripheral neuropathy who had no response to amitriptyline after four weeks were randomised to transcutaneous electrotherapy or control or amytriptylline for 12 weeks. Symptomatic improvement occurred in 12 of 14 in the TENS group ($p < 0.03$) suggesting TENS may be a useful adjuvant treatment to conventional treatment for peripheral neuropathy.

Recently, a new technique of high frequency muscle stimulation was compared to TENS in a randomised trial of people with type 2 diabetes with peripheral neuropathy (n = 41). Improvements in self-reported pain on a ten-point visual analogue scale was higher in the high frequency group, 80 per cent compared with 33 per cent in the TENS group and persisted for several days after treatment (Reichstein and Labrenz 2005).

A number of other neuropathy treatments are advertised in various general magazines but no information is provided about their mode of action, safety, efficiency or benefit. These include HeatEater™ gel innersoles marketed to reduce the burning pain of peripheral neuropathy by cooling the feet and increasing circulation. WALL insoles, which claim to increase walking comfort and provide arch support and cool the feet, which in turn may exercise easier. Since many patients report relief from walking on cold smooth surfaces the HeatEater™ gels may provide relief for some people.

Gastroparesis

Autonomic neuropathy affects a number of body functions including gastric emptying and gut motility. It is common, occurring in 30–40 per cent of people with diabetes, under-diagnosed and produces a range of signs and symptoms (Vinick *et al.* 2000; Aly and Weston 2002). Onset is usually slow with mild symptoms or present with functional abnormalities. The gastrointestinal tract is commonly affected, but age and medicine-related gastrointestinal problems can occur in people with diabetes and these problems are likely to be exacerbated if autonomic neuropathy is present (Spallone and Menzinger 1997).

Delayed gastric emptying that causes bloating and a feeling of fullness, nausea and vomiting and postural hypotension cause discomfort. Conventional management therapies include medications such as Metoclopramide, antibiotics such as tetracycline or trimethoprim to treat bacterial overgrowth and cholestyramine to chelate bile salts, which reduce gut motility and managing postural hypotension using medicines such as Fludrocortisone. Insulin/oral agents may need to be adjusted frequently.

Complementary approaches include dietary advice to eat small meals and easily digested foods and in some cases choosing gluten-free foods. Probiotics, particularly lactobacillus strains, relieve bowel irritability and constipation. Avoiding substances that constrict blood vessels such as smoking and caffeine, drinking herbal teas such as peppermint, ginger or chamomile to relieve nausea and using abdominal compresses or massage to help reduce abdominal discomfort can provide relief.

Vascular ulcers

Vascular ulcers are venous or arterial in nature or a combination of both. They often require frequent dressing changes, often over a long period of time. The underlying cause of the ulcer must also be treated to prevent recurrences and regular foot care instituted. Improving blood glucose control, rest and antibiotics may be necessary. Vascular ulcers often cause significant pain of themselves and pain occurs during due to the dressing changes. Conventional analgesia does not always control the pain (Kane *et al.* 2004) and complementary pain management techniques may help relieve pain alone, or as adjunctive therapy.

Kane *et al.* conducted a small pilot study in people having frequent wound dressing changes. The therapies consisted of lavender or lemon essential oil odours, relaxing music or preferred music and a control condition. Pain was not reduced during the dressing changes but there was a significant reduction in pain after the dressing change for lavender essential oil and relaxing music. Kane *et al.* suggested commencing these therapies earlier before the dressing was changed and using them as adjunctive therapies.

Essential oils such as lavender have also been shown to reduce agitated behaviour in people with dementia, especially when combined with massage. Field (2002) noted sleep improved following massage to relieve pain. Since there is an association between diabetes and dementia and vascular disease, essential oil massages may help reduce pain by direct analgesic effects, through touch, and by reducing agitation, which in turn make procedures easier and less painful.

Foot ulcers are a serious complication of diabetes often associated with high health costs and significantly impact on quality of life and lead to depression (Vileikyte 2001). Foot ulcers affect 2–3 per cent of people with diabetes per year and 85 per cent of non-traumatic lower limb amputations are due to foot ulcers, half of which are a consequence of diabetes (Vileikyte 2001). Thus stump care as well as foot care is an important aspect of diabetes management.

Headaches or migraine

Headaches are one of the most common types of pain and have a range of causes, some of which are serious and life-threatening such as intracranial bleeds, others result from referred pain from paravertebral joint displacement. Headaches can occur after severe hypoglycaemic episodes and persist after the blood glucose level is raised. Approximately 30 per cent of headaches do not respond to medications (Headache website 2003). There are several types of headaches including migraine, which is often triggered by certain foods and food additives.

Essential oils have been shown to be useful at the aura stage to reduce the severity of the headache by early treatment, to manage the acute episode and to support recovery after the pain subsides (Betts 2003). However, strong smells and food sometimes trigger headaches, in which case essential oils may be contraindicated. A supercritical carbon dioxide feverfew extract (MIG-99) 6.26 mgs three times per day for 16 weeks effectively relieved migraine in a double-blind trial (n = 170). Migraine frequency reduced in the feverfew group from by 1.9 episodes per month compared to 1.3 in the control group (Diener 2005).

The headache-relieving potential of eucalyptus and peppermint essential oils was compared in a double-blind randomised cross-over placebo trial (n = 32) using four different doses of peppermint and/or eucalyptus oil in ethanol applied to the forehead and temples. Electromyographic measurements of temporal muscle activity, contingent negative variation, mood states, and sensitivity to mechanical, thermal, or ischaemic-induced pain were measured at baseline and after treatment. Combination eucalyptus and peppermint together increased cognitive performance and relaxation. Eucalyptus alone had no significant effect. Peppermint alone had an analgesic effect. Commercial preparations of peppermint and lavender such as 'Migrastick' are available but limited research supporting the effectiveness was identified. Anecdotally individual patients report Migrastick helps them control mild to moderate headache especially after hypoglycaemia.

Pain associated with musculoskeletal disease

The musculoskeletal system includes the bones, joints, ligaments, tendons and muscles. Problems affecting these structures are very common across all age groups and can affect normal activities and psychological well-being. They include both acute and chronic conditions and pain, local or transferred, is a common feature of both. Bone pain is different from other pain and is often deep, dull or 'boring' in nature. Rest and sometimes immobilisation relieve most musculoskeletal pain when a fracture is present. A steady increasing pain may indicate the pressure of osteomyelitis, malignancy or neurovascular complications.

Sensory disturbance such as burning, tingling or numbness may occur as a result of pressure on nerves, for example, carpal tunnel syndrome. Posture and gait changes and deformity such as ulnar deviation of the fingers in rheumatoid arthritis may be present. Muscle wasting and muscle spasm also occur and increase the pain.

Management depends on the cause and includes diet to eliminate allergenic foods, and supplements such as silenum, vitamin E and zinc to reduce free radicles and manganese, vitamins C and B_5 exercise to encourage joint mobility and flexibility and increase muscle strength and conventional medicines depending on the cause. Herbal therapies include anti-inflammatory herbs such as Bromelain, ginger, tumeric, *Panax ginseng*, and licorice, which reduce inflammatory mediators, Glucosamine, which may be effective alone or enable lower doses of NSAIDs to be used. Glucosamine does not appear to cause hyperglycaemia. However, allergic skin reactions do occur in susceptible people when glucosamine is derived from seafood (Australian Adverse Drug Reactions Bulletin 2005). Patients should be advised to read product labels carefully. Non-pharmacologic therapies include massage, distraction, relaxation, acupuncture, stretching, mineral baths or packs over the affected joints and contrast hydrotherapy.

Emotional pain

Emotional pain can be due to a number of factors and lead to anxiety and depression. Prolonged emotional pain or stress compromises the immune system and leads to physical illness. Emotional status can be closely linked to an individual's spirituality, self-concept and self-worth and manifest as a number of emotions such as fear which can affect self-care and metabolic control. Stress management, counselling, relaxation, meditation, and guided imagery to help foster positive thinking can be beneficial.

15.7 Summary

Pain management in diabetes may be overlooked because of the focus on metabolic control. More research is needed into the efficacy and benefit of complementary therapies in the management of pain in people with diabetes. However, many pain management therapies can be effectively and safely incorporated into conventional management regimens to improve the physical and psychological comfort of the person with diabetes.

References

Abuaisha B, Costanzi M, Boulton A. Acupuncture for the treatment of chronic painful peripheral diabetic neuropathy: a long term study. *Diabetes Research in Clinical Practice*. 1998: **39**(2); 115–121.

Acute pain Management Guideline Panel. *Acute Pain Management: Operative or Medical Procedures and Trauma*. Clinical practice guideline number 1. US Department of Health and Human Services, 1992.

Alternative Medicine Alert. Coenzyme Q_{10} 2(12): S1, 2003.

Alternative Medicine Alert. Facts about cancer pain. Part 2: non-drug treatments for pain. 8(3), S1–S4, 2005.

Alvara M, Julka I, Marshall H. Diabetic peripheral neuropathy: effectiveness of electrotherapy and amitriptyline for symptomatic relief. *Diabetes Care* 1998: **21**(8): 1322–1325.

Aly N, Weston P. Autonomic neuropathy in older people with diabetes. *Journal of Diabetes Nursing* 2002: **6**(1): 10–14.

Anon. Migraine, the doctor responds. *Aromatherapy World* 1992: Spring: 25–26.

Australian Adverse Drug Events Bulletin. Skin reactions with glucosamine. 2005: **24**(6).23.

Australian Department for Health and Ageing. *National Strategy for the Quality Use of Medicines*. Canberra. http://www.health.gov.au/haf/nmp/advisory/pharma.htm, 2002.

Baldry P. *Acupuncture, Trigger Points and Musculoskeletal Pain*. Edinburgh: Churchill Livingstone, 1993.

Betts T. Use of aromatherapy (with or without hypnosis) in the treatment of intractable epilepsy in a two year follow up study. *Seizure* 2003: **13**(8): 534–538.

Bonica J. History of pain concepts and therapies. In: *The Management of Pain* Vol. 1. New York: Lea & Fabbiger, 1990.

Braun C, Bearinger L, Halcon L, Pettingell S. Adolescents' use of alternative therapies for pain relief. *Journal of Adolescent Health* 2005: **37**: 76.

Breen J. Transitions in the concept of chronic pain. *Advanced Nursing Science*, 2002: **24**(4): 48–59.

Campbell J. Pain, the 5th vital sign. Presidential address. American Pain Society, November 11 1995, Los Angeles.

Chaitow L. *Holistic Pain Relief*. London: Thorsons, 1993.

Chen C-Z, Pon Y-C, Yu J. Immediate effects of various physical medicine modalities on pain threshold of an active myofascial trigger point. *Journal of Musculoskeletal Pain* 1993: **1**(2).

Cherkin D. Randomised trial comparing traditional Chinese medical acupuncture therapeutic massage, and self-care education for chronic low back pain. *Archives of Internal Medicine* 2001: **161**: 1081–1088.

Ching M. Contemporary therapy: aromatherapy in the management of acute pain. *Contemporary Nurse* 1999: **8**: 146–151.

Coccheri S. Changes in the use of health resources by patients with chronic phlebopathies after thermal hydrotherapy. Report from the Naiade project, a nation-wide survey on thermal therapies in Italy *International Angiology: a Journal of the International Union of Angiology* 2002: **21**(2): 196–200.

Diener D. Feverfew extract reduces migraine frequency. *Cephalagia* 2005: **25**: 1031–1041.

Donowitz M. Arachidonic acid metabolites and their role in inflammatory bowel disease. *Gastroenterology* 1985: **88**: 580–587.

Dossey B, Keegan L, Guzzetta C, Kolkmeier C. *Holistic Nursing: A Handbook for Practice*. Aspen, MD: Aspen publishers, 1995.

Dunning T. Applying a Quality Use of Medicines framework to using essential oils in nursing practice. *Complementary Therapies in Clinical Practice*. 2005: **11**: 172–181.

Dworkin R. Advances in neuropathic pain. *Archives of Neurology* 2003: **60**(11): 1524–1537.

Edworthy S. How important is patient self-management? *Balliere's Clinical Rheumatology* 2000: **14**(4): 704–714.

Fenwick C, Stevens J. Post operative pain experiences of central Australian Aboriginal women. What do we understand? *Australian Journal of Rural Health* 1998: **12**: 22–27.

Field T. Massage therapy research methods. In: Lewith G, Jonas W, Walach H. (eds), *Clinical Research in Complementary Therapies*. Edinburgh: Churchill Livingstone, 2002, pp. 263–280.

Ghen M. Treating diabetes mellitus. *American Journal of Natural Medicines* 1998: **5**(8): 18–21.

Ghosh J, Myers C Jr. Arachidonic acid metabolism and cancer of the prostate. *Nutrition* 1998: **14**: 48–57 [editorial].

Goodheart G Jr. *You'll Be Better: The Story of Applied Kinesiology*. Self-published, Geneva, OW: AK Printing, 1980.

Gruener D. New strategies for managing acute pain episodes in patients with chronic pain. *Medscape online* 13.9.2004: 2–4.

Haetzman M, Elliott B, Smith B, Hannaford P, Chambers W. Chronic pain and the use of conventional and alternative therapy. *Family Practice* 2003: **20**(2): 147–154.

Headache Australia website. http://www.headacheaustralia.org.au/what_is_headache/prevalence _and_cost_of_headache (accessed July 2003).

Hallberg L, Carlsson S. Coping with fibromyalgia. *Scandinavian Journal of Caring Science* 2000: **14**(1): 29–36.

Hawthorn J, Redmond K. Pain causes and management. *Pain Management Nursing* 1998: **5**(4): 137–143.

Han J, Stegen K, De Valck C. Influence of breathing therapy on complaints, anxiety and breathing pattern in patients with HVS and anxiety disorders *Journal of Psychosomatic Research* 1996: **41**(5): 481–493.

Hong C-Z, Chen Y-N, Twehouse D, Hong D. Pressure threshold for referred pain by compression on trigger point and adjacent area. *Journal of Musculoskeletal Pain* 1996: **4**(3): 61–79.

International Association for the Study of Pain Subcommittee on Taxonomy. Pain terms, a list with definitions and notes on usage. *Pain* 1986: **8**: 249.

Jakobsson U. Pain management among older people in need of help with activities of daily living.

Jablon S, Naliboff B, Gilmore S, Rosentha, M. Effects of relaxation training on glucose tolerance and diabetic control in type II diabetes. *Applied Psychophysiology and Biofeedback* 1997: **22**(3): 155–169.

Kaada B, Torsteininbo O. Increase in plasma beta endorphins in connective tissue. *General Pharmacology* 1989: **209**(4): 487–489.

Kane F, Brodie E, Coull A, Coyne L, Howd A. *et al.* The analgesic effect of odour and music upon dressing change. *British Journal of Nursing* 2004: **13**(19): 54, 56, 58.

Kiser R. Acupuncture relief of chronic pain syndrome correlates with increased plasma meta-enkephalin concentrations. *Lancet* 1983: ii: 1394–1396.

Koch T. Peppermint oil and irritable bowel syndrome. *American Journal of Gastroenterology* 1999: **93**: 2304–2305.

Kolansinski S. Magnets for musculoskeletal symptoms. *Alternative Medicine Alert* 2005: **8**(5); 53–55.

Kuznetsov O. The use of cryomassage in the rehabilitative treatment of patients with duodenal peptic ulcer at the polyclinic stage. *Voprosy Kurortologii, Fizioterapii, i Lechebnoi Fizicheskoi Kultury* 2000: **2**: 24–26 (in Russian).

Lane J, McCaskill C, Ross S, Feinglos M, Surwit R. Relaxation training for NIDDM. Predicting who may benefit. *Diabetes Care* 1993: **16**(8): 1087–1093.

Lum L. Hyperventilation syndromes. In: Timmons B, Ley R. (eds). *Behavioral and Psychological Approaches to Breathing Disorders*. New York: Plenum Press, 1994.

Mancini S. Clinical, functional and quality of life changes after balneokinesis with sulphurous water in patients with varicose veins. *Zeitschrift für Gefasskrankheiten. Journal For Vascular Diseases* 2003: **32**(1): 26–30.

McCaffery M, Beebe A. Pain: a clinical manual for nursing practice. *Mosby Year Book* 1989: **55**: 7.

McCaffery M, Rolling Ferrell B. Patient age. Does it affect your pain control decisions? *Nursing 91* 1991: **September**: 44–49.

McGrady A, Bailey B, Good M. Controlled study of biofeedback-assisted relaxation in type 1 diabetes. *Diabetes Care* 1991: **14**(5): 360–365.

Melzack R, Wall P. Pain mechanisms: a new theory. *Science* 1965: **150**: 971–979.

Merskey H, Bogdus N, (eds) *Classification of Chronic Pain* 2nd edn. Seattle: ASP Press, 1994, pp. 209–214.

Miller K, Perry P. Relaxation technique and post operative patients undergoing cardiac surgery. *Heart and Lung* 1990: **19**(2): 136–146.

Morgan J Using relaxation to manage post operative pain. *The Canadian Nurse* 1984: **15**.

Morelli A, Seaborne D, Sullivan S. Human reflex modulation during manual massage of humans triceps surae. *Archives of Physical Medicine and Rehabilitation* 1991: **72**: 915–919.

Murphy-Ende A. Mind, body and soul: learn how assessment and education can stop cancer pain. *Oncology Issues*, 2003: **18**(5): 32–28.

Moncada S. Leucocytes and tissue injury: the use of eicosapentenoic acid in the control of white cell activation. *Wiener Klinische Wochenschrift* 1986: **98**(4): 104–106.

Naliboff B, Tachiki K. Autonomic and skeletal muscle responses to neuroelectrical cutaneous stimulation. *Perceptor Motor Skills* 1991: **72**(25): 575–584.

National Health and Medical Research Council (NH&MRC). *Acute Pain Management: Information for General Practitioners*. Canberra: NH&MRC, 1999.

National Heart Foundation. Psychosocial risk is significant risk for coronary heart disease. *Medical Journal of Australia*. 2003: **178**: 272–276.

National Institute of Health. Technology Assessment Statement: Integration of behavioural and relaxation approaches into the treatment of chronic pain and insomnia. 1995: October 1–18, 1–34.

Ornish D, Scherwitz L, Billings J, Brown S. *et al.* Intensive lifestyle changes for reversal of coronary heart disease. *Journal American Medical Association* 1998: **280**(23): 2001–2007.

Power I, Colvin L. Management of acute pain – part 1. *Australian Doctor Supplement* 2001: **March 9**: I–VIII.

Pryor J, Prasad S. *Physiotherapy for Respiratory and Cardiac Problems* 3rd edn. Edinburgh: Churchill Livingstone, 2002.

Rampes H, James R. Complications of acupuncture. *Acupuncture Medicine* 1995: **13**: 26–33.

Reichstein L, Labrenz S. Effective treatment of symptomatic diabetic polyneuropathy by high-frequency external muscle stimulation. *Diabetologia* 2005: **48**: 824–828.

Roth T The impact of disturbed sleep on pain. *Medscape* http//:www.medscape.com/viewarticle/506217 (accessed October 2005).

Saeki Y, Tanaka Y. Effect of inhaling fragrances on pricking pain. *International Journal of Aromatherapy* 2005: **15**: 74–80.

Schmaden K. Epidemiology and impact on quality of life of postherapeutic neuralgia and painful diabetic neuropathy. *The Clinical Journal of Pain* 2002: **18**: 350–354.

Seyal M. Increased excitability of the human corticospinal system with hyperventilation. *Electroencephalography and Clinical Neurophysiology/ Electromyography and Motor Control* 1998: **109**(3): 263–267.

Shekelle P. Spinal manipulation for low back pain. *Annals of Internal Medicine* 1992: **117**: 590.

Sidall R. Patients switch on to pain relief. *Doctor*. 1991: **23**: 36.

Simons D, Travell J, Simons L. *Myofascial Pain and Dysfunction: the Trigger Point Manual*, Vol. 1: *The Upper Extremities*, 2nd edn. Baltimore, MD: Williams and Wilkins, 1999.

Sinclair D. Chronic non-cancer pain basics for the primary care physician. *American Health Consultants Primary Care Report* 2002: **8**(8): 63–74.

Snow A, Hovanec L, Brandt J. A controlled trial of aromatherapy for agitation in nursing home patients with dementia. *Journal of Alternative and Complementary Medicine* 2004: **10**(3): 431–437.

Spallone V, Menzinger G. Autonomic neuropathy; clinical and instrumental findings. *Clinical Neuroscience* 1997: **4**(96): 346–358.

Spencer J, Jacobs J. *Complementary and Alternative Medicine: An Evidence Based Approach.* St. Louis: Mosby, 1999.

Spinella M. *Concise Handbook of Psychoactive Herbs.* New York: Hawthorn Herbal Press, 2005.

Standish L. One year open trial of naturopathic treatment of HIV infection. *Journal of Naturopathic Medicine* 1992: **3**(1): 42–64.

Stevenson C. Non-pharmacological aspects of acute pain management. *Complementary Therapies in Nursing and Midwifery* 1995: **1**: 77–84.

Van Dixhoorn J, Duivenvoorden H. Efficacy of Nijmegen questionnaire in recognition of the hyperventilation syndrome. *Journal of Psychosomatic Research* 1985: **29**: 199–206.

Vansteenkiste J, Rochette F, Demedts M. Diagnostic tests of hyperventilation syndrome. *European Respiratory Journal* 1991: **4**: 393–399

Vickers A. *Massage and Aromatherapy: A Guide for Health Professionals.* London: Chapman Hall, 1996.

Vileikyle L. Diabetic foot ulcers: a quality of life issue. *Diabetes Metabolism Research and Reviews* 2001: **17**: 246–249.

Viniik A, Stansberry K, Pittenger G. Diabetic neuropathies. *Diabetalogia* 2000: **43**: 957–973.

Walther D. *Applied Kinesiology Synopsis.* Pueblo, CO: Systems DC, 1988.

World Health Organization. *Viewpoint on Acupuncture.* Geneva: WHO, 1979.

Wright J. *Reflexology and Acupressure.* London: Hamlyn, no date.

Yoon-Hang Kim. Efficacy of acupuncture for treating back pain. *Alternative Medicine Alert* 2004a: **7**(7): 73–78.

Yoon-Hang Kim. Mindfulness meditation and chronic pain. *Alternative Medicine Alert* 2004b: **6**(8): 33–35.

16 Manipulative Therapies

Russell Banks

16.1 The Origins of Chiropractic Therapy

Four professional groups have used manipulation as one of their therapeutic tools in the past 100 years. The medical, chiropractic, osteopathic and physiotherapy professions have been the major groups involved and most have published peer-reviewed articles and clinical insight into the associated benefits and risks. Manipulation, as a main therapeutic tool, became more widely known with the formation of the Chiropractic Profession in 1895 following Daniel D. Palmer's successful manipulation of a janitor, Harvey Lillard, suffering from hearing loss. Palmer established a school to teach his manipulation methods based on his theory that health depends on effective functioning and coordination of the nervous system. Palmer, in collaboration with his son Bartlett J. Palmer, also proposed the mechanism of an innate force or intelligence that suggest the body recognises inappropriate body function or disease and coordinates an appropriate response to remedy the situation.

They proposed that the bony malposition of vertebra in the spine created poor perception, interpretation, and poor correction of dysfunction in these tissues. Chiropractors were taught to take X-rays of the spine and analyse them to identify subluxations (Schofield 1968). Chiropractors still commonly believe that malposition is a sign of a spinal lesion but they also accept that movement dysfunction is an important requirement.

16.2 Osteopathic Beginnings

In 1874 Still suggested that: 'The living blood swarmed with health corpuscles, which were carried to all parts of the body. Interference with that current of blood and you steam down the river of life and land in the ocean of death' (Still 1908).

The first American School of Osteopathy began in Kirksville, Missouri, in 1892. Still followed the principle that manipulating the spine would allow the blood to flow through arteries and enrich the tissues with health-giving blood

Complementary Therapies and the Management of Diabetes and Vascular Disease   Editor Trish Dunning
© 2006 John Wiley & Sons, Ltd.

(Stoddard 1969; Kron 2003). The confidence and conviction of Still's approach were welcomed at a time when pharmaceutical treatment was not based on scientific testing. Complications of conventional medical treatment and a lack of understanding of disease processes led to a search for alternative treatments.

Both chiropractic and osteopathic theories are based on the premise that spinal manipulation could restore health by re-establishing the normal physiological processes of organs and restoring the ability of the immune system to deal with natural stresses including infection.

It appears that practitioners of both therapies initially believed that treating the spine was a complete treatment, separate from surgery and good nutrition.

16.3   Relationship among Chiropractors, Osteopaths and the Medical Profession

The medical profession have used spinal manipulation as a therapy over the centuries, however, such use waned when the osteopathic and chiropractic professions promoted their underlying explanatory philosophy that manipulation could be used as a complete approach to health care. Kleynhans (1990) suggested that this chiropractic philosophy was an attempt to distinguish chiropractors from other professions; perpetuate chiropractic's existence; utilise professional-specific terms that were not used by other professional groups; provide an alternative explanatory model of disease to the prevailing medical model.

Osteopaths are treated as doctors in the USA where their training includes medicine, prescribing medicines and surgery. In Australia, they are not permitted to prescribe or perform surgery, thus the main focus is on manipulation and mobilisation and other complementary therapies. As a result, the integration of chiropractic into conventional health care, scientific investigation of the therapies, and the development of an acceptable therapeutic approach have been impeded, intellectual processes stagnated and believers and non-believers polarised (Kleynhans 1990).

Both the chiropractic and osteopathic professions initially alienated the medical profession, largely by promulgating Palmer's dogma about such theories as vitalism developed to explain assumptions that were never scientifically validated (Kleynhans 1990). Palmer encouraged practitioners and the public to accept his chiropractic principles in the same way religious leaders expected their parishioners to follow rules or a specified framework for living. He even conducted his own radio broadcast on 'the big idea' (Peters and Chance 2001).

16.4   Principles of Manipulative Therapies

Manipulation and other therapies such as mobilisation are now accepted treatments for pain management but their benefits with respect to most organic conditions remains unproven. However, there is no evidence that they will not have a small effect by improving the circulation or nervous system coordination (Budgell 1999).

Joint sounds

Manipulation was defined in various ways throughout the last century. Most commonly, the term refers to the procedures that produce or attempt to produce an audible sound, known as cavitation. Recently, there is a growing appreciation of a stepped grading of manipulation/mobilisation from grade 1 in the joints range of motion through to joint cavitation.

Many joint sounds occur normally during daily activities and manipulation. Sandoz (1969, 1975) reviewed the literature with regard to a traction force on a metacarpophalangeal joint (undertaken initially by Roston and Haines 1947) and was able to place a clinical relevance to the observations. He noted that joint separation was minimal unless the cavitation occurred. Once cavitation occurred, joint separation, from a neutral position through to the end of range of motion, could be easily undertaken with little applied traction (Sandoz 1969).

Most of the following comment is my own interpretation based on logical extension of the information. A refractory period of approximately 20 minutes occurs in which the joint returns to the premanipulated state after which the joint can be cavitated again (Sandoz 1969, 1975). The passive, and to a lesser extent, active range of motion increases following manipulation. After cavitation, the joint is more easily taken to the ends of the joint's range of motion. It then is inherently less protected from forces applied but the joint is also more easily stimulated from a mechanical sensory perspective. After manipulation, mobilisation or exercise appears to optimise the benefits of movement on mechanoreceptors (Meal and Scott 1986, Brodeur 1995).

Sandoz argued that cavitation with joint manipulation is normal rather than pathological and that its occurrence, or return of joint cracking, after a period of absence and after manipulation, is a positive sign of improvement (Sandoz 1969, 1975). Cavitation appears to be inhibited by hypertonic or spastic muscles, the presence of pain, inflammatory processes in surrounding tissues, joint structural changes in osteoarthritis, some undefined individual tendencies, and atmospheric changes (Sandoz 1969). Brodeur (1995) proposed that the cavitation sound is due to elastic recoil of the synovial capsule as it snaps back from the capsule/synovial fluid interface, which creates gases between the capsule and synovial fluid. Cascioli *et al.* (2003), on analysis of intra-articular gas bubbles, found no evidence of gas in the joints following cavitation. There is obviously more need to research into this mechanism.

How is manipulation undertaken?

Spinal joint manipulation can be performed in any direction to achieve an effect. It is my experience that gapping or inducing a traction force on the joints using the opposite facet joint as a pivot-point in which the section of the spine is stretched is most effective. Alternatively, it appears that the joints can be slid in relation to one another or even levered to gap in the ipsilateral joint to the contact hand. This is much the way that many people can cavitate their metacarpophalangeal joints by opening up the joint on the ipsilateral side adjacent to the pivot.

Mobilisation procedures are similar to manipulation although they are generally applied in a series of repetitions with less force. Mobilisation has many benefits for the spine, including stretching the muscles, increased mechanoreceptor stimulation and subsequent muscle relaxation and an increased range of motion. The methods used to achieve mobilisation vary from slow stretching force simply through range of motion, through to quickly applied force similar to manipulative cavitation. The mechanisms by which mobilisation and manipulation may be beneficial are identified in Table 16.1.

Table 16.1 Mechanisms by which manipulation is effective and an explanation of how it could help manage specific conditions.

Mechanisms by which manipulation might be helpful	Explanation as to how it could help
1. Stimulating mechanoreceptors	Manipulation increases joints motion, stimulates the mechanoreceptors, and inhibits nociceptor transmission to the thalamus at first synapse in the spinal cord at the dorsal root ganglions (gate control theory of pain). The hypoalgesic effects of manipulation are related to central nervous system activity (Mohammadian *et al.* 2004).
2. Relaxating muscles	Spinal manipulation produces almost instantaneous relaxation of local muscles possibly as a reflex response to stretching certain muscles around the spine. Alternatively it may be due to the spine being bombarded with proprioceptive information.
3. Balancing autonomic output	Manipulation can alter autonomic output. Pain causes increased sympathetic output. Thus, manipulation can restore the balance between the sympathetic and parasympathetic systems (Spiegel 2003). Somatoautonomic reflexes exist and can affect the cardiovascular, digestive, urinary, endocrine and immune systems (Budgell 2000).
4. Altering muscle coordination	Smooth muscle movement depends on the coordination of agonist and antagonist muscles, which is controlled by the nervous system, which checks outcome against need, performs more movement and checking (Hodges 2003). Pain can significantly alter muscle control (Barr 2005). Manipulation may re-establish effective coordination of apposing muscles. The joints are less likely to be injured when the nervous system

functions optimally. Return of normal proprioceptive compared to nociceptor input can prevent some injuries. This is one of the principles of rehabilitation exercises and core stability.

5. Altering muscle tone resulting in altered posture

Diminished proprioceptive afferents and increased pain afferents l result in broad areas of muscle weakness and changes the way the body parts can be held or maintained, thus posture can be altered. Therefore, manipulation can contribute to improve posture due to more effective muscle function.

6. Reducing mechanical stress due to improved joint position

Pain can induce altered posture due to an inherent desire to seek relief from pain. Altered posture can place additional stress on joints in proximity to an affected joint/s due to the altered body position. For example if the muscles in the leg cannot maintain foot supination due to pain on maintenance of normal foot alignment, the knee tends to become valgus in orientation put strain on the knee and cause pain. Manipulation can reduce stress on joints and reduce inflammation and pain.

7. Reduced mechanical stress due to improved joint mobility

Manipulation can improve movement in the spinal joints and reduce mechanical stress on nearby joints. Systems within the body where there is shared responsibility for motion or maintaining integrity of the tissues requires all the components to perform, otherwise other components take over particularly in the spine with regard to motion. If one of the intervertebral segments has a reduced range of motion, the neighbouring segments will have increased movement to accommodate for the deficiency. Manipulation can restore joint mobility and reduce stress.

8. Correcting fixated joints in a non-neutral position

Improved joint movement enables joints fixated in a non-neutral position to find a neutral position again. The range of motion of a joint refers to the movement available to a joint on either side of a neutral position. When a joint becomes fixated or its movement is restricted, it may be fixed in a non-neutral position. Theoretically, if the

Table 16.1 (Continued)

Mechanisms by which manipulation might be helpful	Explanation as to how it could help
	motion to that joint is re-established, the joint position will be able to return to a neutral position. Manipulation can be very effective at restoring structural relationships among joints. Chiropractic 'subluxation' is based on this concept.
9. Reducing degenerative changes to the spine	Reducing mechanical stress on the spine can reduce joint inflammation and pain and subsequently, degenerative changes in the spine. Manipulation can reduce mechanical stress on the spinal joints, which subsequently reduces or eliminates inflammation in the mechanically challenged joints. It also reduces the subsequent degenerative changes that occur as a result of stress.
10. Reduced swelling around intervertebral foramina in the spine	Inflamed facet joints in the spine can cause swelling in the adjacent section of the spinal canal and reduce the canal space. Although the reduced canal space may not cause any initial symptoms because the body adjusts, when swelling from an inflamed joint complicates the situation, radicular pain often occurs. Manipulation can reduce/resolve joint inflammation with subsequent resolution of the radicular pain and nerve root compression symptoms. Therefore, less mechanical stress on the spine help resolve inflamed joints and swelling involving the intervertebral foramina in the spine.
11. Freeing intra-articular anatomical entrapments	Facet joints, proximal radioulnar joints, and femorotibial joints can have anatomical structures that can be freed from pressure by manipulation. Many joints in the body have meniscus or anatomical structures that enable them to function effectively and distribute compressive forces or assist with lubrication. These structures can become trapped. Manipulation can free the trapped structures as long as they have not become chronically inflamed or scarred.
12. Muscle relaxation may resolve peripheral nerve compression syndromes	Muscle relaxation can resolve peripheral nerve neuralgia or paraesthesias such as greater occipital neuritis, scalenus anticus and piriformis syndrome. Restoring proprioceptive input and reduces muscle tension and improves or resolves syndromes including scalenus anticus syndrome and greater occipital neuritis. When the thoracic multifidus muscle is allowed to relax following manipulation paraesthesia over a patch near the spine can resolve, a syndrome called notalgia paresthetica (Leibsohn 1992: Massey 1998).

Manipulation using mechanical devices

The Activator

Mechanical manipulation devices are sometimes used by preference and appear to achieve good results in a variety of disorders (Polkinghorn 1995, 1998). These devices include the Activator®, an instrument that was designed to apply very rapid force over a relatively small area and is easily accepted by most patients. The Activator® is usually applied to vertebral processes to stimulate the joint without causing cavitation to muscles. Following a brief contraction, muscles tend to relax.

The Activator®, pictured in Figure 16.1 delivers a reproducible force and has similar characteristics to manual procedures but the duration of the force is brief and, while the force is directed through a small contact, allows the impact to be significant while there are negligible dangers overall (Kawchuk and Herzog 1993). Sometimes the Activator® is effective when other procedures are unsuitable, or

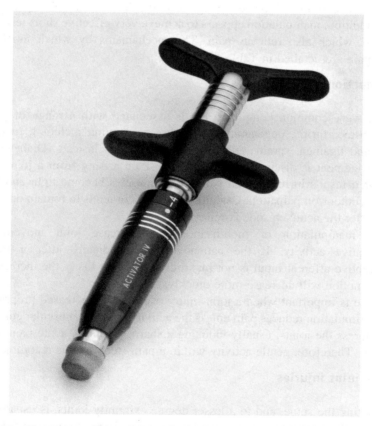

Figure 16.1 Illustration of the Activator 4 Instrument chiropractors use for specific and safe manipulation. Reproduced with the permission of Dr AW Fuhr and Activator Methods International Ltd.

when the patient does not respond to manual manipulative techniques. Some chiropractors use a patient analysis system to determine when the Activator® is indicated.

Mechanical treatment tables

Mechanical treatment tables with various sized sections and mechanisms that allow the surface where the patient lies to drop away on pressure from the practitioner are also used. The distance of drop is only 1–2 cm but provides enough stimulation to achieve joint cavitation more easily or additional stimulus to the manual pressure applied to the spine. Generally, these procedures are undertaken in a neutral position with the patient lying prone or on their side.

Proposed mechanisms of action of manipulation

Many advantages of manipulating the joints and particularly the spine have been proposed. These include increasing mechanical receptor stimulation that tends to block the transmission of nociceptor signals to the thalamus and thus perception of pain. In addition, manipulation appears to achieve very effective short-term muscle relaxation, which also relieves pain. The mechanisms by which manipulation relieves pain are detailed in Table 16.1.

Pain reduction

Pain is a very common complaint and is associated with a range of problems such as osteoarthritis, degenerative disc disease, trauma including to the joint capsule and ligament sprains and less commonly muscle tears. Diabetes-related pain management is discussed in Chapter 15. Pain arising from a joint or other tissue often results in myofascial pain where muscles become tight and have an irregular contour on palpation. Often the muscle pain tends to remain and become chronic after the acute episode is relieved.

Spinal manipulation or mobilisation can increase joint movement and proprioceptive activity. If the patient rests immediately after a treatment, proprioceptive afferent input is not maximised and it is likely the increased joint range of motion will decrease more quickly.

Exercise is important when a joint injury occurs. The increased proprioceptive afferent stimulation reduces pain unless the activity involves muscular contractions that compress the joints, usually inducing a sharp, pinching, acute pain at site of the injury. Therefore, gentle activity within a pain-free range is recommended.

Treating joint injuries

Manipulating the spine, and to a lesser degree extremity joints, is usually safe in a patient with an injury as long as the injured tissue is not strained in the process. In the cervical spine, the joints typically become compressed on lateral flexion of the ipsilateral side, which causes the person to limit the range of motion and acute, sharp pain. In addition, cervical spine extension and ipsilateral rotation result in inflammatory pain. Rotation puts pressure on the ipsilateral facet joints because of coupling (ipsilateral lateral flexion induced by rotation) in the cervical spine, and rotating the spine causes lateral flexion on the same side. Where this distinct pattern is not present, it is likely that significant muscular pain is present. Joint injuries uncommonly result in cord or nerve compression. The nerves within narrowed intervertebral foramina or canal can be compressed due to inflammation and swelling or if trauma has resulted in fracture or dislocation. Any neurological compression signs should be evaluated carefully and referral to a neurologist and/or for additional tests such as CT scans and MRI are appropriate. Spinal manipulation in the circumstance of nerve compression is inappropriate until clarified and specialist advice obtained.

Manipulation, in a cervical facet joint injury is usually toward the contralateral side using rotation or contacted on the contralateral side using lateral flexion. The force should be directed to the joints where movement is restricted, which are often adjacent to the inflamed and injured joints. If the patient experiences acute pain when they are being prepared for manipulation, it is likely that the mechanical forces applied to the spine are inducing compression of inflamed joints or are inducing stretching of damaged muscles or ligaments. In this case an alternative therapeutic approach should be used that does not induce pain. Further investigation or referral is not normally appropriate in this instance. The thoracic spine joints are less likely to be compressed in a relatively flexed position or using rotational techniques. The lumbar spine joints are often aggravated by trunk rotation in one direction more acutely. This usually allows a rotational manipulative technique to be applied, especially if combined with an element of flexion, which tends to reduce joint compressive forces.

In the spine, the injured joint is not always the joint that is restricted in movement. Manipulation can be applied to the fixated joint, while not imparting significant force on the injured joint. If an acromioclavicular joint is inflamed, it is almost impossible to manually manipulate that joint without causing short term acute pain. The Activator® device might be used in this situation if the motion is restricted.

The least possible amount of manipulation should be undertaken to improve the range of motion within the joint. The presence of osteoarthritis significantly restricts the return to normal pain-free movement. Once movement is regained, the joint should be left to function normally. If the joint is continually manipulated, (often noted in patients who use self-manipulation) swelling and joint instability can result (Brodeur 1995). Mild inflammatory pain can result and the patient might request manipulation on a frequent basis to obtain temporary relief but can result ultimately in no long-term benefit. Sometimes joint stiffness returns after a manipulation and might be due to fibrotic changes due to past injuries or the early stages of degenerative conditions such as arthritis. In these patients, manipulation may be needed over an extended period of time (even years) but should only be attempted each time on the basis of a thorough physical examination and as infrequently as possible.

16.5 Indications for Manipulation

Assessing the patient to determine whether manipulation is indicated involves
assessing: posture; position of the joints (alignment); degree of joint stiffness and
range of movement; muscle tonicity; muscle weakness; the possible benefits and
risks of manipulation (see Table 16.2).

Posture

Assessing posture enables the practitioner to view the areas of the body where
muscles are hypertonic. This could indicate malalignment or scoliosis (hypertonic
paraspinal muscles on the convex side of a spinal curve) or be a result of overuse
or increased need. Hypertonicity in the muscles of the upper trapezius and levator
scapulae usually indicates the head is being carried anteriorly and increased work
is demanded on these muscles.

Postural assessment includes gait and movement. Gait can indicate muscle
strength, particularly of the foot and leg and possibly other muscles and balance
and upper limb mobility. Asking the patient to undertake specific activities and
checking for coordinated and smooth movements helps detect movement disorders.
For example, asking the patient to move slowly from a sitting to a supine position
without the practitioner holding their feet can help determine their ability to
eccentrically use abdominal muscles. Asking the person to rise from supine to
sitting position tests muscular control and the integrity of the lower back joints
because the muscles of the lower back and trunk compress most joints in the lower
back when undertaking this activity. Inflamed joints cause significant pain and
inhibit a smooth transition.

Table 16.2 Possible benefits and risks of manipulation.

Tiredness
Headaches
Hypoesthesia
Hyperesthesia
Paresthesia associated with muscle compression syndromes
Decreased muscle strength
Muscle pain and myofascial trigger points (tight and tender)
Organic function disturbances, including:

- tendency to constipation (Leboeuf-Yde 1999)
- indigestion and heartburn (Bryner 1996)
- lack of visual acuity (Stephens 1997)
- lack of concentration.

Joint injuries especially acute traumas
Postural disturbances such as chin protraction
Possible benefits with epilepsy (Alcantara 1998, Pistolese 2001)

Abnormal joint position

In some instances joints in the spine appear to be in an abnormal position or out of alignment. While the spinal segments do vary and are not always symmetrical, abnormal position can indicate relatively fixed movement between adjacent segments (Walker and Buchbinder 1997), which improves after the spine is manipulated. Unequal leg length has been attributed to these positional changes (Knutson 1997).

Joint stiffness

Joint manipulation is only indicated when joint dysfunction or stiffness is present. The degree of limitation can be assessed in relation to different planes of movement (Dishman 1988). For example, there movement may be restricted in an intervertebral segment where the person cannot rotate the joint in one direction but other movements are not restricted. In these circumstances a rotational manipulation or mobilisation procedure may help restore movement and normal function.

Joint restriction can be local or general due to generalised muscle contraction or stiffness, osteoarthritis. When the causative process is generalised, the limitations in movement can be diffuse, limited in more than one direction and involve several segments of the spine. Various unsmooth movements can be detected when assessing how the spine moves and the extremity joints including crepitation and fine vibrations, which may indicate joint degeneration when they occur in several joints. Crepitations are often audible and patients describe them as 'rice bubbles'. The cause of these vibrations is not clear. One common assumption is that they occur as a result of wear and tear of articular cartilage or insufficient synovial fluid. Cracking sounds are common during joint assessment and are caused by cavitation as the joint stretches. Cavitation must be differentiated from the repetitive clunking sound of muscles, tendons or ligaments flicking over the top of bony processes.

Muscle hypertonicity

Muscle hypertonicity, tightness and tenderness are particularly common signs of joint dysfunction in the spine and extremities. The muscles usually become indurated or nodular due to pain in nearby joints or increased and extended use. Hypertonicity in paraspinal muscles that may be assessed by using surface EMG studies can produce an apparent malposition or lump over the vertebral transverse process, but this prominence is often reduced or alleviated almost immediately after manipulation (De Vocht et al. 2005).

Muscle weakness

Muscle weakness is another important sign of joint dysfunction and pain. Muscle weakness almost always occurs as a result of pain. Testing muscles and comparing the two sides of the body is important to make an accurate diagnosis. Muscles weakened by joint pain do not necessarily relate to one myotomal level. Weakened muscles occur generally all around the painful joint. It is possible that all muscles that are innervated by levels of the spine that have corresponding afferents from the inflamed joint may be subsequently weaker. Manual therapists use diagnostic assessment modalities such as radiographs, ultrasound, and CT and MRI scans. Very occasionally radioisotope bone scans might be undertaken to clarify underlying pathology.

16.6 Potential Benefits of Spinal Manipulation

Table 16.2 lists a variety of problems known to respond to manipulation. A trial of manipulation, mobilisation and massage techniques should be considered in people with diabetes, particularly when they have spinal pain or stiffness (Gross *et al.* 1996; Gross *et al.* 2004). Manipulation and mobilisation effectively reduce neck and back pain (Koes *et al.* 1993). A trial of manipulative treatment for diabetics with lower back pain appears to be indicated.

Headache relief

Headaches are a commonly experienced complaint. Diabetics suffer headaches at least as commonly as the general population. Chiropractors, osteopaths and other manipulators successfully treat headaches and migraines (Parker *et al.* 1978; Bronfort *et al.* 2001; Boline *et al.* 1995; Tuchin *et al.* 2000). Recent research into migraines appears to indicate that the caudal end of the trigeminal nucleus (where the cervical and trigeminal nuclei overlap) is likely to be the point from which migraines originate (Goadsby 2005). This activity subsequently can spread to the cortex, causing a wave of cortical electrical depression and protein loss into cortical tissues that induces pain. Depression of the cortical neural activity appears to induce the premigrainous aura and visual symptoms. Depending on what areas of cortex are involved, there may or may not be symptoms consistent with a recognisable prodrome (Buzzi *et al.* 2005).

It is important to acknowledge the possibility that initial excitement of the trigeminal nucleus could come from upper cervical afferent nerve bombardment of the caudal end of the trigeminal nucleus. Cervical spinal manipulation appears to reduce the frequency and pain intensity of attacks in a significant portion of migraine sufferers (Parker *et al.* 1978).

Spinal stiffness

In addition to pain relief, patients commonly seek treatment to increase mobility in the spine. In middle aged and older patients, reduced mobility, particularly neck mobility, can be very inconvenient and possibly dangerous, for example, checking for cars when driving. Mobility and neck rotation frequently improve following manipulative therapies. The improvement ranges from minimal to significant. The degree of improvement may depend on muscular activity associated with reduced range of motion: the more muscular restriction present, the better the chances of improvement.

Improvement in neurological function may also occur; if pain is reduced and proprioceptive sensation improved, neurological function can be restored, particularly autonomic function and may include vertigo. Changes may be subtle such as small changes in vascular perfusion, or more obvious improvement in balance and well-being. Type 2 diabetics usually are of the age where joint stiffness and osteoarthritis are present. Improvement in joint function will often improve regional muscle strength and general well-being.

Neuropathies

A number of different neurological conditions commonly occur in people with in diabetes. Spinal pain and osteoarthritis in the spine and extremity joints can be reduced by manipulation or mobilisation (Shekelle et al. 1992; Frost et al. 2004). Murphy (1994) suggested that myofascial dysfunction may play a role in susceptibility to diabetic polyneuropathy and treating dysfunctional conditions may lead to improvement in neuropathic pain and associated dysfunction. A "T4 syndrome" that presents with nocturnal or early morning paresthesia in a glove-like distribution may respond well to upper thoracic manipulation (DeFranca and Levine 1995). People with diabetes are no more likely to have a T4 syndrome, but they can present with neurological changes that could very well be explained by a less serious condition such as the T4 syndrome or perhaps a radiculopathy. Referral to a neurologist or musculoskeletal practitioner for clarification is prudent.

Hypertension

Hypertension is a common complaint in people with diabetes. Pain and discomfort from any physical ailment or illness can elevate systolic blood pressure. Some manipulative therapists suggest manipulating the spine can reduce blood pressure (Spiegel et al. 2003; Knutson 2001), and others disagree (Goertz 2002). Research demonstrates conflicting findings. Soft tissue manipulation has been shown to reduce plasma fibrinogen, a marker of increased parasympathetic activity (Driscoll et al. 2000; Budgell 2000). Lowering blood pressure by relaxing the plantar fascia relieves pain and reduces blood pressure as a secondary effect.

Manipulation of the thoracic spinal region has been recommend for lowering blood pressure (Spiegel et al. 2003). It is likely that a diminished excitation of the thoracic cord due to diminishing pain from afferents in this area results in subsequently less sympathetic nerve activity from this part of the spine. However, there is no consensus about which regions are important and some experts indicate both the cervical and lumbar spinal regions are important. Spiegel et al. indicated multiple manipulations were more effective than a single treatment. In any case manipulation should be combined with lifestyle modification and antihypertensive agents in people with diabetes.

Cervicogenic vertigo

Vertigo is another symptom often experienced by people with diabetes (Kraft 1998; Gawron *et al.* 2002). There are many causes of vertigo: Menière's disease, benign paroxysmal positional vertigo, vestibulitis and cervicogenic dizziness, all of which can occur in diabetics. Determining the cause of vertigo is challenging and must be distinguished form hypoglycaemia. Generally vestibulitis follows an upper respiratory tract infection and can be so severe and persistent that the patient is often bed-ridden. Head movements in a single plane often aggravate benign paroxysmal positional vertigo (BPPV). For example, patients often find they experience short episodes of vertigo when they rise quickly from a supine position to a sitting position. Menière's disease can be associated with tinnitus and gradual hearing loss and is less specific with regard to the direction of movement that exacerbates the vertigo than BPPV.

Cervicogenic dizziness and vertigo can occur when a patient has stiff cervical joints. It is likely that the sensory mechanoreceptors in the spine, that normally transmit information movement from joints in the neck to the brain, which matches with the information from the visual cortex and vestibular nuclei in the pons, are affected and result in less afferent information from the spine. If the afferent input from joints is disturbed due to increased or decreased joint function, vertigo sometimes occurs. Many people with diabetes have cervical spondylosis and while manipulation cannot reverse these degenerative changes, it can improve function enough to reduce the episodes of vertigo. The onset of cervicogenic vertigo can be sudden if dysfunction occurs suddenly or fluctuates. Movements that aggravate the vertigo occur in multiple planes. Manipulating the cervical spine often helps in the acute stage but multiple treatments may be required for optimal benefit (Kessinger and Boneva 2000; Bracher *et al.* 2000).

Intestinal motility

Decreased intestinal motility often occurs in association with lower back pain and sometimes following trauma to sacral nerves. It has been my experience that manipulation to relieve lower back pain often improves intestinal motility. Constipation is a significant problem in older people, many of whom are diabetic. Interestingly, patients have reported immediate relief from lower back pain after significant bowel movements.

Massage

Massage is one of the most commonly applied therapies for musculoskeletal pain and can be combined with manipulation (Preyde 2000) because the muscles can remain hypertonic and nodular for some time after the joint inflammation resolves. In addition, the 'aching, tight' muscular pain can be significant. In the case of a torticollis, the pain from muscles often dominates the acute inflammation of cervical facet joints. In diabetics where manipulation is appropriate, massage, discussed in Chapter 13, is most beneficial.

Core strengthening exercises

Enhancing core strength and stability has gained much support in the last decade. The principle being increased strength and coordination of the small muscles around the spine is essential to normal spinal function and stability. It provides a strong foundation to support the function of the extremities and thus usual activities of daily living (Hodges 2003; Barr *et al.* 2005). Core stability is the underlying principle of Pilates exercises. Coordinating muscle function so they react and keep changing actions according to need, enables the body to cope with changing forces during daily tasks (Moore 2004). Core strengthening is beneficial for a number of diabetes-related conditions. For example, after lower limb amputation to balance the asymmetrical forces and stress on the body and strengthen the supporting muscles.

Balancing uneven leg lengths

A small percentage of people have anatomical or effective leg-length discrepancies including patients with hip prostheses or leg prosthesis (following amputation), past fractures, unilateral foot pronation or foot drop, peripheral neuropathy or those with chronic pain who develop significant ipsilateral pelvic weakness. A diabetic with neuropathy involving the lower limb may develop deficiencies in strength of muscles in the leg and foot that maintain the normal arch within the foot. If foot pronation occurs on one side, asymmetrical leg lengths will subsequently occur. Structural scoliosis can also change the symmetry of the pelvis and cause unequal leg length. In these patients a foot lift can be worthwhile. People adapt to differences in leg length and inserting foot lifts to correct asymmetry can unexpectedly increase the deformity in the spine, therefore, corrections should occur in small increments. Once structural and symptomatic improvement occurs, a more durable insert could be obtained.

16.7   Risks and Complications Associated with Manipulative Therapies

All therapeutic interventions are associated with a degree of risk and manipulative procedures are no exception. Most of the adverse events associated with manipulation are minor and include local discomfort, tiredness and nausea (Senstad *et al.* 1996). The four significant complications of manipulation and mobilisation are:

1. vertebral artery dissection or damage;
2. disc prolapse or deterioration;
3. osteophytic or vertebral process fracture of osteophytes;
4. damage to epiphyseal centres.

The greater the force used on the spine, the higher the risk of complications.

Arterial dissection or disruption

Although rare, arterial dissection or occlusion involving either the vertebral artery or carotid artery is the most significant adverse event associated with manipulation (Smith *et al.* 2003; Haneline *et al.* 2003). Vascular incidents are more frequent in the 38–41 age range and appear to be unrelated to atherosclerosis. There is a growing body of evidence that individual risk factors such as elevated homocystine levels may increase the risk (Rosner 2004). Homocystine $> 10.2\mu$mol/L doubles the risk of vascular complications of manipulation possibly due to disruption of the structure of collagen and elastin in the arterial wall. Most authors have found that homocysteine levels are slightly elevated in type 1 and type 2 diabetic patients (Hofmann *et al.* 1998).

At present, the major indicator of risk of vascular disruption/destruction is unusually strong, persistent neck pain and/or unusual persistent headache present on one side only. It may be possible to auscultate bruits because vascular disruption may occur in both vertebral and carotid arteries. The manipulative force to the neck can be enough to change the underlying pathology from partial to irreversible disruption and cause a stroke. In the case of unusual neck pain, particularly in middle-aged people, manipulation may be contraindicated, or a more conservative approach using mobilisation initially should be considered (Hurwitz 2005).

Many people with type 2 diabetes are over 50 years of age and may suffer chronic or fluctuating neck pain. These patients appear to have fairly small risks of vascular disintegration even though they have high risk of atherosclerosis and stroke unless glucose is well controlled.

Intervertebral disc damage

Intervertebral disc problems are another quite rare but significant complication of spinal manipulative procedures. Vertebral disc problems can present with neurological deficits such as sensory changes or paresthesia or muscular weakness following a myotomal pattern. Vertebral disc pain is often deep-seated and aching in nature whereas radiculopathy causes relentless, strong, shooting pain within the affected limb (Bergmann and Jongeward 1998). While manipulative techniques are not a contraindication for patients with disc lesions, a small proportion deteriorate, and sometimes a major prolapse into the spinal canal affecting nerve roots and ascending and descending tracts within the cervical spine and cauda equina of the lumbar spine, occurs (Haldeman and Rubinstein 1992a). Manipulating the cervical spine toward the side of the radiculopathy is more likely to aggravate the problem. Fortunately, the intervertebral discs become dehydrated in most patients over 50 years of age and are less likely to prolapse. Diabetics with neurological deficits due to nerve root compression from disc pathology and radiculopathy should be not manipulated or the choice of technique should be a low force procedure. Referral is appropriate to a practitioner who will consider these risks and has a repertoire of techniques that would enable appropriate care.

Fractures

Fractures can occur if excessive force is used or if the patient has fragile bones and disease processes such as tumours, osteogenesis imperfecta, osteochondromatosis, Gaucher's disease and Diffuse idiopathic skeletal hyperostosis (DISH) (Mody *et al.* 1988; Maskery and Burrows 2002). Conditions such as a hemangioma are unlikely to be damaged by outside forces. Osteoporosis weakens skeletal bones. Manipulative procedures performed on compression fractures can increase pain and prolong disability (Haldeman and Rubinstein 1992b). Most vertebral fractures occur when the vertebral bodies are compressed. Very few manipulative procedures involve significant compression type forces. Bony processes such as the transverse processes can break, but do not affect spinal segment stability and are rare. DISH occurs almost three times as often in people with type 2 diabetes (Sahin 2002) but is usually a stable, solid deformity of the spine (Mody *et al.* 1988). However, DISH is associated with an increased incidence of unstable spinal fractures (fracture of the bony bridging) (Mody *et al.* 1988; Maskery and Burrows 2002). Considerable care must be exercised when manipulating patients with advanced DISH. Mobilisation procedures using low force techniques may be appropriate.

Manipulation and Children

Manipulation appears to be effective in children (Hayden *et al.* 2003) although while epiphyseal damage has been proposed, I could not find any literature to support this possible complication. In addition, the compressive forces on epiphyses are minimal with most manipulative techniques. Children generally respond quickly because of their excellent healing capacity, however, manipulation should be used sparingly and specifically. There is little evidence that children benefit from regular manipulation as a preventative measure.

16.8 Summary

Manipulation and mobilisation procedures can have a role in the management of people with diabetes primarily to manage pain and improve gait and muscle strength and mobilisation to improve the ability to exercise and undertake activities of daily living and quality of life. Improvements in these areas may improve patient mobility and exercise participation and have secondary benefits for blood glucose and lipid levels as well as blood pressure.

References

Alcantara J, Heschong R, Plaugher G, Alcantara J. Chiropractic management of a patient with subluxations, low back pain and epileptic seizures. *Journal of Manipulative and Physiological Therapeutics* 1998; **21**(6): 410–418.

Barr K, Griggs M, Cadby T. Lumbar stabilization: core concepts and current literature, part 1. *American Journal of Physical Medicine & Rehabilitation* 2005; **84**: 473–480.

Bergmann T, Jongeward B. Manipulative therapy in lower back pain with leg pain and neurological deficit. *Journal of Manipulative and Physiological Therapeutics* 1998; **21**(4): 288–294.

Boline P, Kassak K, Bronfort G, Nelson C, Anderson A. Spinal manipulation vs. Amitriptyline for the treatment of chronic tension-type headaches: a randomised clinical trial. *Journal of Manipulative and Physiological Therapeutics* 1995; **18**(3): 148–154.

Bracher E, Almeida C, Almeida R, Duprat A, Bracher C. A combined approach for the treatment of cervical vertigo. *Journal of Manipulative and Physiological Therapeutics* 2000; **23**(2): 96–100.

Briggs L, Boone W. Effects of a chiropractic adjustment on changes in pupillary diameter: a model for evaluating somatovisceral response. *Journal of Manipulative and Physiological Therapeutics* 1988; **11**(3): 181–189.

Bronfort G, Assendelft W, Evans R, Haas M, Bouter L. Efficacy of spinal manipulation for chronic headache: a systemic review. *Journal of Manipulative and Physiological Therapeutics* 2001; **24**(7): 457–466.

Bryner P, Staerker P. Indigestion and heartburn: a descriptive study of prevalence in persons seeking care from chiropractors. *Journal of Manipulative and Physiological Therapeutics* 1996; **19**(5): 317–323.

Budgell B. Spinal manipulative therapy and visceral disorders. *Chiropractic Journal of Australia* 1999; **29**(4): 123–128.

Budgell B. Reflex effects of subluxation: the autonomic nervous system. *Journal of Manipulative and Physiological Therapeutics* 2000; **23**(2): 104–106.

Buzzi M, Moskowitz M. The pathophysiology of migraine: year 2005. *Journal Headache Pain*, Published online (accessed 13 May 2005).

Cascioli V, Corr P, Till A. An investigation into the production of intra-articular gas bubbles and increase in joint space in the zygapophyseal joints of the cervical spine in asymptomatic subjects after spinal manipulation. *Journal of Manipulative and Physiological Therapeutics* 2003; **26**(6): 356–364.

De Franca G, Levine L. The T4 syndrome. *Journal of Manipulative and Physiological Therapeutics* 1995; **18**(10): 34–37.

De Vocht J, Pickar J, Wilder D. Spinal manipulation alters electromyographic activity of paraspinal muscles: a descriptive study. *Journal of Manipulative and Physiological Therapeutics* 2005; **28**(7): 465–471.

Dishman R. Static and dynamic components of the chiropractic subluxation complex: a literature review. *Journal of Manipulative and Physiological Therapeutics* 1988; **11**(2): 98–107.

Driscoll M, Hall M. Effects of spinal manipulative therapy on autonomic activity and the cardiovascular system: a case study using the electrocardiogram and arterial tonometry. *Journal of Manipulative and Physiological Therapeutics* 2000; **23**(8): 545–550.

Frost H, Lamb S, Doll H, Taffe Carver P, Stewart-Brown S. Randomised controlled trial of physiotherapy compared with advice for low back pain. *British Medical Journal*. Published Online at bmj.com doi:10.1136/bmj. 38216.868808.7C, 2004.

Gawron W, Pospiech L, Orendorz-Fraczykowska K, Noczynska A. Are there any disturbances in vestibular organ of children and young adults with Type 1 diabetes? *Diabetologia* 2002; **45**(5): 728–734.

Goadsby P. Migraine pathophysiology. *Headache* 2005; **45** (Suppl 1): S14–S24.

Goertz C, Grimm R, Svendsen K, Grandits G. Treatment of hypertension with alternative therapies study: a randomised clinical trial. *Journal of Hypertension* 2002; **20**: 2063–2068.

Gross A, Aker P, Goldsmith C, Peloso P. Conservative management of mechanical neck disorders: a systemic overview and meta-analysis. *British Medical Journal* 1996; **313**(7068): 1291–1296.

Gross A, Hoving J, Haines T, Goldsmith C, Kay T, Bronfort G. A Cochrane review of manipulation and mobilization for mechanical neck disorders. *Spine* 2004; **29**(4): 1541–1548.

Haldeman S, Rubinstein S. Cauda equina syndrome in patients undergoing manipulation of the lumbar spine. *Spine* 1992a; **17**(2): 1469–1473.

Haldeman S, Rubinstein S. Compressive fractures in patients undergoing spinal manipulative therapy. *Journal of Manipulative and Physiological Therapeutics* 1992b; **15**(7): 450–454.

Haneline M, Croft A, Frishberg B. Association of internal carotid artery dissection and chiropractic manipulation. *The Neurologist* 2003; **9**(1): 35–44.

Harris W, Wagnon R. The effects of chiropractic adjustments on distal skin temperature. *Journal of Manipulative and Physiological Therapeutics* 1987; **10**(2): 57–60.

Hayden J, Mior S, Verhoef M. Evaluation of chiropractic management of pediatric patients with low back pain: a prospective cohort study. *Journal of Manipulative and Physiological Therapeutics* 2003; **26**(1): 1–8.

Hodges P. Core stability exercise in chronic low back pain. *Orthopedic Clinics of North America* 2003; **34**: 245–254.

Hofmann M, Kohl B, Zumbach M, Borcea V, Henkels M, Amiral J, Schmidt AM, Fiehn W, Ziegler R, Wahl P, Nawroth P. Hyperhomocysteinemia and endothelial dysfunction in IDDM. *Diabetes Care* 1998; **21**(5): 841–848.

Hurwitz E, Morgenstern H, Vassilaki M, Chiang L. Frequency and clinical predictors of adverse reactions to chiropractic care in the UCLA neck pain study. *Spine* 2005; **30**(3): 1477–1484.

Kawchuk G, Herzog W. Biomechanical characterization (fingerprinting) of five novel methods of cervical spine manipulation. *Journal of Manipulative and Physiological Therapeutics* 1993; **16**(5): 573–577.

Kessinger R, Boneva D. Vertigo, tinnitus, and hearing loss in the geriatric patient. *Journal of Manipulative and Physiological Therapeutics* 2000; **23**(5): 352–361.

Kleynhans A. Where chiropractic and philosophy meet. *Journal of Australian Chiropractors' Association* 1990; **20**(4): 129–134.

Knutson G. Thermal asymmetry of the upper extremity in scalenus anticus syndrome, leg-length inequality and response to chiropractic adjustment. *Journal of Manipulative and Physiological Therapeutics* 1997; **20**(7): 476–481.

Knutson G. Significant changes in systolic blood pressure post vectored upper cervical adjustment vs resting control groups: a possible effect of the cervicosympathetic and/or pressor reflex. *Journal of Manipulative and Physiological Therapeutics* 2001; **24**(2): 101–109.

Koes B, Bouter L, van Mameren H, Essers A, Verstegen G, Hofhuizen D, Houben J, Knipschild P. A randomised clinical trial of manual therapy and physiotherapy for persistent back and neck complaints: subgroup analysis and relationship between outcome measures. *Journal of Manipulative and Physiological Therapeutics* 1993; **16**(4): 211–219.

Kraft J. Hyperinsulinemia: a merging history with idiopathic tinnitus, vertigo and hearing loss. *International Tinnitus Journal* 1998; **4**(2): 127–130.

Kron J. Osteopathy. *Complementary Medicine* 2003; **Sep/Oct**: 22–27.

Leboeuf-Yde C, Axen I, Ahlefeldt G, Lidefelt P, Rosenbaum A, Thurnherr T. The types and frequencies of improved nonmuskuloskeletal symptoms reported after chiropractic spinal manipulative therapy. *Journal of Manipulative and Physiological Therapeutics* 1999; **22**(9): 559–564.

Leibsohn E. Treatment of notalgia paresthetica with capsaicin. *Cutis* 1992; **49**(5): 335–336.

Maskery N, Burrows N. Cervical spine control: bending the rules. *Emergency Medicine Journal* 2002; **19**(6): 592–593.

Massey E. Sensory mononeuropathies. *Seminars in Neurology* 1998; **18**(2): 177–183.

Meal G, Scott R. Analysis of the joint crack by simultaneous recording of sound and tension. *Journal of Manipulative and Physiological Therapeutics* 1986; **9**(3): 189–195.

Mody G, Charles R, Ranchod H, Rubin D. Cervical spine fracture in diffuse idiopathic skeletal hyperostosis. *Journal of Rheumatology* 1988; **15**(1): 192–131.

Mohammadian P, Gonsalves A, Tsai C, Hummel T, Carpenter T. Areas of capsaicin-induced secondary hyperalgesia and allodynia are reduced by a single chiropractic adjustment: a preliminary study. *Journal of Manipulative and Physiological Therapeutics* 2004; **27**(6): 381–387.

Moore M. Upper crossed syndrome and its relationship to cervicogenic headache. *Journal of Manipulative and Physiological Therapeutics* 2004; **27**(6): 414–420.

Murphy D. Diagnosis and manipulative treatment in diabetic polyneuropathy and its relation to intertarsal joint dysfunction. *Journal of Manipulative and Physiological Therapeutics* 1994; **17**(1): 29–37.

Owens E, Hart J, Donofrio J, Haralambous J, Mierzejewski E. Paraspinal skin temperature patterns: an interexaminer and intraexaminer reliability study. *Journal of Manipulative and Physiological Therapeutics* 2004; **27**(3): 155–159.

Parker G, Tupling H, Pryor D. A controlled trial of cervical manipulation for migraine. *Australian & New Zealand Journal of Medicine* 1978; **8**(6): 589–593.

Peters R, Chance M. Chiropractic in Australia 1905–1945, The Searby Saga: a story of hardships and determination. *Chiropractic Journal of Australia* 2001; **31**(1): 17–32.

Pistolese R. Epilepsy and seizure disorders: a review of literature relative to chiropractic care of children. *Journal of Manipulative and Physiological Therapeutics* 2001; **24**(3): 199–205.

Polkinghorn B. Chiropractic treatment of frozen shoulder syndrome (adhesive capsulitis) utilizing mechanical force, manually assisted short lever adjusting procedures. *Journal of Manipulative and Physiological Therapeutics* 1995; **18**(2): 105–115.

Polkinghorn B. Treatment of cervical disc protrusions via instrumental chiropractic adjustment. *Journal of Manipulative and Physiological Therapeutics* 1998; **21**(2): 114–121.

Preyde M. Effectiveness of massage therapy for subacute low-back pain: a randomised controlled trial. *Canadian Medical Association Journal* 2000; **162**(13): 1815–1820.

Rosner A. Commentary: spontaneous cervical artery dissections and implications for homocysteine. *Journal of Manipulative and Physiological Therapeutics* 2004; **27**(2): 124–132.

Roston J, Haines R. Cracking in the metacarpophalangeal joint. *Journal of Anatomy* 1947; **81**.

Sahin G, Polat G, Bagis S, Milcan A, Erdogan C. Study of axial bone mineral density in postmenopausal women with diffuse idiopathic skeletal hyperostosis related to Type 2 diabetes mellitus. *Journal of Women's Health* 2002; **11**(9): 801–804.

Sandoz R. The significance of the manipulative crack and of other articular noises. *Annals of the Swiss Chiropractors' Association* 1969; **IV**: 47–68.

Sandoz R. Some physical mechanisms and effects of spinal adjustments. *Annals of the Swiss Chiropractors' Association* 1975; **VII**: 91–141.

Schofield AG. *Chiropractice*. Surrey: Biddles, 1968.

Senstad O, Leboeuf-Yde C, Borchgrevink C. Side-effects of chiropractic spinal manipulation: types frequency, discomfort and course. *Scandinavian Journal of Primary Health Care* 1996; **14**: 50–53.

Shekelle P, Adams A, Chassin M, Hurwitz E, Brook R. Spinal manipulation for low-back pain. *Annals of Internal Medicine* 1992; **117**(7): 590–598.

Smith W, Johnston S, Skalabrin E, Weaver M, Azari P, Albers G, Gress D. Spinal manipulative therapy is an independent risk factor for vertebral artery dissection. *Neurology* 2003; **60**(9): 1424–1428.

Spiegel A, Capobianco J, Kruger A, Spinner W. *Heart Disease*. Baltimore, MD: Lippincott Williams & Wilkins, 2003.

Stephens D, Gorman F, Bilton D. The step phenomenon in the recovery of vision with spinal manipulation: a report on two 13 year olds treated together. *Journal of Manipulative and Physiological Therapeutics* 1997; **20**(9): 628–633.

Still A. *Autobiography*. Kirksville, Missouri, 1908.

Stoddard A. *Manual of Osteopathic Practice*, 2nd edn. London: Hutchinson, 1969.

Tuchin P, Pollard H, Bonello R. A randomised controlled trial of chiropractic spinal manipulative therapy for migraine. *Journal of Manipulative and Physiological Therapeutics* 2000; **23**(2): 91–95.

Walker B, Buchbinder R. Most commonly used methods of detecting spinal subluxation and the preferred term for its description: a survey of chiropractors in Victoria, Australia. *Journal of Manipulative and Physiological Therapeutics* 1997; **20**(9): 583–589.

Wingfield B, Gorman R. Treatment of severe glaucomatous visual field deficit by chiropractic spinal manipulative therapy: a prospective case study and discussion. *Journal of Manipulative and Physiological Therapeutics* 2000; **23**(6): 428–434.

Index

Note: Figures and Tables are indicated by *italic page numbers*; 'CAM' means 'complementary and alternative medicine'

DATE DUE

MAR 1 9 2008